MORBID THOUGHTS AND THE DOMINO EFFECT

ACKNOWLEDGMENTS

Hello to all who are reading this. My name is Perry Muse, and I am the author.

First and foremost, I want to thank God for putting the idea of this book into my mind and guiding me as I wrote. I never thought of writing a book about my life until it came to me in a dream. Even then I was skeptical. Now I understand why God put it in my heart to write.

Next, I want to thank my wife. She endured 30 years of what is in these pages, and I could not have done it without her. She alone knows the struggles, dark times, and pain. She was my light, comfort, and motivation.

Thanks to my closest friends and family for their support through all of this. Again, they were my motivation and support mechanism.

I am eternally grateful to Rochelle Beckstine. Before this project she did not know me. However, she agreed to help me from beginning to end. Rochelle never gave up on correcting my bad grammar, but more importantly, she helped bring my words to life and gave them color with her own personal gift of writing. I give her a lot of credit and will forever be indebted.

I want to thank the doctors, nurses, surgery staff, physical therapy personnel, and medical staff that have worked on me, treated me, and helped heal me time and time again. You are my heroes.

I specifically want to thank Dr. Charles Famoyin, Dr. Rick Kind, Dr. Richard Ballard, Dr. Mahdi Taha, and Deanna Hensley, APN, Dr. Naveen Raj, Dr. Gregory Stewart, Dr. Michael Wells, and Dr. Jonathan Nesbitt. This is the "A Team" of people who went above and beyond to help me. I consider them all to be much more than medical personnel.

Thanks to Max at Comitic Software for allowing me to quote some of the messages in my "Daily Horoscope" app. These were more than coincidental, but more importantly, they inspired me and lifted me up when I was battling the morbid thoughts.

Special thanks to Pamela at Delaney Designs. I called her with my concept for the cover. It must have sounded quite odd, but she took time to listen, ask questions, and understand the critical points of the concept. Her work was expedient, and very well done. She never hesitated to go back months later to tweak the design. Thank you so much.

Thanks to Rachel Bostwick on Fiverr for the incredible video trailer. You exceeded my expectations and were a pleasure to work with. I can't stop watching it!

Special thanks to Alanna Rupert & Ezekial Cooper for putting their artistic talents to work for me to display.

Lastly, I want to thank my boss, Erik. He trusted me and believed in me when I went through multiple surgeries and treatments in a very few years. He could have replaced me, and I would have supported him in doing so. But instead, he supported me and allowed me to work from afar and fight the good fight. I love my job and returning to work at 100 percent was a daily source of motivation. I will never forget your support.

Dedicated to

My beloved wife, **Nila Muse**

•

Love is patient. **Love** is kind.

It does not envy; it does not boast; it is not proud.

It does not dishonor others; it is not self-seeking; it is not easily angered;
it keeps no record of wrongs.

Love does not delight in evil but rejoices with the truth.

It always protects, always trusts, always hopes, always perseveres.

Love never fails.

And now these three remain: faith, hope, and love.
But the greatest of these is **Love**.

•

Corinthians 13:4–8,13 (CEV)

TABLE OF CONTENTS

PROLOGUE

Four months ago, the C-bomb dropped on Nila and me.

Fast forward to me, dreaming. I was having a discussion with a man. I had no idea who this gentleman was, but we were acquaintances in the dream.

"You have cancer, and I believe it has likely spread," he said flippantly. In my head, I already knew this, but he seemed to be telling me for the first time. My thoughts and fears droned large in my head as he loudly buzzed out his next words about treatment and whatnot. Eventually, he noticed my silence.

He asked, "So, what are you doing these days?"

I responded, "Just trying not to let cancer kill me."

The gentleman chuckled slightly at my answer and said,

"Why Perry, you're already dead; you just haven't finished the book yet."

The mind has a way of generating dark thoughts and dreams when one feels life is threatened. My mind has always been quite imaginative anyway. Dealing with **cancer** definitely consumes your thoughts and has a way of realigning priorities. It tests relationships, mental fortitude, and physical endurance.

Morbid Thoughts is a memoir full of true stories, unexpected dreams, and thoughts that passed through my mind while trying to beat cancer. It is meant to paint an accurate picture of the events and battles that were endured. I hope this is entertaining, but mostly helpful and informative to someone else who may be fighting the good fight. One can laugh or be depressed. I did both.

A LITTLE BIT ABOUT ME

I never put much faith in astrology signs, but, as I mentioned before, when you are facing death, you find faith in many ways. I am a Sagittarius, and I fit every description of what a Sagittarius is. A person's identity is all part of their cancer battle; it all comes into play as a part of the whole domino effect that is a cancer battle.

My life has been influenced by so many. I was heavily influenced by the women in my family. I still look up to my grandmother, mother, sister, and wife. These are the people I credit with molding my personality and outlook. I draw wisdom, strength, humility, courage, and faith from these influential figures.

So, what does it mean to be a Sagittarius? I will share the answer as the book moves along. All of my Sagittarian tendencies played a big part in my cancer battle, so I realize that personality and attitude determine our life and the happiness we gain from it.

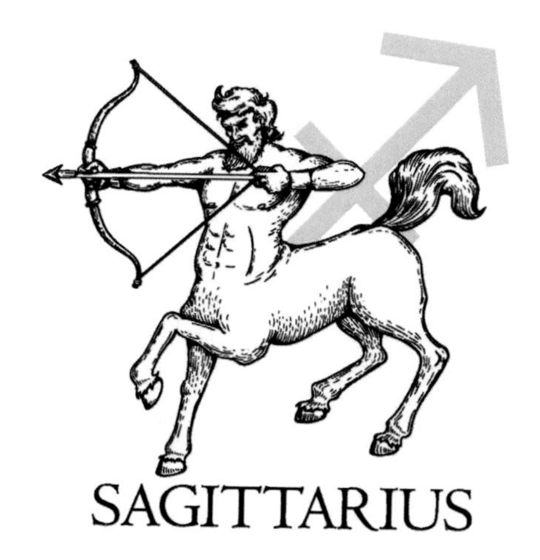

Chapter 1

BEFORE THE DAWN

Sagittarius is the most brutally honest of the Zodiac.

It was July 2017. I was the vice president of manufacturing and general manager of a thirty-nine-year-old corporation. I oversaw two manufacturing plants. We were wrapping up our third consecutive record-breaking year in the history of the company. I had a great wife, four kids, three dogs, and a cat. The kids were all grown, so Nila and I had the house to ourselves. We'd moved to Johnson City, Tennessee, eight years ago, so I could start our new plant and get it running. Nila loved the area, as did I, so we relocated.

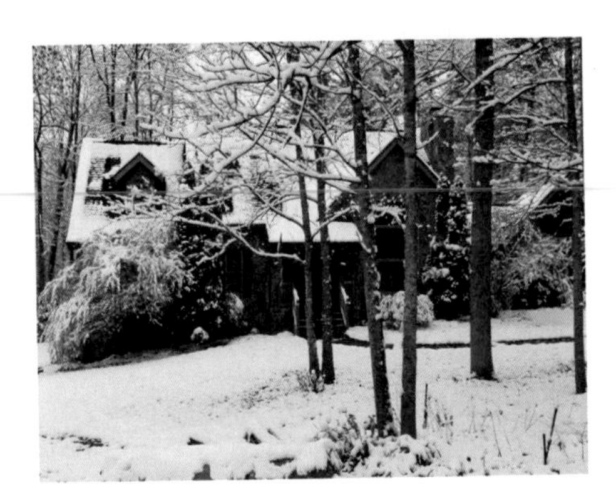

Our house on a snowy day

We often told people that we "lived in the forest." There was an unoccupied lot on one side that was completely wooded. It had a lot of tall pine trees that all leaned heavily in the direction away from our house. It was an odd sight and, for all of the years we had lived there, we always marveled at the trees' resiliency on windy days. The creaking was loud and could be heard indoors on windy days as the trees were tested, bending and swaying. Sometimes it sounded like a heavy wooden door in a castle, slowly opening, with huge hinges in dire need of oil.

Behind the house was a large forest. We lived in harmony with deer, chipmunks, squirrels, and other wildlife. Well, actually, Sparky hated the squirrels, and they just tolerated him! The dogs loved to roam the woods. During the winter, we could stand on the upper deck and watch them for a couple of hundred yards.

The house itself was two and a half levels, part rock and part stucco with two-inch wood strips that made the house look like a cottage in the forest. When we had visitors, the most common remark was, "Wow, I didn't even know this place existed." That was how we liked it.

During this time, it wasn't uncommon for me to get tired. My job was stressful. I am a true, 100 percent Sagittarius. This means I am a perfectionist, among other things. Constantly seeking perfection can take its toll. However, in the summer of 2017, I was a little more fatigued than normal. I took steps to address the situation that included diet change, mattress change, exercise, etc. None of these seemed to be working. I was drinking 5-Hour Energy shots routinely because they didn't give me the jitters or make me crash. My sex drive was taking a nosedive, and my work was starting to suffer.

Finally, on July 10, 2017, I decided something was wrong. By 2:00 p.m. in the afternoon every day, I was so sleepy that I couldn't stay awake at work. I started having to call Nila to come pick me up for fear I couldn't stay awake if I were to drive home.

I pulled into the parking lot of my regular walk-in medical care facility. I sat there for a moment and, in true Sagittarian style, decided this *must* be something I could fix. Why did I need to pay someone to tell me to take some supplements, or increase my cardio, or blah blah blah? Then I thought, "Oh well, I am here, so I might as well go in."

For the first time ever, I met a physician assistant named Deanna Hensley. She was... is...amazing. She ordered a blood lab to find out why I was so chronically fatigued. The next day Deanna called me with an unnerving sense of urgency and despair in her voice.

Deanna informed me that my prostate-specific antigen (PSA) was high, which was an understatement.

I asked, "What does that mean?"

She did not answer my question.

Instead, she said they were going to "rush" getting me an appointment with a urologist.

I thought, "Homework."

I was in my mid-fifties and had had plenty of experience with doctors. I'd had eleven surgeries. I said Deanna was and is amazing, and this is why. Throughout this process, she followed what was happening with me. She actually called me to check in and get updated on how I felt and to tell me what was next! How many people can say that? It was a first in my lifetime. She was a Christian and *always* told me she prayed for me regularly. The depth of her care made my heart swell.

I found out that the normal PSA range is .1 – 4. My PSA was one seventy-nine! This indicated that I had prostate cancer. As time passed and I did more research, I spoke with guys who once had prostate cancer, making me realize that my PSA was unknown territory to most.

"Way to go, Sagittarius; you just had to outdo everyone" was an initial thought. "No one will beat your high score!"

But this is something you don't want to beat everyone at. Low score wins.

Everyone I spoke to was quick to point out the success rate of beating prostate cancer.

"Only three out of a hundred men die from prostate cancer," they said.

As with most statistics, I found there were variations behind the numbers. We were encouraged to hear prostate cancer survivors tell us what a simple process it was.

"Thirty days of radiation that each take about five to ten minutes. This kills the cancer on the outside of the prostate. Then they will plant a radiation seed inside of the prostate, and it kills the internal cancer. No side effects, no fatigue. They will prescribe you Viagra, and everything will be fine." But none of these stories came from someone with a one seventy-nine PSA. It meant I had a fight on my hands. I just didn't know how long and dirty of a fight it would be. It was all beginning to sink in.

I received the call for my appointment with the urologist. I had a couple of weeks to ponder things before my visit. It was the downtime when I allowed the negative guy on my shoulder to speak to me, and I became really low.

There was a poem that I come across that spoke to my spirit. Although this poem is about the author's wife's battle with Alzheimer's, I related to many of the lines.

DO NOT ASK ME TO REMEMBER

By Owen Darnell

Chapter 2

IT'S A DOG'S LIFE

Sagittarians are deep thinkers. They will want to examine who the other person is and where they are going and can see the end with a clarity that others mostly lack.

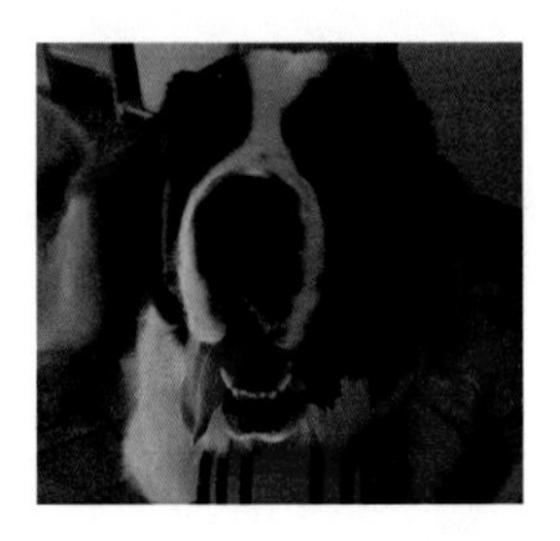

Our Saint Bernard, Thor

The life expectancy of dogs varies. There are multiple factors that come into play. For example, breed, climate, food, and exercise, to name a few. We had always been a family of animal lovers, but especially dogs. We had a Papillon (Sparky), a seven-year-old Saint Bernard (Sebastian), a one-year-old Saint Bernard (Thor), a fourteen-year-old Maine Coon cat (Mr. Mitten), several fish, and two love birds (Fred and Daphne).

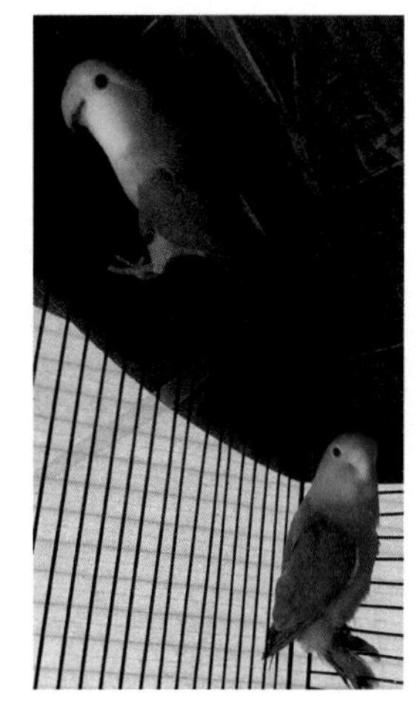

Fred & Daphne

The love birds were named after the characters from *Scooby-Doo*. However, I have no idea why they are called love birds. Quite frankly, they are mean to each other. We had specifically picked these two out based on observations by the manager that ran the pet store. He was confident the pair was a male and female. Plus, they were always together in the big cage.

One day I went to our cage and noticed something odd about Daphne. I had a difficult time locating her legs, and she was using her beak to move from spot to spot. Upon closer observation, I realized one of her legs was nothing more than a nub! Evidently, Fred had bitten off one of her legs! It was a terrible event, no doubt. Since that time, Fred has always sat tight against Daphne, holding her against the cage so she can sleep.

It has been a couple of years, and they are both still doing fine.

I always joke and say, "After Fred bit her leg off, he probably told her, 'Bitch, you have one more chance!'"

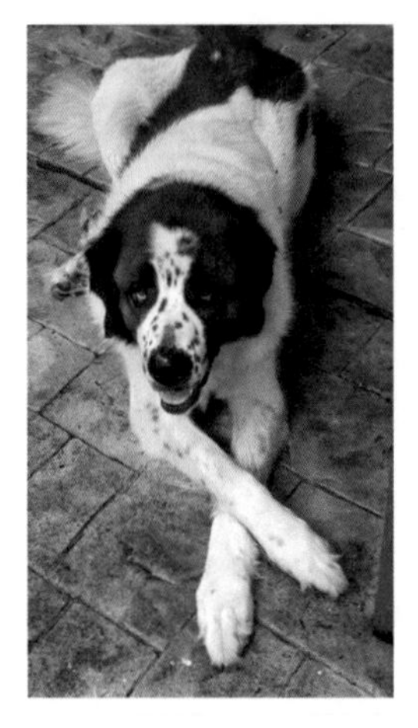

Sebastian

We found out quickly that Saint Bernards are our favorite breed of dog to own. Sebastian had always been very calm. The only time he ran was when we pulled into the drive. Even then, it was more of a trot than a run. One of our kids nicknamed him Lurch from the TV series *The Addams Family* because he quietly snuck up on everyone. He then gently slipped his head beneath their hand to invoke the petting process. We referred to it as the never-ending head rub because he would follow you wherever you walked, keeping his head positioned perfectly under your hand.

Sebastian's calm demeanor and loving disposition were very welcome after I got the news. Petting him seemed to make things slow down and removed the chaos that was my mind's thoughts. It was very therapeutic and made me wonder why I had never made him a therapy dog. Sebastian and the patients would both experience benefits. We always told folks at the dog park that Sebastian was there for the people, and Thor was there for the dogs.

So, in 2018, Sebastian and I were certified by the Alliance of Therapy Dogs. About a year later, we were further certified for the R.E.A.D. program. That was where we went to the library, and children took turns reading to Sebastian. The program is targeted to help children who are not interested in reading and struggle with reading comprehension. It is an amazing program. Children who participate for one year increase their reading comprehension by three to four levels!

Sparky was a Papillon, which is French for butterfly. When observed from behind with his ears raised, you could see the obvious butterfly shape of Sparky's ears, especially as the ear fringe developed and grew. He was an alpha male and stayed inside, but he was an avid hater of squirrels and loved to ruin their day. Speedy Gonzales was no match for that dog.

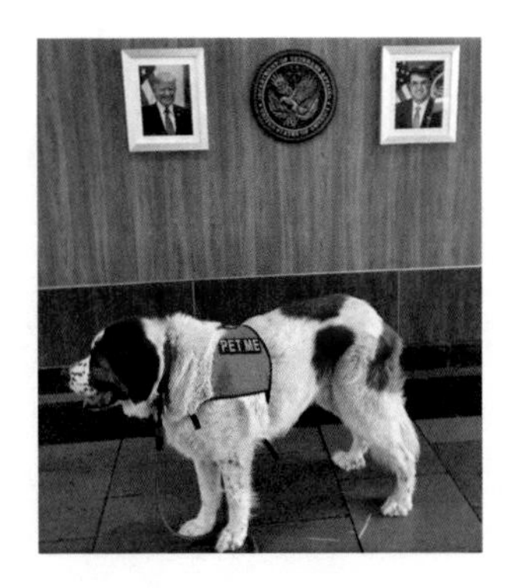

Sebastian at the VA

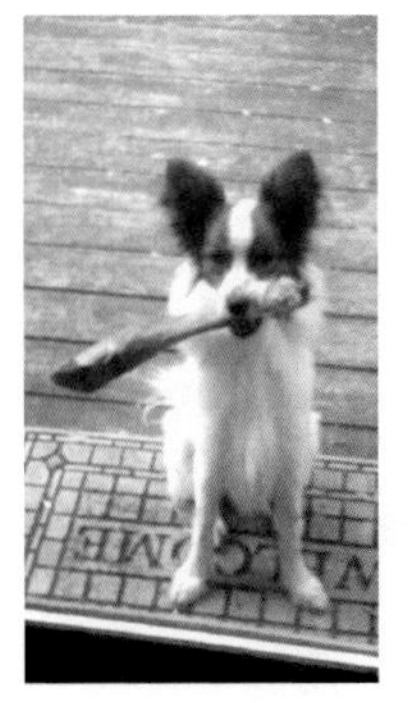

Sparky

Sparky was fast and agile. If ever you watch the agility competition portion of dog shows, you will find Papillons almost always win their class. Sparky was a rare long-legged red Papillon. His long legs only increased his athleticism. He had never caught a squirrel (and hopefully never would) but had been within inches many times, jumping over five feet onto a tree trunk only to be slightly out jumped at the last minute.

Our Maine Coon, Mr. Mitten

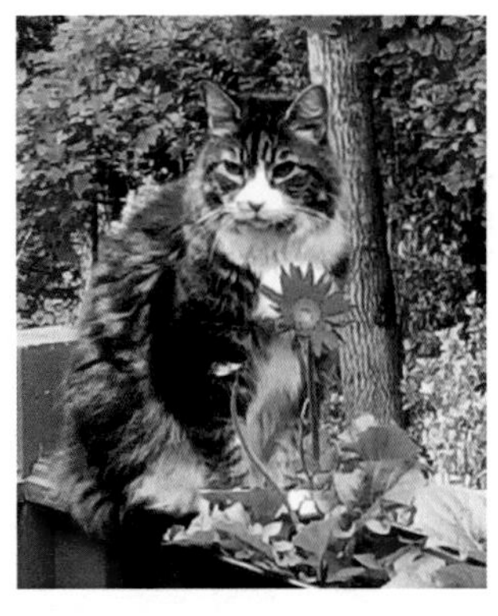

Mr. Mitten weighed about twenty pounds, the same as Sparky. He was about fourteen years old and was one of seventeen cats we had once! I didn't want *any* cats after a terrible experience in my past. Our youngest son, Jeremy, brought home a cat he had already named Atreyu. Before I knew it (or before we could get her fixed), she had kittens. Two females for a total of three. Then, they all had kittens at the same time! *We had seventeen cats*! They had to be separated. The moms were stealing one another's kittens. Each of the three litters looked identical to me. That was when I said, "Enough! Pick one!"

Our five-year-old daughter Alanna picked and named Mr. Mitten.

He was the best cat in the world. This is a picture of Mr. Mitten sitting in Alanna's shoe when he was little. Remember, Alanna was only five. And Nila is holding Mr. Mitten as a full-grown cat—he covered her entire top half! He was a huge cat!

Mr. Mitten at eight weeks old

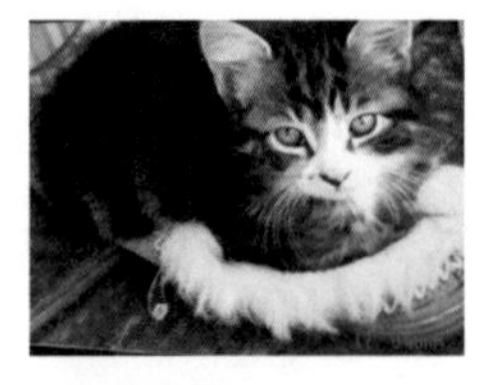

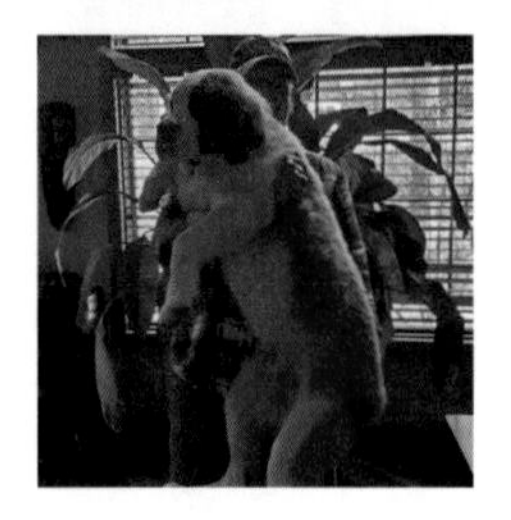

Thor at twenty weeks old

Mr. Mitten, full grown

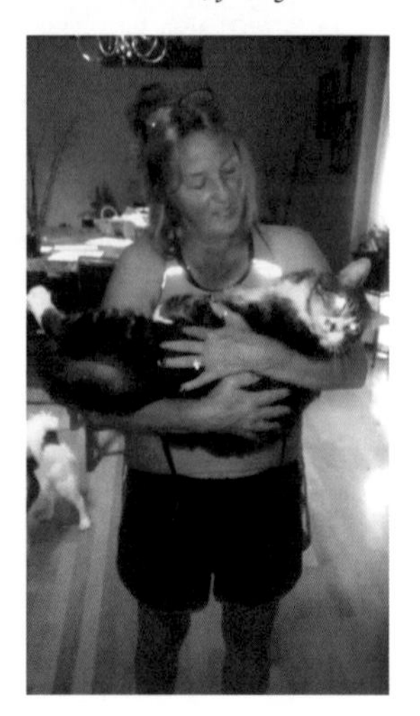

Thor was the polar opposite of Sebastian in every way except loving all people. He grew at a rate of five pounds per week and was...is...always high energy. To say that Thor ran more in one day than Sebastian did in three years was *not* an exaggeration.

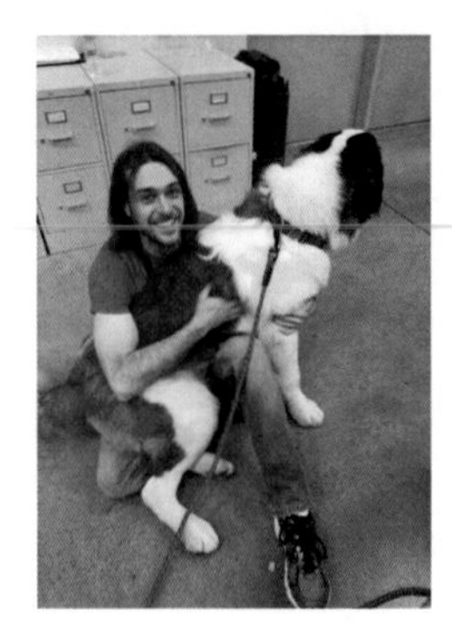

Joey Blessing with Thor at Lowe's

We took Thor to the local Lowe's at nine weeks old, and he was an automatic hit with the employees. We took him there regularly after that, and the employees started texting their coworkers, "Thor is here!" On our trips to Lowe's, Thor's biggest fan was Joey Blessing, who always dropped whatever he was doing and dashed to Thor. The picture was taken one day when Joey was working.

Thor did not know his own size. In January 2018, he was fourteen months old, weighed a hundred and thirty pounds, and still thought he was a lapdog.

But pets are a comfort. As I became sick and tired, I noticed Sparky made it a point to always sit as close to me as possible. It was heartwarming how he would gently put his front paws on me and slowly, cautiously walk his way up my chest so as to be able to give me loving licks on the ear, his favorite spot. Then, he would curl up close and stay there until I got up. Then our Maine Coon, Mr. Mitten, would come sit on my lap several times each evening. Just on my lap.

It got my attention. It wasn't abnormal to be loving, but the animals stuck to me like a magnet then and still do. I'm sure they knew something was wrong. It broke my heart that my sickness seemed to concern them so.

Even now, I often worry about the day I will lose my animals. Saint Bernards typically live nine years. We researched the breed thoroughly and control their growth by not overfeeding. They tend to grow faster than their joints can handle. We feed the dogs high-end food with plenty of vitamins, high protein, and glucosamine. We give them glucosamine supplements, as well. You can stretch out their life span to twelve years, which is still a short amount of time.

When I realized how my mind worked on such morbid thoughts, especially when alone, I asked Nila not to leave me by myself. However, it is impossible not to be alone sometimes. One day I was sitting on the patio. Nila had gone inside for something. Sebastian had lurched over, and I was giving him a good head rub. Thor was running around doing puppy stuff, and I began to think about Sebastian getting older. He was seven years old. Subconsciously, I think we got Thor because Sebastian was aging.

Then it hit me... "My dogs may very well outlive me."

During this time, the lyrics to this song really touched my heart. They are so very true.

I LOVE MY DOG

Cat Stevens 1967

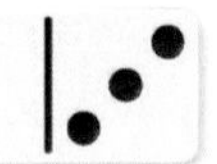

Chapter 3

INSULT TO INJURY PART I

Sagittarius individuals are very fun-loving, and they can make even a boring activity an interesting one.

In June 2017, I noticed I was having pain and discomfort in my left shoulder. As time passed, the pain ramped up. I was not a stranger to shoulder pain...or pain in general. To date, I had had eleven surgical procedures and other injuries that did not require surgery.

I attended college at the University of West Georgia in Carrollton, Georgia, as a jazz performance major. Like a lot of Southern boys, I played sports throughout middle and high school. I realized at an early age that I was too small to think about sports as a long-term career choice.

I started playing trumpet in the fifth grade. My dream was to play saxophone because it was my mom's favorite. (It turns out it was my wife's favorite, as well.) However, during instrument tryouts, the instructor and I found my hands were too small to reach around the sax. When I picked up the trumpet, I was able to immediately play a note—G. That was it. My parents and I were told that I was a natural for the trumpet, and the saxophone was history.

By the eighth grade, I was promoted to high school band, and by the ninth grade, I was lead trumpet. In high school, I continued playing basketball and baseball, but I felt like football would have been a death sentence, considering my undersized stature.

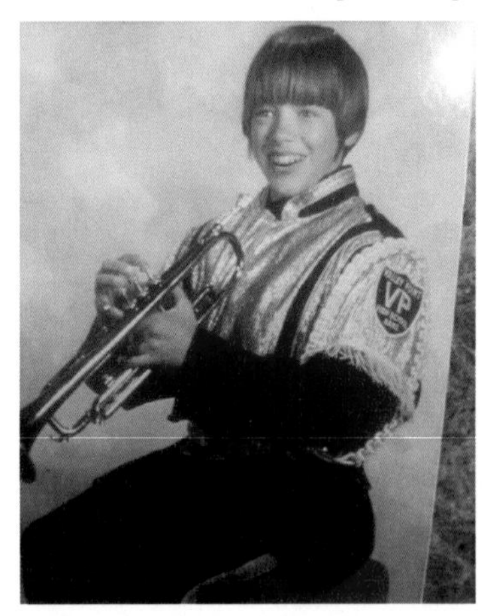

Perry, eighth grade

My dedication to music paid off with a great scholarship to West Georgia, and I loved playing in the jazz band. We would travel to perform at schools for recruiting and played at the local watering hole sometimes. I worked at Pizza Inn to make some pocket money. However, being a jazz performance major had its downside. I was required to take piano, music theory, private lessons, and all of the normal classes everyone else took. It was a power load every semester.

It was December 1979. My friend and I had spent the past couple of weeks binge listening to Pink Floyd's new double album, "The Wall," since it had hit the shelves of the local music store on November 30.

One evening it was around dusk and rainy. I had left my work uniform at the dorm, and my friend was taking me back to retrieve it. We went a "new, shorter" way that was unfamiliar. The road we were on intersected with another road in the middle of a long, sweeping curve. Unbeknownst to us, a wreck earlier in the day had taken out the stop sign. It appeared the oncoming car was not maintaining its lane, and panic set in.

We were going about fifty-five miles per hour, and the other car was estimated to be doing the same. Both vehicles tried to swerve to miss the other, and we collided...headlight to headlight. I had tried to fasten my seat belt when we left Pizza Inn, but the passenger side belt was broken. We were in one of the vans where the engine was in a compartment between the driver and passenger. There was a wooden drink holder mounted firmly on top.

Upon contact, I became a projectile. My left side bounced off the drink holder. My knees broke through the dash, and I began my headfirst flight through the windshield. I continued across the hood of the other car and violently crashed into their windshield back first. The windshield gave way, and my flight suddenly stopped inside the other car. The windshield was between the two other passengers and me.

I pulled myself out, rolled off the hood and onto the pavement. The wet pavement and cold rain were soothing, but the pain was excruciating.

The driver of the car I landed in had been killed instantly. The passenger, his wife, died later that evening.

My friend driving the van was not injured.

I was certain my ribs were broken. I was telling myself, "Don't breathe too deeply. There is surely a jagged rib bone that will puncture your lung."

When I arrived at the hospital, after the terribly painful ambulance ride, the nurse requested a urine sample. As I began to fill the cup while lying on the gurney, all I saw was blood. At that point, I almost passed out. My left kidney was lacerated in several places. Nothing broken, including my ribs. I had quite the knot on my head.

I remember waking up in the hospital and seeing a lot of family in the room. It startled me because I knew that for some of them to be there, it must be serious. "Oh crap, I must be dying." I was overcome by pain. The nurse hit the button to release the morphine, and I fell fast asleep again.

"After all of that, little did I know it would be just another brick in the wall."

My two years at West Georgia College were tainted by my car accident. My lengthy time in the hospital and inability to play my trumpet cost me my music scholarship. I would have no degree. There would be no more performing. I moved back to Dalton, GA, and went to work at McDonald's. I spent a lot of my free time playing basketball with some people I still call friends.

Basketball was a true love of mine. However, I was really short, so I worked hard at the game. Dr. J (Julius Erving) was my hero. My dad put up a basketball goal, and that is where I spent countless hours. The dirt was uneven, but it only helped to hone my dribbling skills. I spent every available minute either practicing my trumpet or developing my basketball skills. The trumpet came easy; the basketball would require some fancy ball handling, speed, and hang time to avoid blocked shots.

I learned early on in my basketball days that the shorter one is, and the higher a person jumps, the farther the return to earth can be. What goes up must come down. When you couple that with doing so at high speeds, it equates to twisted, rolling ankle sprains. It's a stretch to say I might have been five six, most likely less.

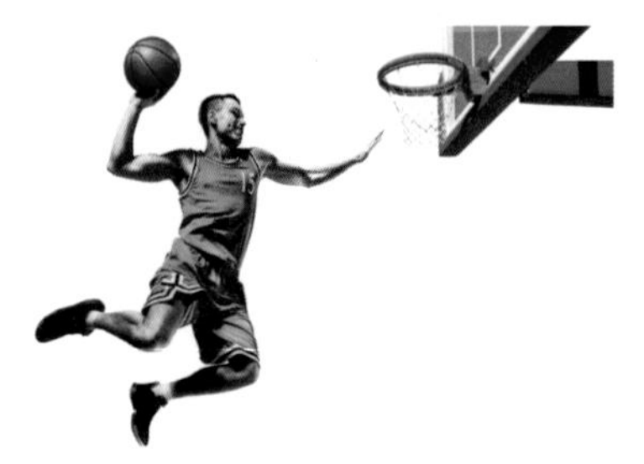

I developed the vertical leap to a point where dunking a volleyball was possible. The volleyball was lighter, smaller, and provided more grip than a basketball. At five six (maybe), that left another four feet, six inches to the rim. Then, add a few more inches to get the volleyball to clear the rim. Hopefully you get the point. I was running as fast as possible—leaping, dunking (sometimes), and then letting gravity suck me back down to the hardwood floor.

When I rolled my ankle (usually in my white Converse All Stars), it was wickedly painful. Almost immediately, a softball-sized knot appeared, and a beautiful shade of purple bloomed across my ankle. Last time I counted my sprained ankles, I was about thirty, and it was the right ankle, leading ten to left ankle eight.

Sports are important to me. In my early thirties, I played men's league softball. My position was shortstop, just like in youth baseball. I played three to four times a week on various teams. Nila always came to watch, and I loved to try to impress the love of my life sitting in the stands, always yelling for me.

But organized sports weren't the only sports I got passionate enough about to land in the emergency room or in a splint. Once I was playing horseshoes, and one shoe got caught on a tree limb. I know what you're thinking...weird, right? The pits were not in the best location. I jumped to grab the shoe, landed awkwardly (alcohol may have been involved), and rolled my ankle.

This one was pretty bad. I already knew the drill. I went to the hospital; they X-rayed the ankle, put an air splint on, and sent me on my way to heal. It was my right ankle again.

The day after the ankle finally healed and I was freed from the cast, I played in a softball tournament. It was a Saturday morning. My very first time at bat, I hit a ground ball to third base. I took off running, trying to beat the throw. As I stretched on the final stride, I knew it was going to be close. My right foot hit the bag, and something terrible happened. First base popped up out of the ground, leaving a hole. My ankle crashed and rolled through the hole; the pain was unbearable.

I felt broken, just like Pantera's song "I'm Broken." Sometimes I needed that song. Sometimes I still do.

I'M BROKEN

Pantera 1994

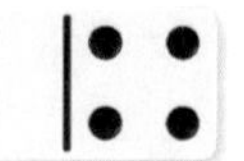

Chapter 4

SOCKS FOR A SQUID

Sagittarians love their jobs, and so they work very hard and push themselves to the max.

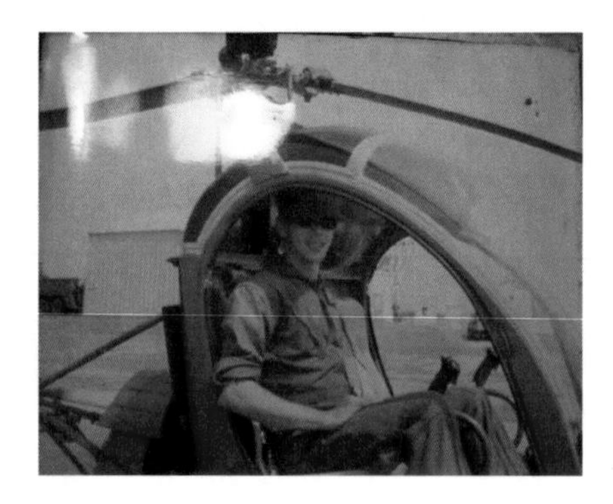

Perry in US Army flight school, 1982

How does one go from college scholarship student with a future in music to being a basic Joe? It is easier than you think, and there were not that many choices.

First, I was in a head-on collision where I incurred severe injuries (I wasn't driving, and the seat belt wasn't working). Thus, I lost my scholarship because I had to take time off due to my injuries—the diaphragm, lips, jaw, and neck muscles all play a critical role in trumpet playing; mine were recuperating.

So, I went home and got a job working at McDonald's. (It is amazing the things I learned that I still practice today. One example? Clean as you go. I cook often, and usually when I am finished with a meal, I also have a clean kitchen.) I worked my way up to swing manager and really loved my job. It is truly some of my best memories. However, I hooked up with the wrong crowd and made some mistakes that got me into trouble. I went before a judge, and he gave me five choices. Four of them were Army, Navy, Air Force, or Marines. The fifth choice was much less desirable.

I went into the army and excelled in basic training, but I lacked discipline. I went on to AIT (advanced individual training) and became a helicopter crew chief. From there, I found a pathway to flight school. Warrant Officer Candidate Flight school was, and still is to this day, the hardest thing I had ever done.

On hell day, or day one, the Training, Advising, & Counseling (TAC) officers' job was to break us and get as many as possible to quit. They were damn good at their job! We had spent two weeks in "snowbird" status, prepping all our clothes, etc., for start day. So, hell day began abruptly at 4:00 a.m. For three hours, we ran, did push-ups, chin-ups, log drills, and more. Yes, it crossed my mind to walk away. We were then turned loose and required to put on our class A's and report to the chow hall in seven minutes.

We ran into the barracks to find everyone's entire belongings piled in the center of the floor. We just started grabbing stuff and putting it on. No time to measure where the metal pins went. We couldn't find enough dammits (a cap that goes over the pin to hold it on). We were lucky to find our name tags.

We fell into line and double timed it to the chow hall. In the distance, I could hear the TAC officers screaming because we were late. A naval transfer couldn't find a tie. It was chaos. We couldn't show up and not be in uniform. "All for one, and one for all" was literally on a sign hanging ten feet from us. I quickly removed my socks and made a makeshift tie. I had to tie it around his belt to hold it in place, so it sort of, kind of, maybe at a glance, looked like a black tie.

After breakfast, we had to fall into formation for an inspection. When the TAC officer got to our navy mate, he began to rip him verbally about his uniform. He took special pride in humiliating this sailor who had transferred into army flight school. It took longer than I expected, but he finally got to the tie.

"I don't know how in the hell you squids tie your ties, but that will *not* fly here in the United States Army Aviation School!" he said.

Of all the WOCs (warrant officer candidates) in my flight, they chose me to step out of line and fix his tie. Of course, I failed. I had already done my level best to make my socks look like a tie before we arrived. The TAC officer had little patience and moved me as he told everyone within a block how incompetent I was.

Then it happened. He figured out it was a pair of socks! He shared the news with his fellow TAC officers, and they all joined in verbally demolishing this poor navy guy.

“Pull up your legs,” said the TAC officer to the navy recruit first.

To their surprise, he had socks on. That turned their attention to everyone else on the flight.

“Pull up your pant legs!” the TAC officers shouted at the rest of us.

When they saw my ankles were bare, it was impossible for them to contain their outbursts of laughter. They stepped around the building to hide the entertainment value this situation provided.

As I waited for them to return from the side of the building, I was sure my flight school time had ended on hell day, but not because I quit—because my socks were around some squid’s neck.

When the TAC officers returned, we had the remainder of our inspection. The average number of demerits was in the twenty thousand range. Each one thousand demerits required writing an official military letter to explain. This, of course, would have to be done during the brief personal time we got each evening.

I proudly received twenty thousand demerits, but I was also awarded ten thousand merit points for exceptional courage. I had found my calling.

At the end of school (one year), we were marched into a room and sat down. On the board were different helicopters with numbers beside them: Chinook -1, Scout -5, Cobra -3, etc. The number was how many of each were available for our graduating class. The order to pick was determined by where you finished school among your peers.

Flight school was more than flying. It was a degree in aerodynamic engineering and everything that was required to be an officer in the United States Army. The entire time I was in flight school, it was my goal to finish high enough to pick a Cobra. The Apache helicopters were not out yet. I wanted to fly something that had guns, so I could shoot back! And when the day came, that is exactly what I picked.

The army was tough on my first marriage. It takes a special wife to endure. The time came when I was given the choice of staying in the army and getting a divorce or getting out and staying married. I had two small children, so I gave up the army. It seems it didn’t matter, for the marriage still failed, and we divorced. I regret to this day leaving the army. However, I met my soul mate in 1991 and married her. That was twenty-eight years ago, and I will choose Nila over Uncle Sam every time!

Written by Perry Muse

Ten years after starting flight school, this song hit the radio. I have always thought of my journey, including my current one, and how the lyrics to this song applied to my life.

LEARNING TO FLY

Tom Petty And The Heartbreakers 1991

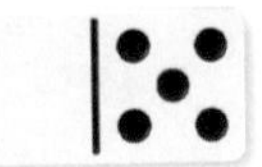

Chapter 5

INSULT TO INJURY PART II

Sagittarians are wild, independent, fun, friendly, and outgoing. They are considered the wild children of the zodiac. One will always find them with a zest for life and a curiosity level that is wild.

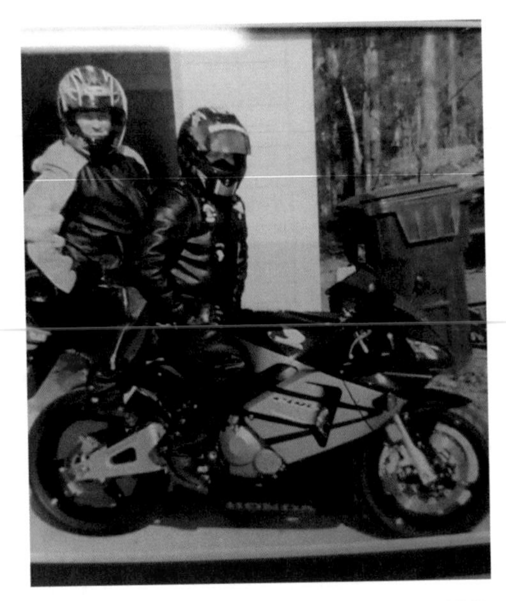

Nila and I in 2009 on my Honda CBR600RR

Excerpt from the movie "Ford vs Ferrari"

Nick Miles was on the track, preparing for the 1966 Twenty-Four Hours of Le Mans. This is a conversation between him and his son Peter at turn eight.

Peter: "What are you doing?"

Nick: "See that crack (pointing to the crack in the track)? That's my mark at turn eight."

Peter: "How do I slow down?"

Nick: "Push the brakes and downshift (demonstrating with his hands)."

Peter: "But you'll be doing a hundred and fifty miles per hour! So, how will you see it?"

Nick: "When you go fast, everything else slows down. You don't do that (cupping his hands around his face); you do this (opening his cupped hands to allow all of his peripheral vision). And then you see everything. You have to be kind to the car. You feel this poor thing groaning underneath you. If you're going to push a piece of machinery to the limit and expect it to hold together, you have to have some sense as to where that limit is."

In 2009, our eldest son, Shane, was in the US Army and owned a beautiful black and silver Honda CBR600RR. Most know this type of bike as a "crotch rocket" and for good reason. When he deployed, I eagerly took it off his hands. After flying helicopters in the US Army, a "cruiser" just wasn't going to scratch my itch. Growing up, I remember my mom saying many times that I was a "thrill seeker." She was correct. Remember that Sagittarians are the wild children of the zodiac, always curious, with a zest for life.

Over time I learned the art of riding a crotch rocket; I loved plugging in my earbuds, turning on some heavy metal, and experiencing all the bike had to offer. I lived several miles from a friend, the perfect distance for a great ride. To start with, I turned my iPod to Judas Priest. I opened the album Angel of Retribution, scrolled down to the song "Hellrider," and off I went. My perfect ride always included Interstate 75. Each time I made the trip, it was a challenge to beat my best time. Once I made the trip from exit to exit before the song ended. It was a 15.6-mile trip, and Hellrider was a six-minute, twenty-three-second song. You do the math.

Once off the interstate, it was a short distance and a left-hand turn onto a long and winding, dead-end road. There was a section of sharp curves, a long straightaway, and more curves. No houses, no worry of children or cars pulling out in front of me. A section of road made for me and my CBR.

On August 11, 2009, I made the trip once again. This time I was followed by my wife Nila in our family vehicle. I didn't attempt to break any records that day! She had recently found out I could ride wheelies. When she saw it firsthand, she made it clear she never wanted to see it again. On the CBR, I would pop the wheelie in second gear at about twenty-five to thirty miles per hour. It took no time at all to be at eighty miles per hour!

As we took the left onto the road made for riding, I decided to pull a little prank. When we got to the first set of curves, I gunned it. My intention was to whip through the curves, gas it on the straightaway, and disappear into the second set of curves before she came out of the first set. Don't ask why—I still don't know what prompted me to do this.

As I cleared the first set of curves, I gassed it. Then, I started watching my rear-view mirror because, of course, I wanted to make sure my poorly devised plan was working. So far, so good. Then I lifted my eyes from the mirror to look ahead at what should have been a desolate section of road. Standing in the middle of the road was a dog. I remember the puzzled look of the dog as I came screaming out of the curves, heading straight for it. I instinctively leaned right, and my bike left the road.

The road had been recently paved with asphalt, so the shoulder was pretty high with a steep, four-foot red dirt bank leading to tall, unkempt grass. My speed pushed me beyond the four-foot bank and the grass line. It was eerie. The section of the road where I crashed had been viciously cleared of all life for thirty yards from the road to a tree line where towering oaks and maples competed with sparse pines. Perhaps someone had foretold of a crash on this part of the road? There was also a huge, gaping sinkhole halfway between the shoulder of the road and the wood line. As I wickedly fishtailed, I vividly remember feeling grateful my ride didn't end in that gaping sinkhole.

I thought, "Death may be better than any other outcome if the crash happens here."

I fought for control of my bike into and out of the slide, and my efforts were rewarded when I felt the bike begin to move for me instead of against me once again in the grassy area just before the trees. Immediately, I was thinking about getting safely back onto the road. Because of my training in the army, I'd learned how to slow things down. When a situation became chaotic, I was now able to slow things way down. Don't ask me how. I believe the gift had always been there to some degree. Perhaps it is exactly as Nick Miles described it to Peter *in Ford vs Ferrari;* sometimes when you go very fast, everything actually slows down, and you see everything.

After the army, I was fully aware of this potential. I know I have often been able to slow things down and don't even realize it until the event is over. Then, I am able to recite what occurred in great detail. This situation was no different.

In this situation, I quickly saw that a telephone pole was in my path to the road. Strangely enough, this telephone pole was closer to the edge of the road than any I had seen before. Actually, it was closer than any I have seen since, as well. Making the challenge greater was the fact that it was on the four-foot steep bank. I did my absolute best to miss the pole to the left, hoping the angle was right to keep the newly paved edge of the pavement from sending me airborne or jerking the handles from my grip, and you know I was gripping tight!

At the last moment, I realized I wasn't going to clear the telephone pole, or at least I was going to graze it. I released my right hand from the throttle and tucked it close to my chest. I had stayed on the gas, partially for momentum, partially from adrenaline and thinking less about the throttle and more about the telephone pole.

In retrospect, that's funny. I was wearing a red, black, and white PowerTrip jacket. One of the patches read, "Less brake, more throttle." It should have read, "Less telephone pole, less throttle."

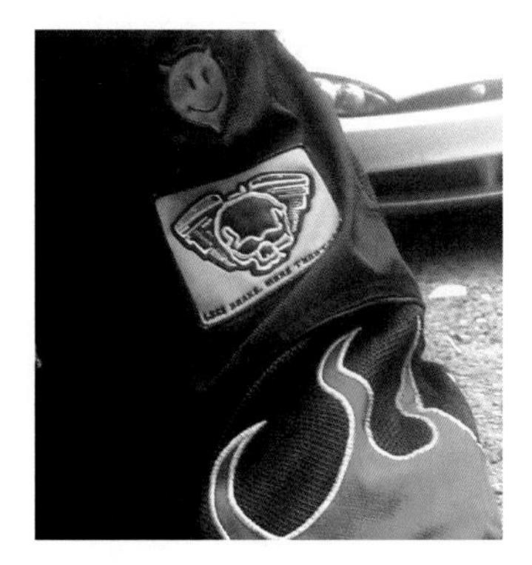

Patch on left sleeve of PowerTrip jacket

When I released the throttle, I also snuggled my right leg in as tight as possible to the bike. I didn't want the telephone pole to rip me off the bike. The last thing I did before contact was look down at the digital speedometer. The number I saw was a hundred and ten.

Needless to say, I clipped the telephone pole with a tremendous jolt.

Unfortunately, my best-planned scheme to miss the pole did not take the handlebar into consideration. The right side of the front forks hit first. This turned the wheel and jerked the left handle from my grip. Remember, I let go of the right to protect my hand and arm. Next, the gas tank section and right handle and throttle caught the pole. As you might imagine, my right leg and foot were caught in between. I say the motorcycle "clipped" the pole, but considering part of the pole was removed, perhaps that was understated.

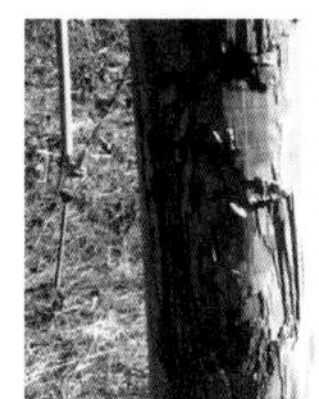
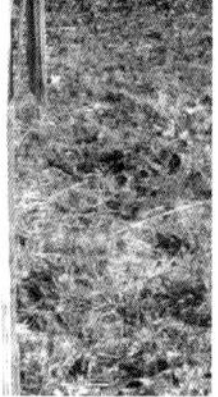

Damaged telephone pole from wreck

The impact had a ricochet effect that sent me back onto the street, riding with no hands. I vividly remember the handlebars "tank slapping"...left side, right side, left side. There was no saving it at this point, and I made the decision to bail.

I dove off the left side. I remember thinking, as the pavement flew toward my face, "I never wanted to ever have to do this." As I hit the pavement and began my violent tumble down the street, I was greatly concerned about the bike running over me. Flip-flop, bounce, roll, and a sudden loud grinding sound. No music in my ears for this ride! Just an incredible grinding sound in stereo. I was sliding facedown, no longer flip-flopping.

I looked up to see where the bike happened to be. I was leading the race, but not by a comfortable margin. I watched the bike wobble and slam violently onto the pavement, only to bounce right back up and keep following me. Later, we found the left foot peg broken off and planted firmly into the new pavement.

I quickly thought of my hands and fingers. I felt I needed to ball up my fists to prevent breaking all of them. As I did, the violent flipping, flopping, and rolling resumed. Then, the stoppage again, and nothing but the sound of my helmet grinding, face first, on the pavement. This time when I looked up to see where the bike was, I saw it trail off the road. It was the same direction as the initial swerve when I was on board, except this time it began to flip end over end.

Each time, the bike seemed to bounce higher until it vanished up in the trees. Again, I was concerned about my hands and fingers. The bike was no longer a concern. Again, I started the violent flip-flopping. This time, since I was no longer thinking about being run over by the bike, I remember thinking, "Wow, I'm going to make it through this and not even be hurt. You managed not to kill yourself again somehow."

Just as abruptly as it all started, it all stopped. One hundred and ninety-two feet from where I dove off, I came to rest on the shoulder of the road with my head on the pavement. For the first time since it all began, I felt all of the damage on my body.

I thought, "This may have been a showcase of my worst judgment, but I had all of my gear on, thank God. A top-shelf KBC helmet, PowerTrip jacket, gloves, pants, and boots."

When Nila came out of the curves, I was already flip-flopping down the road. The bike had disappeared. She was frantic.

When she reached me lying on the asphalt, in typical fashion, I calmly started giving her orders.

"Take off my helmet; it's smothering me," I told her from the ground.

She debated with me, trying to convince me that I should not move. But I repeated my demands over and over again until she started working on me. The face shield was gone from my helmet, so she didn't understand how I could be smothering, but I didn't even realize it was gone!

Once the helmet was gone, I wanted more help to remove gear.

"Now, take off my gloves," I told Nila.

I had no idea that the back of my left hand was resting on my forearm. Apparently, my left hand and arm were what I used when I hit the pavement.

You see, at this moment in my head, I was living in a land where, during my recent accident, I had looked like Superman, flying off my bike to safety. Yet, now I've gained perspective, and I'm sure anyone who saw my accident would have said it looked more like a cowboy being thrown from a bull, with the fresh pavement kicking me down the road.

After the gloves were gone, I told her to remove my jacket and place it under my head as a pillow. Nila's main point was the uncertain state of my left wrist, which was clearly broken (the doctors later described it as "powdered"). However, I was still oblivious to my hand lying back on my forearm.

"Take off my jacket! When EMS shows up, they will take scissors and cut this $350 PowerTrip jacket off me!" I argued just as strongly.

She removed the jacket, called my friend for a bottle of water, and then called 911. My bike had gone twenty-six feet up into the trees!

In the hospital, I was given morphine shots at close intervals. Then, a friend from school came in, rolling some type of machine. My immediate observation was the metal mesh sleeves. It looked like the woven sleeves that I remembered playing with as a kid. I would put a finger into each end and try to pull them out. He asked my wife if I had been given morphine.

Nila said, "Yes, three in the last forty-five minutes."

"That won't be enough," Bobby said.

When the time arrived, he placed my fingers into each mesh sleeve. He strapped down my arm across my bicep. The monitor behind it was turned on, and I could see the two bones in my wrist. They were completely broken and no longer aligned; they had slipped down alongside one another. I was fascinated.

Meanwhile, I was asking Bobby how his mom and family were. He stepped behind the machine and began to pull the wrist in opposite directions in order to get the bones back in line. I screamed and tried to reach him and force him to stop. He was quite experienced and made sure nothing was in reach, including himself. Nila had to leave the room.

Once Bobby cranked my wrist to where the bones were no longer alongside one another, he carefully reached over and used his hands to do the final alignment. To date, this was the greatest pain I had ever experienced. Once during the procedure, the nurse walked by, opting not to come in.

Later, she asked, "Are you okay? Because I heard you screaming like a little girl." I was too exhausted to respond. It was rhetorical anyway. She knew I wasn't okay.

Internal monologue: "Perry, you are an idiot. You really thought, 'Wow, I'm going to make it through this and not even get hurt'?"

In total, I had a torn right bicep. My right foot got squeezed between the bike and the pole, so it tried to separate my foot from my leg. Torn ligaments. My left elbow had slammed the pavement hard enough for a fracture and a fluid pouch that was close to tennis ball sized. Broken left wrist (plate and ten screws). All of the flip-flopping knocked many ribs out of place. To this day I still must use a foam cylinder to roll on and pop them back in. It is a painful reminder daily of the wreck back in 2009.

We left the hospital around 3:00 a.m. I refused to let them admit me. There was nothing a nurse was going to do that Nila couldn't do. At 8:00 a.m., I made her drive me to the chiropractor.

"Just do what you can, Doc," I told him.

After the chiropractor, I had Nila take me to work. She pushed me in on my new set of wheels. I remember hating being in a wheelchair.

"Who ever thought I would trade in a CBR600RR for a stupid wheelchair?" Thinking about it now, there are probably a lot of people who knew me well enough that would have taken that bet and won.

I remember feeling this sense of pride the day the telephone pole was replaced. I never dreamt a crotch rocket could do enough damage to a telephone pole to warrant replacement. But we Sagittarians don't typically do things half-assed.

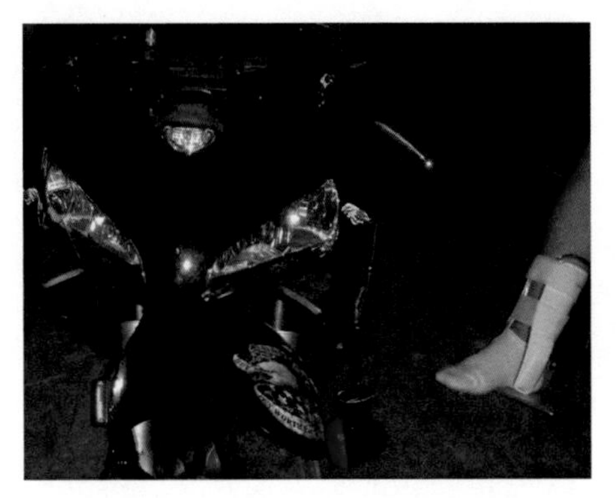

Handlebars straight, but not the front wheel

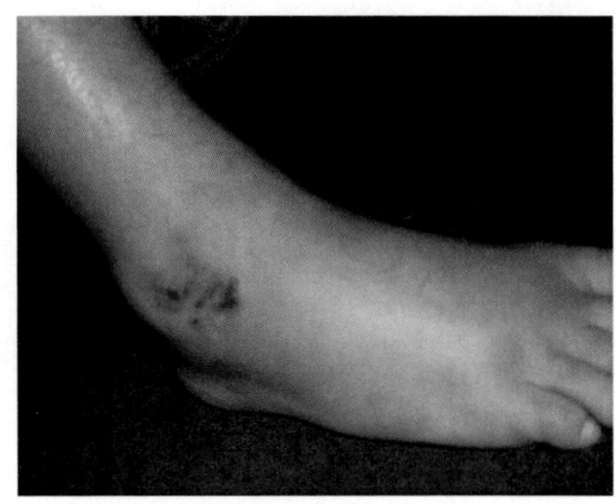

Right ankle

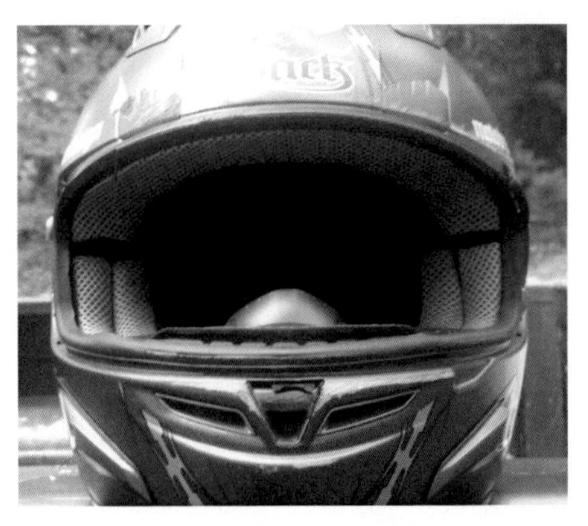

Front view of KBC helmet with abrasion marks

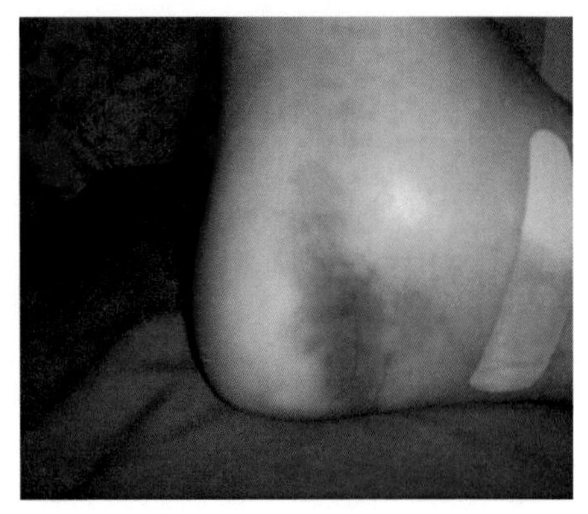

Right heel

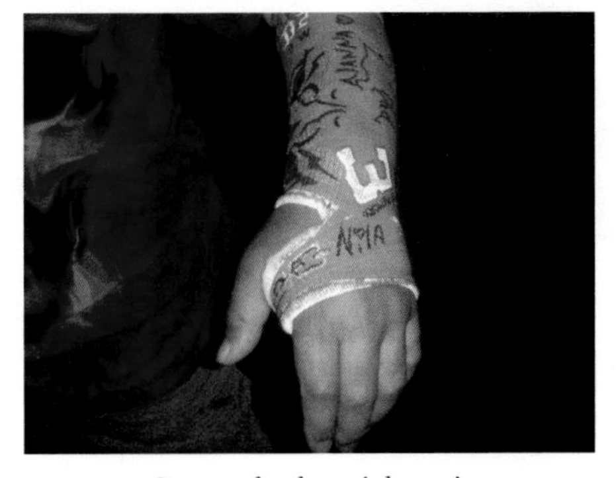

Cast on broken right wrist

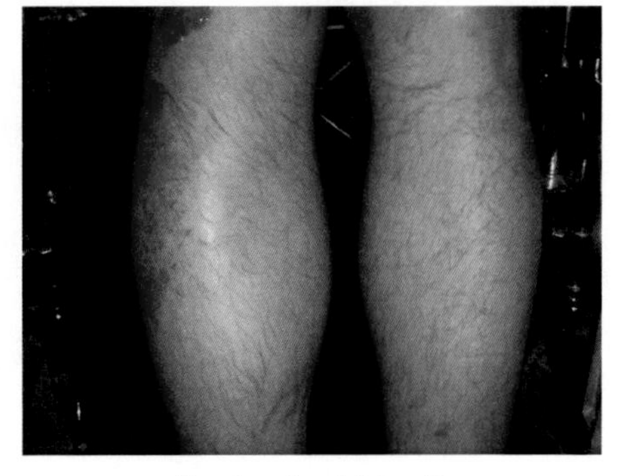

Road rash, right calf

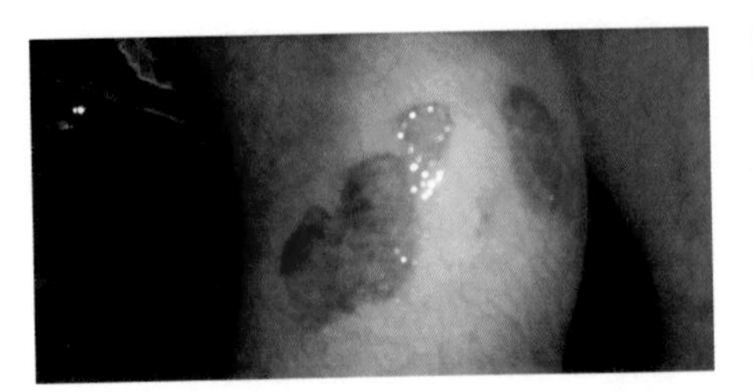

Road rash, right knee

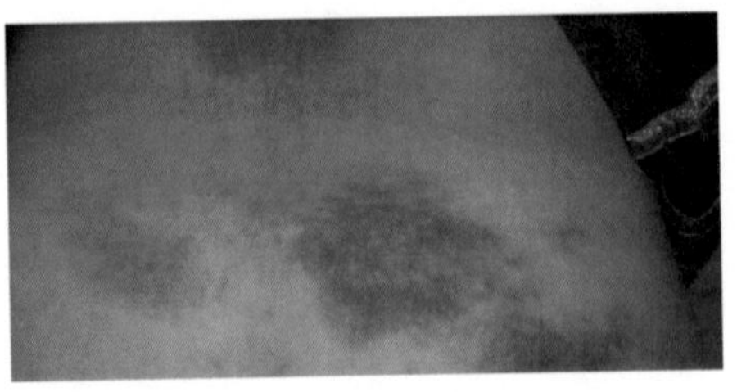

Bruises on back and buttocks

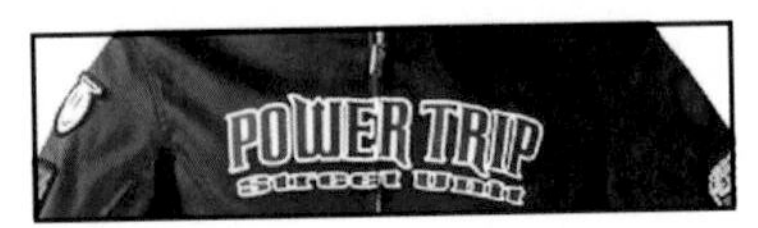

PowerTrip Jacket

The PowerTrip jacket had an emoji on each side. One had a halo; the other had horns. I pulled the one with horns off and gave my jacket to a rider who didn't own one. I told my story and asked him to promise to always wear it for safety.

My "power trip" was over. When I was riding my motorcycle, I felt unstoppable, invincible, and free. I could see every little rock on the road even when I was flying at a hundred miles per hour. Cars would try to change into my lane, and I would kick their doors. I was arrogant to think that I would never crash, and nothing would ever happen to me. I was lucky it didn't happen when I was on the highway as I kicked someone's door. When my bike fishtailed in the dirt, and I did my dance with the asphalt, I was humbled.

The motorcycle wreck was one of many times I probably should have died. I heard this song at a friend's house one day, not long after the accident. The lyrics seem to have been written especially for me.

AND THE WORLD KEEPS SPINNING

Glen Campbell 1970

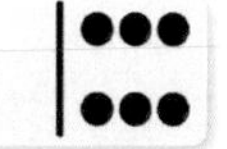

Chapter 6

NEWTON'S 3RD LAW

Sagittarians need a career that provides them with plenty of freedom and excitement. But for Sagittarians, it is hard to focus on one thing as they have a lot of interests and love to explore new things.

In chapter 3, right before we took a journey back in time to my army days and my motorcycle accident, I told you my left shoulder ached. To be clear, the pain in my left shoulder radiated throughout my neck and back so that I had to turn my entire body to see right or left. I couldn't even walk my dog. I had stubbornly ignored it to this point because a doctor who treated me for my motorcycle crash had told me that my motorcycle injuries would reoccur as rheumatoid arthritis; that is what this felt like—pain in places where I had motorcycle injuries.

So, I felt like my left shoulder ached a lot, but not intolerably. The primary issue was raising my arm or trying to lift anything. Thor was a big puppy at nine months old. He was rambunctious and as strong as an ox. It was extremely disappointing that I was unable to play with him. Growing at a rate of five pounds per week, he was quickly becoming a big dog. He would hurt me due to no fault of his own, and I couldn't bear the pain. He looked at me with those big, beautiful, droopy eyes, and I could read his thoughts: "Why won't you touch me? Why won't you play?"

I tried to treat the shoulder without medical intervention, of course. My subconscious attitude of being a seasoned medical expert only prolonged the pain and made the situation worse. July 20, 2017: the day I found out I had cancer (not officially, but I was told my PSA score), my shoulder pain took a backseat. The realization of what my PSA test result really meant began to sink in.

The dark cloud started to form around my thoughts: "Has the cancer spread throughout my body? Could it be in my shoulder?"

For many, the full focus would turn to the cancer. As a Sagittarius, a singular focus is almost impossible. My mind was in turbo mode, making the mental to-do list.

- Call the family
- Call my boss
- Power of attorney
- Update will
- Make a list of all accounts, usernames, passwords
- Schedule a family weekend at home
- Check beneficiaries
- Check Aflac policy for cancer coverage
- Do intense research on prostate cancer with high PSA
- Get urologist referral appointment
- Put Foam Products contingency plan together
- Hug Nila tight
- Pray

The list was constantly being updated and prioritized. Addressing the shoulder pain did not make the list. At least not in the top twenty-five. I decided not to make my cancer news public. Not yet. Even when the time came, I was unsure about how public I was willing for it to be. The constant questions about how I was feeling or the pre-judgment of how I looked or acted on a given day didn't need to be piled on my plate.

The whispers among friends and coworkers, "Did you see Perry today? He isn't looking well. I believe he has lost a lot of weight. Do you think we will get a new boss? Let's not bother him with emails or phone calls. He appears to have enough going on."

Formally stated, **Newton's third law** is: "For every action, there is an **equal and opposite reaction**." The statement means that in every interaction, there is a pair of forces acting on the two interacting objects.

For me, cancer was the action, and all the things that happened as the result of cancer that would not have happened otherwise were the reactions. So, Newton's Law could be aptly seen in my life through all of the things that happened as the result of cancer that would not have happened otherwise, including anemia, diaphragmatic plication, fatigue, low testosterone (<2.4), SED rate, C-reactive protein, rheumatoid factor, depression, digestive issues (milk, ice cream), and gas (in the chest that felt like the onset of a heart attack). Sir Isaac Newton wasn't cogitating cancer when he inspired the scientific community with his third law of motion or when he developed the infinitesimal calculus. But in 2021, I am still experiencing the reactions from cancer's initial action. I prefer to call it the domino effect.

My initial research revealed the cancer diagnosis would lead to an immediate Lupron injection. These injections would likely be routine and quarterly. Lupron reduces the testosterone in the body, which feeds the prostate cancer. Eliminating testosterone starves out the cancer. I became anemic. In my routine blood test, my hemoglobin (or hematocrit) was flagged as very low.

The main protein in the red blood cells is the hemoglobin. It is the part that carries oxygen and delivers it throughout your body. Any diagnosis of anemia means that the hemoglobin levels are low as well. If it gets too low, tissues and organs can become starved for oxygen. Some of the symptoms of anemia, like fatigue and pain, happen because the body's organs are not getting what they need to perform.

Because of the anemia, I was originally prescribed iron tablets (ferrous sulfate). It was a horrible experience because no one bothered to tell me I needed increased amounts of vitamin C to get the iron to absorb. Therefore, the iron was not absorbing, and my anemia was not improving. Actually, it continued to worsen.

If that wasn't a bad enough reaction, the iron caused severe constipation, and the stomach pain was unbearable at times. This is when I found Dr. Famoyin, a hematologist and oncologist. A hematologist specializes in the diagnosis, treatment, and prevention of diseases of the blood, including cancerous and noncancerous disorders that affect the individual components of blood (such as white blood cells, red blood cells, or platelets) or the organs that produce them (including the bone marrow and spleen). Hematology is a subspecialty of internal medicine that often overlaps with oncology (the study of cancer).

I was scheduled to have iron infusions given intravenously (IV). I would go to Dr. Famoyin three times a week for six weeks. Each infusion lasted a few hours. At first, I didn't realize they were putting Benadryl in the IV cocktail. This was due to some people's allergic reactions. It made me sleepy. After my iron infusions laced with Benadryl, Nila would drive me home, and I would go straight to bed to finish my Benadryl nap. Once I figured out what was going on, I had them omit the Benadryl, and I was able to return to work. It was very important for me to return to work and fulfill my obligations.

"I surely don't need both cancer and an unemployment check," I thought.

By the time I started with the infusions, I began to notice dry, white spots on my skin, the corners of my mouth, my earlobes, my penis, and my eyes.

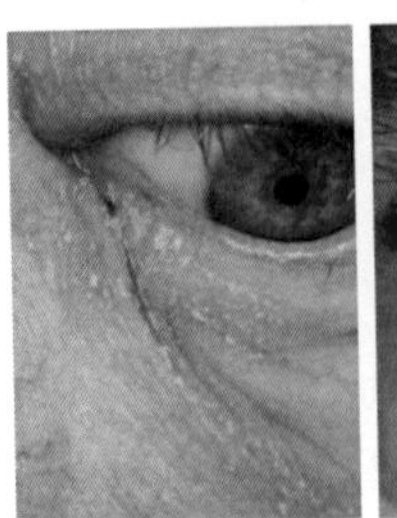
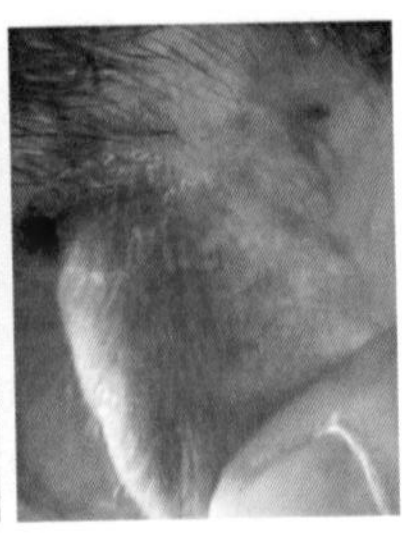

Psoriasis on eye / face

Psoriasis on ear

The dry skin would crack and burn. In the shower, the dry skin washed away and left pink, raw skin beneath. Regular lotion didn't really help. Not long term. I finally bought some cream, Gold Bond psoriasis relief, designed especially for psoriasis. It worked the best. But that didn't explain why I suddenly had psoriasis.

"So, cancer isn't enough? I need psoriasis, as well?"

My body was falling prey to Newton's Law...my cancer had affected my blood cells, and it seemed to me rather suddenly that the rest of my body felt like it was falling apart. My hematologist explained to me that since my body was unable to get the oxygen it needed due to a lack of hemoglobin, the muscles and tissues were malfunctioning.

"You see, people who usually have glowing, healthy skin who suddenly start to suffer from dryness or flaking skin may also be suffering from an iron deficiency," he said. "Your blood carries much-needed oxygen to all of the cells in the body. When there is an iron deficiency, the body will prioritize vital organs and systems in order to keep you alive. The hair, skin, and nails are often the first parts of the body to exhibit signs of iron loss. Hair that is not fed a steady supply of oxygen will eventually lose moisture and weaken. The skin will become dry and chapped as the cells begin to die from iron deficiency." I took this to mean that people need to pay more attention to their skin and hair. It seems they can be an early warning sign of trouble.

But the cracked and bleeding skin wasn't my only issue; at night my legs would ache. No matter how I tried, I could not get them comfortable. By now I had begun to research and understand the reactions to my body having iron-deficient anemia. My legs? Restless leg syndrome. People with iron deficiency regularly suffer from restless leg syndrome. The syndrome is exactly like what it sounds...people with it feel they must shake, stretch, or otherwise move their legs when sitting or lying down. Some people may also notice an itch or a sensation of crawling along their legs and feet. Many people say restless leg syndrome disrupts their sleep or is worse at night, causing tiredness during the day.

The iron infusions worked. The only problem was that it took six weeks of treatments to get back to a normal level. I immediately made it my goal to recognize the signs and get back to the good doctor for more infusions before I reached this state again.

As for my aching shoulder? I chose to not have any work done to fix it. I visited the orthopedic doctor and was told I had a three-fourths tear of my rotator cuff, possibly more. This was confirmed from an MRI of my left shoulder. Thinking back, I remember the moment it happened. I was walking Thor in the yard on a leash. Unbeknownst to me, the neighbors let their Great Danes out. Thor took off to the left with a huge jerk on my left arm and shoulder.

I wanted to wait until after my prostate surgery and radiation. Honestly, I needed to know what the future held before I committed to that surgery. Who knows? It might not even be worth it.

"I can just see everyone at my funeral, standing around the casket. One of my friends looks to the other and comments that I look good. The other responds by saying, 'I sure am happy he was able to get that shoulder fixed before cancer killed him.'"

The reaction to my decision not to have it fixed? My shoulder froze. (I will explain later.)

When it finally sunk in that I had cancer, there were plenty of things to ponder while lying awake in bed each night. The lack of sleep was not a good prescription for combating the already profuse fatigue. But there was much to be done, and an unknown amount of time to do it. I tossed and turned. Many a night I watched the clock: 12:00 a.m., 1:15 a.m., 2:05 a.m., 3:11 a.m., 4:15 a.m., 5:30 a.m. I would give up and get out of bed. An early start on the to-do list for the day. I spent the night planning it.

"I can sleep when I'm dead."

All my days were filled with fatigue. It was a constant battle to find ways to push through it. Still today, the lyrics to this song describe my daily life.

FATIGUE

Ingrid Dec 2012

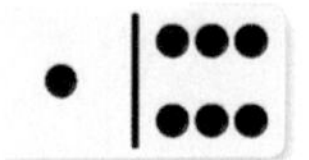

Chapter 7

HOW WE LOST FAMILY FEUD

Sagittarians strongly value their families, though they are rarely close to them. They are honest and straightforward toward their families, even though they are quite complex while expressing their feelings.

It was September. The heat of summer had faded to be replaced by the cooler temperatures perfect for outdoor gatherings and the general enjoyment of life. It seemed like the perfect time to celebrate life. My impending doom only rushed my intentions to gather and to perpetuate family time, whether it be the last time or just another time; who was to say?

Through several visits to the urologist, the one conversation he had avoided was my long-term outlook. He would not tell me about my chances for long-term recovery.

I asked him point blank, "What are my chances of long-term recovery?"

He changed the subject. Or he spoke about my current labs. Because of his avoidance, I felt that gave me the information that I needed to know. I knew that *it* was *BAD.*

So, as a result, I felt compelled to get the family together as soon as possible to explain the details and extent of my cancer. To have a celebration while I still felt well enough.

My prostatectomy surgery was scheduled for October 13. Actually, Friday the 13th.

In my mind, there might not be another time to have this get-together after that surgery.

I've heard of many cases where people pass away without having important conversations. There are arguments and divisions over who gets what, and I wanted to avoid those by getting everything out in the open with a family gathering.

The other thing is that finances were not Nila's strong suit, and she would need some help when I was not around. When I died, there was a $750,000 life insurance policy, whose purpose was to pay off the house and set up a trust for Nila to receive money as long as she wanted to live in the house. I was still concerned that even so, she might need help.

Honestly, Nila will be a mess when I die. If you could see in our home when I was in bed, sleeping for hours upon hours, she was also in bed, sleeping. To an outsider, it would seem like she was the one with cancer because of the way she was reacting through her clinical depression.

Looking back at my intentions for holding the family get-together in September, in the whole big scheme of things, I wanted to tell them about my cancer because they really had no knowledge of the degree of my cancer, and it was time to be 100 percent forthcoming. And I wanted to do it in person, not by phone.

I should also say here that I invited someone else to our celebration. There was a period in my life, when I was recently out of the army and recently divorced, when I was actually homeless. There was a guy that I worked with who I did not know at all. He invited me into his home to stay because he knew I was living out of my car.

It was the most generous gesture I had ever experienced in my life. He had one child and one on the way. He also had an aunt and nephew living with him at the time. I can't imagine someone having such a huge heart as to invite a stranger into his home when he already had a full house. That was in 1990. We are still best friends today. So, I also wanted to invite him and his wife to this event. Not the family get-together but the celebration later in the day. He was as close to me as my biological brother, and I felt it appropriate that they be there.

Shane, our oldest son, arrived from Illinois first on Friday, September 8. He was in the army and served in Afghanistan and Iraq. In Afghanistan, he endured setting up a physical readiness training (PRT) site, and, for nine months, they had no running water or electricity. Shane also lost one of his best friends to a roadside improvised explosive device (IED) in a convoy.

When Shane got out of the army, he was not the same person. He had severe post-traumatic stress disorder (PTSD). I always felt responsible because there was a time when he was in training, and he called me, wanting to get out of the army, and I knew when he went in that it wasn't for him. But I convinced him to stay in. I actually told him, "If you get out of the army, you will likely regret quitting for the rest of your life."

I didn't know this when I was in the army, but once you get out and you have served your time, there is a pride you carry like a banner with you for the rest of your life. Shane did and does carry that pride with him, but he also carries a lot of pain and struggles. In retrospect, I wish I had helped him get out. Shane's nickname in the army was Short Fuse Muse.

Shortly after Shane arrived, more of our kids began to show up. Shane was immediately upset because he thought everyone was showing up without their significant others. I chalked that up to poor communication on my part.

When I married Nila, Shane was five, and she had a child that was four. This weekend was also her child's birthday. To me, it was another reason to celebrate.

Our youngest child is Alanna. She is fifteen years younger than our youngest son, Jeremy. Alanna was going through her own medical problems at the time. She was out of work due to her knee. Steroid shots weren't working, and she had a scheduled surgery. The surgery revealed a lateral tear, shredded meniscus, a tumor under the cap, and one pound of fatty scar tissue, but no cartilage.

Within the first hour of Alanna arriving home, Shane questioned why she wasn't working. Alanna explained that the doctor had put her out of work because her job required her to stand all day and would cause more pain.

Shane's immediate response was, "A doctor's not going to tell you to quit your job. That's a f***ing lie."

Alanna burst into tears and began to yell at Shane.

Nila had to intervene. Alanna was trying to leave the basement, and Shane was following and continuing to berate her. She went upstairs to her old bedroom to be alone. That ended interactions between Shane and Alanna for the rest of the evening.

Shortly after Alanna went upstairs, Jeremy arrived from Georgia. Jeremy is our youngest son. When Nila and I married, the boys were three, four, and five. Having three sons so close in age, we did the best we could, but it was hard, and money was tight—we rented a 1950s trailer to live in; when Alanna came around twelve years later, it was a completely different picture. We leased to own a three-bedroom brick house; plus, in just a few years, we only had one child in the house to provide for, so she lived as an only child while our boys lived as a family of five or even six after Alanna came along.

The boys always made comments about Alanna having it better than them when she grew up. It always broke my heart when they would say that. I wished I could have done better for them. I did the best I could with what I had. Doesn't everyone?

On Saturday morning, we took everyone to breakfast at our favorite local restaurant, Pennyman's. All in all, it was a great breakfast and gave me hope that the mood would be more conducive to a celebration than an argument. After breakfast, we all went out to the rock patio to have our family meeting. I brought a wooden chest that had been padlocked for many, many years, where the kids had stored their own "collectibles." They were anxious to see what was in there. It had literally been twenty years since they had seen them.

I started with the grimmest news. What they had read on Google about prostate cancer might be true about other people's prostate cancer, but not mine. My prostate cancer had spread beyond my prostate. My Gleason score was eight out of ten, which meant that the cancer was very aggressive, like a tiger shark hunting prey. Only this tiger shark was loose in my body somewhere. The cancer was also stage four out of five stages. So, to put it into perspective, if you are in stage five, you are considered terminal.

What they were expecting and what they had heard about prostate cancer was different from what they were hearing from me, so I was staring at shocked faces. They were having their own morbid thoughts. I thought they would have questions for me, but no one was speaking.

The second part of my plan was to discuss my assets and my plans for what would happen after my death. This was a tough conversation for me to have. I really wanted to have this conversation to avoid any family arguments after my demise. I had practiced this conversation fifty times before this day, but as I sat there with them, giving my instructions straight from my memory, it finally hit me that I was talking about my own death. I asked my children to take a walk through the house that weekend and note down furniture or things that they might like to have after Nila and I were both gone.

As I tried to tell the children the best way to do this, Shane interrupted me and said, "This is BS. You need to find another doctor...you need a second opinion."

I told him I planned to do that.

Somber moment, caught off guard. It was clear that the other's minds were off in a million directions...trying to process.

If I were to do it over again, I would share this information ahead of time rather than shock them all at once. It seemed like a good plan at the time, but now I realize the position that I put them in.

We went back to talking about the assets. The main conversation with the boys was what to do with the house.

They said, "We didn't grow up in this house, so it doesn't have any special meaning to us. The best thing to do is just sell it."

Alanna, on the other hand, spent ten years of her life growing up in the house, and she had a different opinion. To this day, we have not resolved how to handle the house.

Shane said he wanted my guns.

Alanna and Jeremy wanted my music collection and my NASCAR collectibles.

Other than that, they just wanted to sell everything.

The next thing we did was decide to open the wooden box and pull out all of the things we had saved for most of the kids' lives (they were collectible items to them).

There were things from the 1996 Olympics in Atlanta that Nila and I attended. We were actually in Olympic Park less than twenty-four hours before the bombing that killed one person and injured eleven others. There was a host of other miscellaneous items important to the boys that they had put in the box. When we opened the box, there was a lot of excitement. As soon as that was over, the mood changed, and the excitement was over.

We had gotten a birthday cookie for the birthday celebration. At that point, Shane went into the house to watch the Georgia Bulldogs football game and to be alone.

Alanna tried to engage Shane with questions, yet his response was similar to the night before, basically cold and angry.

So, the family get-together continued without him.

Steve and Paula, my best friends who took me in when I was homeless, showed up wearing their Tennessee Vols shirts.

When they came downstairs and spoke to Shane, his response was, “Tennessee sucks, and what the f*** are you doing here?”

Steve came to me, hugged me, and asked me if they shouldn’t be there. I told them they were part of my family. Tensions lowered, and as the evening went on, we were able to get everyone together on the patio. We had some drinks, took great pictures, and told many stories.

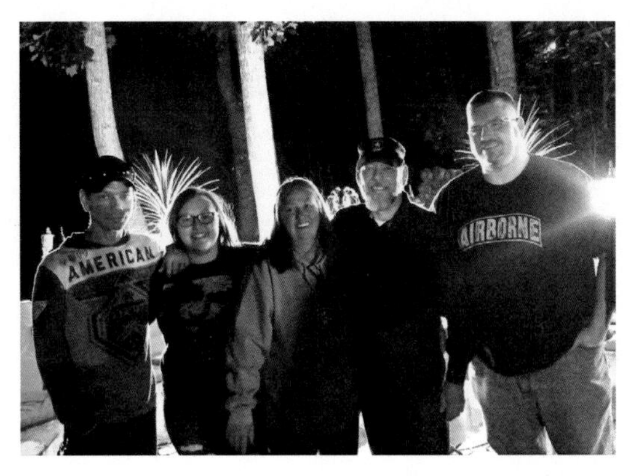

Left to right: Jeremy Muse, Alanna Muse Rupert, Nila Muse, Perry Muse, Shane Muse

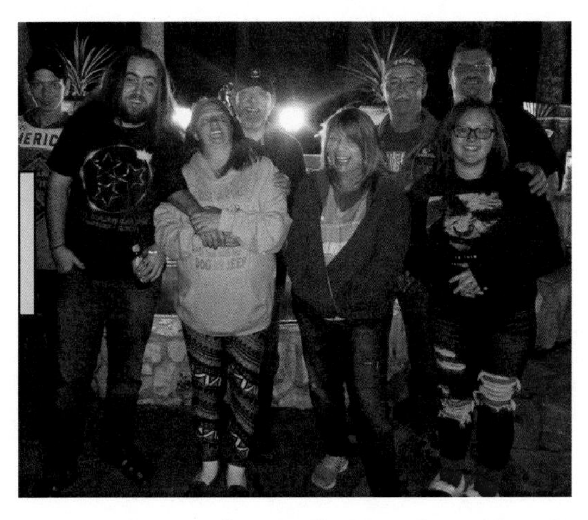

Left to right: Jeremy Muse, Steve Keylon II, Nila Muse, Perry Muse, Paula Keylon, Steve Keylon, Alanna Muse Rupert, Shane Muse

The next morning, Jeremy headed back to Georgia. Cory and Alanna went back home, and, later that day, Shane flew home. Two of my children did not participate in creating a list of things they might want, and the two who did participate wanted very little. Unfortunately, it seemed they valued our lives not at all. No one wanted any of our pictures. What would remain of Nila and me after we were gone?

Shane remained upset, disgruntled, and angry up until the time he left. He seemed fine at the party, but I realized the next day that he was faking it. After he left, he unfriended me on Facebook and blocked my number for several months. Later, I was able to ask him what was wrong with him during that time, and this is what he said: In his mind, the get-together was premature. He vented his anger at Alanna, and it became a petty sibling dispute (in his words). He also did not want to deal with picking over my stuff and tagging it for "later," and he could not come to terms with the fact that I might die.

I take responsibility again for this because I should have been transparent with everyone and told them how grim the outlook was before they showed up. I only had the energy to do the get-together because I was running on 5-Hour Energy drinks and green tea; I was hiding what I really felt like. I did not want them to see their dad dying of cancer. I wanted them to see their old dad. I wanted to have one last party with them—me laughing and drinking with them at a celebration, even if it meant I needed to do it with steroids, meds, and energy drinks to boost me. The contrast between the grim news and what they saw in me at that celebration was confusing to everyone and created the resulting arguments, denial, and pushback. I was even ghosted by my own son. That's how I lost Family Feud.

I truly love my family. I wasn't always the best at showing and telling them, but they are my world. Whitney says it best in the lyrics from this song.

FAMILY FIRST

Whitney Houston 2011

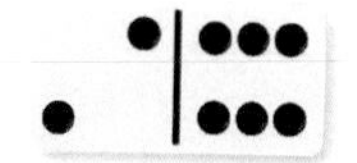

Chapter 8

WHEN ACID WAS A BIG THING

The Sagittarian is an optimist. He loves the world and everything in it. If something doesn't go his way, he knows that he'll still be able to survive without more than a scrape or a bruise.

I was born in 1960, a decade many commonly refer to as "the sixties." Others defined it as the "cultural decade" when many cultural and political trends were set around the world. Old ways were changed, and new ways were taken up. The introduction of the birth control pill and rampant use of certain drugs are just a couple of examples.

The Vietnam War began in 1955. In 1961, seven hundred American advisory forces were sent to Vietnam. By June 1962, that number had risen to twelve thousand. The number grew again to sixteen thousand in 1963. In 1964, Congress authorized President Lyndon Johnson to "take all necessary measures" to protect American soldiers from the "communist Viet Cong." Within days, the draft began.

At home in the United States, the struggle for civil rights drew national attention in February 1960 when four black students sat down at a whites-only lunch counter in Greensboro, North Carolina, and refused to leave. Their movement quickly spread as hundreds of demonstrators went to that lunch counter every day. Across the upper south, tens of thousands packed into segregated restaurants and stores.

In 1964, President Johnson passed a civil rights act prohibiting discrimination in public places. It also allowed the Justice Department to sue states and promised equal opportunities to all. Martin Luther King Jr. was an American Christian minister who became the most visible civil rights activist and leader of the civil rights movement. In 1968, he was assassinated.

Groups began to show impatience with the government and the incremental reforms being passed in Congress. Therefore, they formed counterculture movements, including the civil rights movement, the feminist movement, and the antiwar movement, among others. Student activists became extremely radical. They took over college campuses, organized massive antiwar protests, and occupied parks and other public places in large numbers. Some factions made bombs and set campus buildings on fire.

The counterculture grew more and more outlandish throughout the sixties. A segment of young people dropped out of political life completely. They became known as "hippies." These hippies grew long hair and practiced "free love." Some moved to communes to escape everyday life in the sixties. This is when acid became a big thing.

Lysergic acid diethylamide (LSD), also known conversationally as acid, is a hallucinogenic drug. Effects typically include altered thoughts, feelings, and awareness of one's surroundings. Many users see or hear things that do not exist. Effects typically begin within half an hour of taking the drug and can last for up to twelve hours. LSD is used mainly as a recreational drug or for spiritual reasons. Users commonly refer to using the drug as tripping or getting fried. Sobering from the experience is commonly referred to as crashing, or coming down.

Albert Hofmann first synthesized LSD in 1938. The hallucinogenic effects were not realized until 1943. An oral dose of as little as twenty-five micrograms (a few grains of salt) will produce vivid hallucinations. But acid was made popular by individuals such as psychologist Timothy Leary, who famously encouraged students to "turn on, tune in, and drop out." This was a prominent factor in creating a counterculture of drug abuse that spread from the United States to other parts of the world.

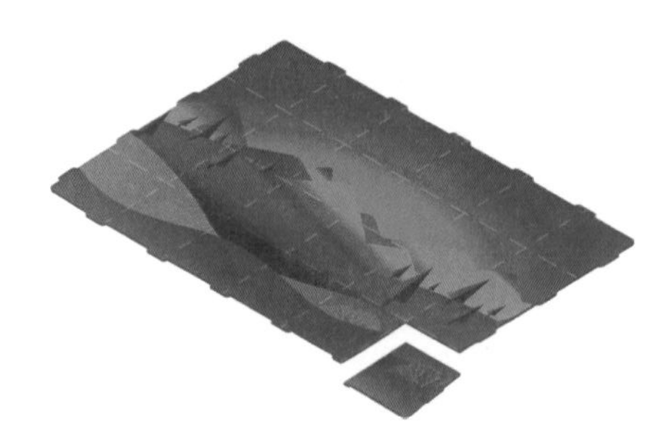

Blotter Acid

Some of the more prominent types of acid were blotter, windowpane, or purple microdot. Blotter was made using a paper sheet and applying droplets of LSD to it. Sometimes the paper had pictures and lines to divide up the doses or hits. Windowpane was similar but used a transparent sheet that could have small gel packs with the LSD inside. Differently, purple microdot was in pill form and colored purple. The shell of the pill encapsulated the LSD.

Psilocybin mushrooms have been used for thousands of years. In 1961, R. Gordon Wasson, a banker and mushroom enthusiast, brought a sample of the mushrooms back to Hofmann from his vacation in Mexico, where he had found an indigenous tribe using them. Psychiatrists, scientists, and mental health experts considered psychedelics like psilocybin to be treatments for a broad range of psychiatric diagnoses, such as alcoholism, schizophrenia, autism, depression, and more. As with LSD, psilocybin mushrooms were declared a Schedule I controlled substance, primarily due to having no accepted medicinal use and due to their high potential for abuse.

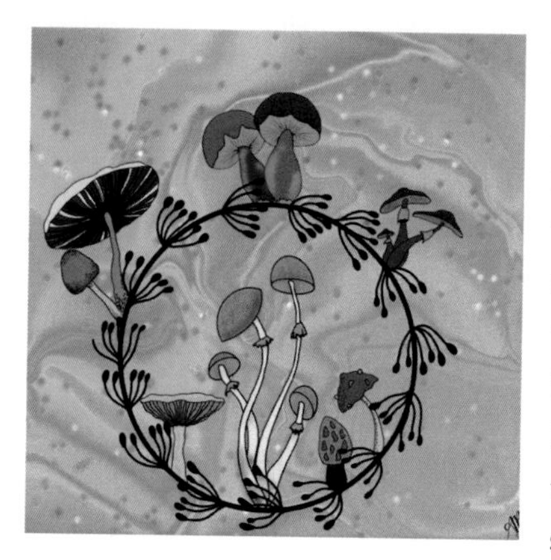

Artwork by Alanna Muse Rupert

Acid became a part of the culture of the sixties. In 1964, the Merry Pranksters sponsored an "acid test" using LSD produced in San Francisco in the first major underground LSD factory. The Pranksters staged a series of events that involved dropping acid (a slang term for taking LSD) accompanied by light shows, film projection, and improvised music. The Merry Pranksters traveled across America in a psychedelically decorated school bus and distributed the acid. Their activities are documented in the book *The Electric Kool-Aid Acid Test.*

Acid also influenced music and art. It was gaining popularity, in part due to bands such as the Grateful Dead and Jefferson Airplane taking part in the acid test. It was also being reflected in creative posters and album art. New genres of music, called psychedelic music and psychedelic rock, tried to create music that described the acid experience.

The sixties were my first decade of life. I remember the Vietnam War. The Vietnam War came to an end, and my father retired from the army after twenty-four years. He also served one term in the Korean War prior to his two terms in the Vietnam War.

I didn't learn about civil rights or dropping acid until much later in life. I do remember being so excited to see my father and the other soldiers coming home. I recall being confused about why the hippies were so angry at them. They threw debris, spit at them, and yelled obscenities at the soldiers as they paraded by from the airplane that brought them home from war. It was my first experience seeing the anger and division in the world I lived in. I was perplexed and disappointed.

In my early years of life, I also recall living in Columbus, Georgia. The year was 1965, and I was five years old. My sister, seven years older than me, was riding me on the handlebars of her bike. The bike got a bit out of control, and I ended up in the ditch. I don't remember the landing, mostly because it knocked me unconscious. I can imagine her panic, especially since I also had a vertical cut in the center of my forehead that was a couple of inches long. For a five-year-old, that was a big cut on the forehead. We all know how much a cut on the head bleeds. So, I was in the ditch, unconscious and bleeding. This would become my first scar.

I loved growing up in the sixties and seventies. In 1976, at age sixteen, I owned a brown Ford Pinto. After basketball practice one day, my friend David was behind me in his Chevelle SS. It was a beauty—marine blue with the iconic white stripes running along the center of the hood and trunk.

As we drove home that day, I was in the lead on a curvy road when David revved his engine and pulled into the right lane. I couldn't believe he thought he could pass me! He didn't know that Sagittarians do not like to come in second! I blocked, punching the engine faster and pulling the wheel to the right so that my car moved ahead of his in the left lane. Only now, I wasn't looking at the lane ahead of me; I was spending most of the time looking in my rear-view mirror.

Suddenly, gravel crunched under my car, and I felt the wheels shift as they sped off the pavement and off the road on the right-hand side. I abruptly jerked the steering wheel to the left, overcorrecting. Now, as if in a dream, I suddenly found myself speeding along in the ditch on the opposite side of the road from the one I had initially run off. The sound of the ditch scouring the driver's side of the Pinto was deafening. The view of the ditch was up close and personal at a foot or so from my head.

The glass broke, shards flying, leaving the driver's window open. Then, the car began to roll. I placed my hand firmly above my head for support. The drive through the ditch and the roll that ensued seemed to last for an eternity. Then, there was a violent change of direction. Looking out of the hole that framed the windshield, I saw the sky, the ground, the sky, and then the ground. My left hand held firmly to the steering wheel, and my right was still planted firmly above my head. Another violent change of direction, and I was rolling again. I was quite the roller coaster enthusiast, and this ride had remarkable similarities. Then, as suddenly as it all began, it stopped.

The brown Pinto sat in a gravel drive just as perfectly as if I had been driving out to the road from the house behind me. I felt my right knee getting sore. And then there was a burning sensation in my right calf. When I looked down, the engine sat in the cab with me, burning through my jeans.

David later said that when I left the ditch, I rolled four times, hit a small tree, flipped end over end two times, hit another small tree, and rolled two last times. When I was finally removed from the car (thanks to the Jaws of Life cutting through the Pinto frame like a giant can opener), I had cut my right knee where it hit the key ring in the ignition and had a slight burn on my calf from the engine.

"I've got to get a Chevelle" was my first thought.

My next car was a burnt orange 1972 Chevelle, and still ranks as my first favorite car I have ever owned. I never wrecked my Chevelle, likely because I never had to worry about finishing second while driving it.

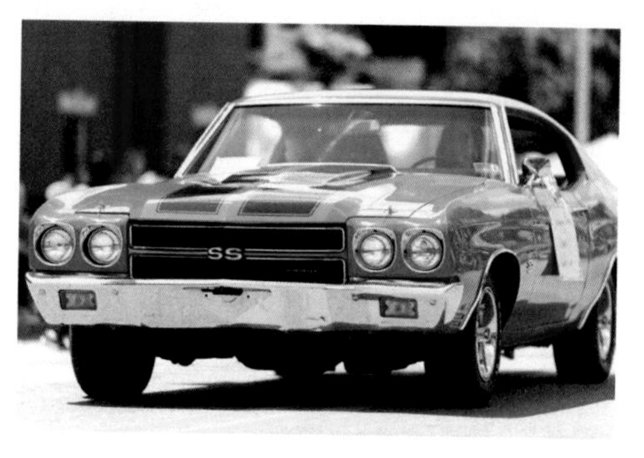

Like driving fast and trying to be the best, my whole life I have enjoyed almost any food I tried. When I was in the army, I had a good friend who was married to a lady from Thailand. She grew her own herbs and peppers. I marveled at some of the tiny peppers.

"How long until they will be grown?" I would ask.

"They are ripe now," she would say.

The dinner she prepared with her homemade peppers and spices was the hottest food I had ever eaten, but I loved it. I quickly understood the frozen mugs of beer that were served just before filling our plates. Whoever coined the phrase "dynamite comes in small packages" must have eaten authentic Thai food!

I took the opportunity to eat Thai food often after my initial dinner experience with the tiny peppers. However, I also enjoyed foods of all nationalities, from Southern home cooking to Italian. As with most youngsters, I never concerned myself with what I ate or drank. I consumed hot wings with a heat index of "torched." I drank my favorite alcoholic beverage, Crown Royal, chilled and without a mixer. I loved barbecue, Cajun burgers with onions, and all things spicy. In fact, when I was stationed at Fort Polk Louisiana, I took full advantage of creole seasoned foods. But, as with many things, my diet would come back to haunt me in a way that eerily connected to the decade I was born into, the sixties, the age of acid trips.

At nearly fifty-seven years old, I was way past due for my first colonoscopy. But that is where life found me on October 2, 2017, just two weeks before my prostate surgery. To this point, I had neglected simple annual blood work that would have detected my prostate cancer five years earlier.

"I've spent all of my free time studying prostate cancer. I don't want to learn about colon cancer too," I thought to myself before my procedure.

The purpose of a colonoscopy is to evaluate the colon for cancerous lesions, identify areas of bleeding, or diagnose other gut-related disorders.

Leading up to the procedure, Dr. Fry recommended specific dietary changes such as no raw fruit or vegetables, nuts, or grains. The day before, I was prescribed a colonoscopy preparation, commonly known as just prep. While different prep types exist, the aim is always to empty the colon of fecal matter, so that a doctor can view it clearly. It is important to hydrate well a couple of days before the prep, as you may dehydrate otherwise. It is also important not to take in any food or liquids that are red or orange. These may give the doctor a false impression of bleeding in the colon. I was instructed to drink part one of the prep the evening before. Part two was to be taken the morning of the procedure. Unpleasant does not begin to describe the experience with the prep.

I was also instructed to stop taking certain medications that could increase the risk of bleeding during my colonoscopy. For me, it was nonsteroidal anti-inflammatory drugs (NSAIDs). Unfortunately, ibuprofen and naproxen, both NSAIDs, were a routine part of my daily life.

"Those pesky ribs will be sore and stiff tomorrow until they shoot me up with the knockout cocktail," I thought.

The morning of October 2, I woke up and drank the second part of my prep. When I arrived for the procedure, I was introduced to the nursing staff who would be in the room with me during the colonoscopy, as well as the anesthesia specialist who would be providing sedation.

Once I was dressed in the fashionable gown, complete with full back access, a nurse inserted an IV into the vein on the back side of my right hand. This is a painful place to get an IV. But it was worth it so I could receive the medications during the procedure. First, a little something to relax me and ensure my stomach remained calm. Later, the cocktail to make me sleep during the intrusion. When the anesthesiologist injected the sedation medication, I began to feel...high. I fought sleep for as long as possible and enjoyed the feeling of inebriation.

"I think I'm starting to trip, man. This is what it must have been like when acid was a big thing. No wonder his name is Dr. Fry," I thought.

The colonoscopy procedure involves inserting a thin scope with a light on the end into the rectum. They look for irregularities in the colon's lining and, if they find anything suspicious, such as a polyp, they might take a biopsy or remove it, if possible.

Ideally, a person's colon prep will be so effective that a doctor can advance the colonoscope far enough into the colon to see where the small and large intestines join. When the doctor has completed the examination, he will remove the scope. The anesthesia professional will stop administering medication, and the person will wake up.

I woke up in a recovery suite. No more tripping, just a groggy, disoriented feeling, like I had just crashed. Soon after, Dr. Fry joined Nila and me to review the results. If the colonoscopy was positive, it would mean cancerous or precancerous cells were present. But Dr. Fry reported everything was fine. No polyps. He showed us pictures taken during the procedure. I was relieved and thanked the doctor. Now, Nila could drive me home.

Slowly, over time during 2017, I found myself needing to consume antacids. I was dealing with heartburn and acid reflux routinely. I began adjusting my diet, but the problem worsened anyway. By mid-2017, I had Tums at home, in both of my offices, in my satchel, and in every vehicle. Some days I carried a pack around in my pocket.

"Please don't tell me I have esophagus cancer. I know it won't be from my prostate cancer. It will be because I torched my throat," I thought.

Shortly after my colonoscopy, it was time to see Dr. Fry again.

Two months after my colonoscopy, on December 5, 2017, Dr. Fry performed an esophagogastroduodenoscopy (EGD). An EGD is a test to examine the lining of the esophagus, stomach, and first part of the small intestine. I was back in the medical center where the colonoscopy had been performed just a few days earlier. The procedure uses an endoscope, which is a flexible tube with a light and camera at the end.

The nurse attached wires to my body that were connected on the other end to a machine to monitor my breathing, heart rate, and oxygen. My IV was inserted into the right forearm, along the inside portion and about midway between my wrist and the fold of my elbow. This was just as uncomfortable as the IV in the back of my right hand, which had stayed sore and bruised for several days. Then, the anesthesiologist came in.

"This is where I get fried!" I thought.

But this time the drug wasn't anything like before, and I just fell asleep.

I felt no pain during the procedure. While I slept, a mouth guard was put in to protect my teeth, and I was rolled onto my left side. The scope was inserted through the esophagus to the stomach and duodenum or the first part of the small intestine. Biopsies were taken to review under a microscope. The procedure was over in about twenty minutes, and I was rolled to recovery.

Dr. Fry sat down and reviewed the findings. This time the report wasn't so positive.

"You have gastroesophageal reflux disease (GERD), which has resulted in Barrett's esophagus," he said. "There is substantial damage that could lead to cancer if not treated immediately. We will send the biopsies off to a lab and have results in a couple of days."

"There's that C word again!" I thought.

GERD is a digestive disorder that affects the lower esophageal sphincter (LES), the ring of muscle between the esophagus and stomach. Dr. Fry explained that I suffered from GERD due to a condition called a hiatal hernia. In most cases, GERD can be relieved through diet and lifestyle changes; however, some people may require medication or surgery.

Barrett's esophagus is a condition in which the flat pink lining of the esophagus becomes damaged by acid reflux, which causes the lining to thicken and become red. Between the esophagus and the stomach is a critically important valve, the lower esophageal sphincter (LES). Over time, my LES began to fail, leading to acid being able to travel from my stomach and causing chemical damage to my esophagus, thus causing me to develop GERD. Months, or years, of acid slipping by the failing LES valve and causing my reflux, and nighttime regurgitation, eroded the lining of my esophagus.

Barrett's esophagus is commonly associated with an increased risk of developing esophageal cancer.

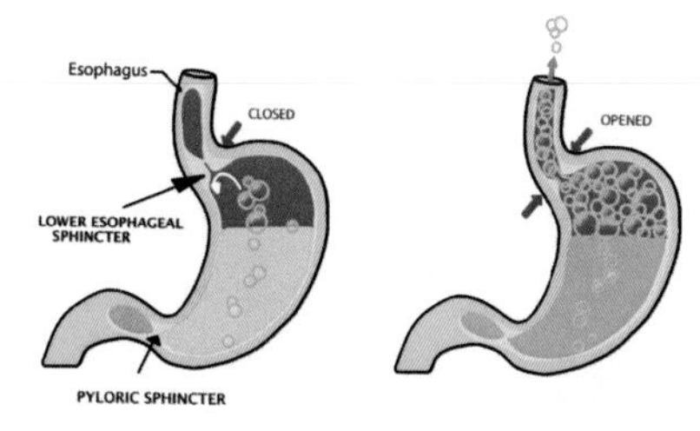

Artwork by Alanna Muse Rupert

The acid in your stomach is a colorless, watery digestive fluid whose main purpose is to break down food. In chemical terms, it is an acid solution with a pH between one and three, consisting mainly of hydrochloric acid (HCl). Neutral is seven. The lower the ph, the more acidic. During the digestive process, stomach acid (or gastric acid) kills bacteria and helps break food down into very small particles of nutrients and substances that can be absorbed through your intestinal walls and ultimately into your bloodstream. The average person's stomach produces about two to three liters of gastric juice per day.

Dr. Fry urged me to change my diet and prescribed 40 mg of Omeprazole daily. I did not hesitate to follow his instructions. I retired from eating Thai peppers, torch-indexed wings, and red sauces. I also weaned myself off fried foods (not 100 percent) unless I controlled the oil. It took discipline to change my habits, but it was far better than the alternative.

"Should I have a Cajun burger with a side of esophageal cancer or some baked chicken?"...my internal dialogue.

My annual follow-up with Dr. Fry showed marked improvement in my Barrett's esophagus symptoms. I still had bottles of Tums everywhere, as a reminder to keep taking my daily pill and to watch what I ate. Fortunately, my biopsies were negative.

LSD was a big thing in the sixties and seventies. But for me, it was a different kind of acid that was a big thing in 2017. One that could have caused another kind of cancer had I procrastinated a little longer, just as I did with my prostate.

Life is short, so the saying goes. When I reflected back on my life after the cancer diagnosis, the lyrics to this song reached out and grabbed me. I think this could be true for most of us.

TIME

Pink Floyd 1973

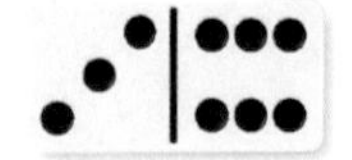

Chapter 9

INVADE, OCCUPY, INFEST, INUNDATE, DEPART

If something bad happens in life, Sagittarians try hard to cover up their emotions and to have a spectacular comeback.

July 28, 2017, was my initial visit to see the urologist.

It had been eighteen days since my visit to Deanna and my first discovery of PSA. The lead-up to the appointment was accompanied by anticipation and anxiety. It reminded me of when Nila and I were younger.

The year was 1997. My employer at the time offered testing and vaccines. I don't recall the specifics. What I do remember is the company nurse contacting me and asking that Nila and I come in to see her. I found it odd and immediately went to her office. She sat across from us and began to explain the reason for calling us in. As she spoke, she began to cry. "Oh my God, did she stumble upon something terminal? Is she about to tell me I have cancer?"

But it wasn't cancer. She explained that I had tested positive for hepatitis C. Hep C is a contagious liver disease spread through contact with the blood of a person who has the virus. It can result in serious liver damage, including liver failure. Remember, this was 1997. There are six genotypes of hep C, and they are all curable today. However, not in 1997.

She began to lay out the rules we must live by: "Perry must not share any of his eating utensils. No one in the family can drink after him. There can be no exchange of bodily fluids. This means even kissing is not allowed. This is very contagious and life-threatening."

Still crying, she apologized again: "I am so very sorry." As though she had given it to me.

Nila and I were shocked and in disbelief. There was no Google to research for us. The nurse made an appointment for us to see a specialist and handed me a paper with all of the rules. Basically, I was to isolate myself. It was three weeks. Three long and excruciating weeks of wondering what would be next. We waited anxiously for a doctor to tell us more about my hepatitis C condition. Finally, the day arrived, and we drove to the office of the specialist.

He was a liver specialist and greeted us in the opposite fashion to the way my company nurse had sent us off. He was jovial and very upbeat. I wasn't in the mood for silver linings and chitchat.

"C'mon, Doc. Let's get to it. Tell me how long until my liver sends up the white flag. I'm sure you know the odds of a transplant and the success rate. Give it to me, so I can get my head wrapped around the options."

Instead, he opened with shocking news of his own: "It's quite common to have a false positive when not testing specifically for hep C. We will run the specific liver test and see what the results tell us."

The test is called a recombinant immunoblot assay (RIBA). The test registers if there are any hep C antibodies. We were stunned and completely unprepared for the doctor's news. I wasn't out of the woods yet, but there was tremendous hope. An hour earlier there had been only impending doom and morbid thoughts. It took several days for the results to come back. The RIBA test revealed it had, in fact, been a false positive.

I cannot begin to explain the heartache that we endured from the moment the nurse began to cry until the phone rang with the message that it had all been a mistake. I still don't understand how this could happen. How can a person be expected to wait, completely segregate from his family, stop working, and not be devastated? How much of a difference would it have made to know about the high likelihood of my diagnosis being a false positive? Plus, I'm sure no one even considered the conversations with my wife while she was hurting and wondering how I might have contracted this. And she was wondering, did I give it to her? What about our three boys?

To say we were devastated is absolutely not an overstatement. And the wait to see the specialist, plus the wait to get that phone call, seemed like an eternity. The days waiting to see my urologist after finding out my PSA number were very similar as far as intensity, anxiety, and an unsure future. But this time, I purportedly wasn't contagious.

I recall watching movies to pass the downtime. Nila and I always made time to have a movie night. We read books together and watched a variety of movies from a broad range of genres. I always loved reading with her. I would read, and she listened. It was like watching a movie, but somehow a little more special...romantic. We would stop and discuss what was happening or what might be coming, like hitting pause on the DVD player.

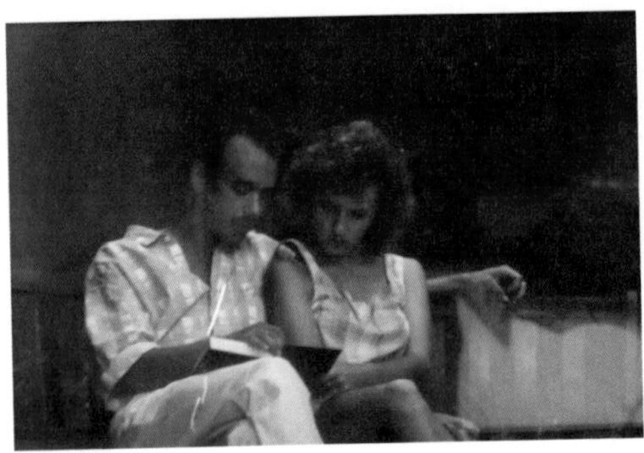

Perry and Nila, summer 1991

In 2017, while we spent time trying to ignore all of the possibilities surrounding my PSA numbers and their implications, it seemed every movie we watched contained a part where one of the characters had cancer. Even when we watched regular television, there were commercials for Cancer Treatment Centers of America, or "if you used product X and have been diagnosed with cancer, call ...." It was impossible to forget about my condition. The whole world was making sure of that.

When we walked into the urologist's large waiting area, it was nearly full. I was surprised to see how good the urology business was! Once we were called back, the nurse took my vitals and processed through the normal questions. When asked about what brought me to their office, I shared that my PSA had checked high.

"What was your PSA score?" she asked.

"One seventy-nine," I say.

She stopped typing on her chart, looked up at me, and said, "Wow, that's high," with a forced positive smile.

Dr. Hinder came in and was gone almost as fast. Like a whirlwind, he brushed by us, giving information, then he was out the door.

"One seventy-nine is a really high PSA. You will start Lupron shots immediately. We will schedule those every six months for the next two years. We will need to get a rush on insurance approval. The shots are around $4,500 each. We need to schedule you for a biopsy to determine your Gleason score and a path forward," he said, and then he was gone.

I felt like a woebegone trailer upturned by the whirlwind—shots that cost $4,500 each? Shots I would need for the next two years?

"Do they plan on me having cancer for two more years? My friend said they would just put a radiation seed in the prostate to kill the cancer from the inside and then give me radiation treatments to kill it from the outside. The cancer will be killing me from the inside if it lasts two more years!"

Deep down I had hoped that perhaps the PSA test results were similar to the hep C. Maybe I had had a false positive because there needed to be a specific PSA test from a specialist. But not this time. One day after my initial visit with Dr. Hinder, they called and confirmed the one seventy-nine PSA.

It wasn't until I gathered all of my medical records to write this book that I noticed little things in the reports. For example, take my first report from my initial appointment with Dr. Hinder. Line #1 states: **cc: I have an elevated PSA**. The report from the day of my biopsy is the same overall format. However, now line #1 states: **I have prostate cancer**.

At 8:30 a.m. on August 8, 2017, about one week since my initial consultation, I had the prostate biopsy performed. The procedure was short and only took about ten to twenty minutes. I was asked to lie on my side and bring my knees to my chest. The area being tested was slightly numbed. A lubricated probe was inserted into the rectum to generate the ultrasound. A small needle was then inserted through the probe to take tissue samples from my prostate. There was some mild pain and discomfort, but it wasn't remarkable. After twelve tissue samples were taken, they were sent to a lab for analysis.

A couple of days later, I was back in the office to discuss the results of my biopsy. The news was grim.

"We use a nationally recognized scale called a Gleason score to determine the size of the tumor within the prostate and the percent of cancer within each biopsy," said Dr. Hinder. "The numbers are added together to equal a single Gleason score. We have determined your score to be between seven and eight out of ten. The higher the number, the more serious, as this means a greater infestation. The average weight of a normal prostate is twenty grams. Your prostate weighs approximately forty grams."

"Before you leave today, you will get your first Lupron shot and continue every six months. There are two options to consider. The first is to have a radiation seed embedded into your prostate, followed by radiation treatments. I do not recommend this option for you," said Dr. Hinder. "Your high Gleason score, plus the size and weight of the prostate, indicates to me the cancer has likely spread outside of the prostate. The second option is a radical prostatectomy. This is where we remove the prostate and follow up with radiation in the nearby areas where the cancer may have spread."

Within ten seconds, I chose the surgery. I didn't have but one choice realistically. The results showed the least percentage of cancer in any biopsy was 70 percent. The most was 100 percent. The 70 percent portions were in the minority.

The official writeup stated, "*The tumor is present in almost every core, documenting bilateral disease, with the highest involvement in the mid portion of both lobes, lesser involvement of the base by volume, and relatively low involvement of the apex bilaterally. I do not see extraprostatic extensions in these biopsies.*"

If I read this before writing this book, I do not recall. Perhaps my mind was overwhelmed. Perhaps I didn't feel the need to read it since Dr. Hinder told me what I needed to know. Either way, as I read this on June 26, 2020, the last statement was unclear. So, while writing this chapter, I looked it up. Remember what Dr. Hinder said, "Your high Gleason score, size, and weight of the prostate indicates to me it has likely spread outside of the prostate." *Extraprostatic (extracapsular) extension of prostate cancer* refers to local tumor growth *beyond* the fibromuscular band surrounding the prostate gland. Extraprostatic extension is associated with a higher risk of recurrence and metastasis and *lower cancer-specific survival* after a radical prostatectomy.

As of this moment, I don't have an answer as to why his report would say there was no evidence of tumor growth beyond the prostate, but Dr. Hinder expressed to me that he thought there was, and he was the medical expert.

It is difficult to consume bad news, especially when the word cancer is involved. But it is important to read the reports and understand what they say. What I researched states prostate cancer spread outside of the prostate and is an extraprostatic extension, and the research clearly tells you it is associated with a high recurrence rate and lower survival, even with prostatectomy surgery.

In my mind, when I left the consultation, I believed my future was a short, dismal one. Maybe it still is. I want to believe Dr. Hinder wanted to assume the worst in order to treat me accordingly and give me the best shot at a positive outcome. That's a wonderful plan, but it would have been nice to know. Perhaps Dr. Hinder told me his plan was to treat the worst possible scenario based on my numbers, and he told me that mixed in with everything else, and I just missed it. It was a lot to consume in a few minutes.

Either way, it was just today (June 26, 2020) that I realized there is a possibility the cancer was not confined to the prostate. Research and ask questions. I left the office in a bit of a daze and don't recall ever reading my biopsy report. I went into another room, where I received my first $4,500 Lupron shot.

"So much for $4,500. This didn't feel any different from the flu shot I got for free at Walgreens, but if it kills cancer, give me two!"

My next step was a bone scan on September 6, 2017. This was a computed tomography scan (CT scan) that created horizontal images of my body using a combination of X-rays and horizontal images. A CT scan shows detailed images of different parts of the body, including the bones, muscles, fat, and organs. My CT scan focused on the abdomen and pelvis areas with and without contrast.

In a CT scan, dense substances like bones are easy to see, but soft tissues don't show up as well. They may look faint in the image. To help them appear clearly, you may need a special dye called a contrast material. Contrast materials block the X-rays and appear white on the scan, highlighting blood vessels, organs, or other structures. I wasn't sure why the bone scan was needed until I researched a little. The bones are greatly affected by prostate cancer. Not only can the cancer spread to the bones once outside of the prostate, but the treatments are also hard on the skeleton.

Nearly all types of cancer can spread or metastasize to the bones, but some types of cancer are particularly likely to spread to bone, including breast cancer and prostate cancer. Bone metastasis can occur in any bone but more commonly occurs in the spine, pelvis, and thigh bones. It can cause pain and broken bones. With rare exceptions, cancer that has spread to the bones can't be cured.

"If my prostate cancer has spread into Mr. Skeleton, the sand is racing to the bottom of the hourglass."

The test wasn't very long. My biggest issue was the hard table. It had been eight years since I flip-flopped one hundred and ninety-two feet down the payment, trying to outrun my bike. The days were rare that I did not need to see my chiropractor or roll on my blue cylinder to pop ribs back into place. I wondered if they would ever just stay put. But for now, it was painful to lie flat on the hard surface for the bone scan.

Once I was able to find some level of tolerance, the table quickly carried me inside of the machine, through the large donut-shaped device. I closed my eyes and rested while listening to all of the unique sounds. I heard slight buzzing, clicking, and whirring sounds as the scanner inside the donut hole revolved around me. Once it was over, the table carried me back out.

I recall it being difficult to rise up from the table. The ribs were quite angry with me. As I struggled to make it to a sitting position, the technician looked on, asking if I needed help, and wearing an expression of helplessness. It made me feel old and far removed from the muscular guy that had lived on Walraven Way only a few years prior.

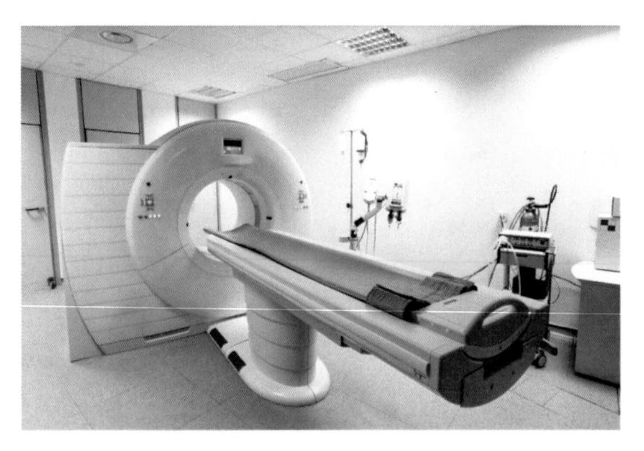

CT /PET machine

Again, we were playing the waiting game. I was trying to focus on work, and I started planning to get things in order while I was out on surgery. I couldn't let my job slip. The sign of a great manager and leader is having structure and personnel in place so you can go on vacation. This wasn't vacation, but I needed things to be in order. By now I had decided to tell the family the whole truth and nothing but the truth. The family get-together was quickly planned, and I began rehearsing how I would share the news. There would be questions, and I wanted to have answers to all of them. I also wanted the news to be shared face to face. They deserved that. Perhaps a celebration afterward.

Meanwhile, the anticipation finally ended. The phone rang, and I finally got some positive news.

"Your bone scan is clear," said a female voice on the other end of the line. (I have no idea who the person was.)

"So," I thought, "if the cancer has spread outside of the prostate, Mr. Skeleton is safe for now."

When I got the news that my bones were safe, but I was going to have my prostate removed, and radiation, I decided to make an appointment with our daughter to have a nice portrait of Nila and me made. I wanted to do all of this while I could still physically do it. Before the weight fell off and Mr. Skeleton became more apparent. When we sat for the picture, I had already lost twenty-five pounds in about six weeks—a radical diet plan I would not endorse; who would?

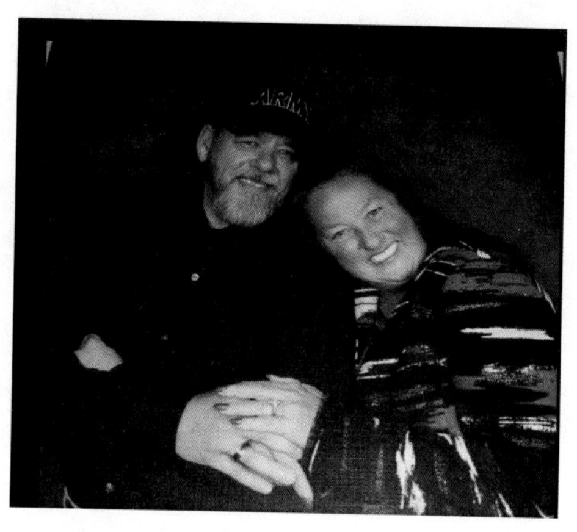

Our portrait taken by Alanna Muse Rupert

I showed up for my surgery at 6:00 a.m. on October 13, 2017. It was impossible not to think about the fact that it was Friday the 13th. I went through the normal preparations and recited my name and birth date a dozen times. I was finally given my first dose of medication to "get me comfortable." Over time and through all of my prior surgeries, I had challenged myself to fight going to sleep. I never fell asleep after the first dose. I wanted to look around and see all that was going on. What did the equipment look like?

The warm air blowing beneath the blanket felt good in the cold surgery room. Half a dozen folks were busy zipping around, getting everything prepped. They were working like machines. I was given the final dose, and a mask was placed on my face.

"Breathe deep," someone said.

The challenge to stay awake grew harder. Gradually, I began losing an understanding of the conversations. I felt removed from the room and off to some adjoining room that echoed with indiscernible sounds. I saw Dr. Hinder and gave in to sleep.

The procedure I had done is called a da Vinci radical prostatectomy. A da Vinci prostatectomy is a procedure that uses a laparoscopic approach and robotics to remove all or part of a man's prostate gland. Surgeons using da Vinci technology may be able to remove your prostate gland through a few small incisions (cuts) or one small incision. During surgery, your surgeon sits at a console next to you and operates using tiny instruments. A camera provides a high-definition, 3D magnified view inside your body. According to the manufacturer, the da Vinci System is called "da Vinci" in part because Leonardo da Vinci's "study of human anatomy eventually led to the design of the first known robot in history."

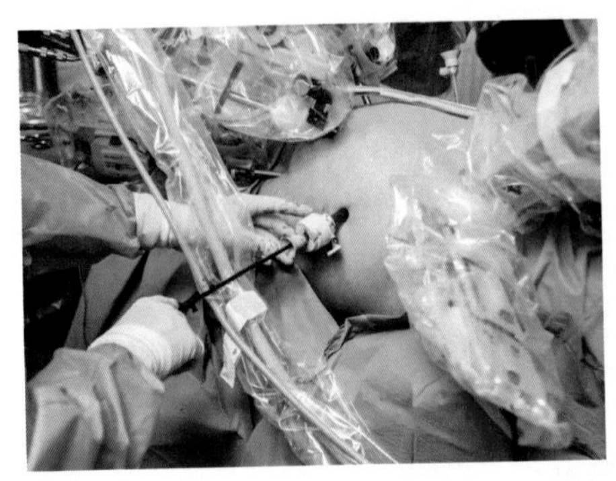

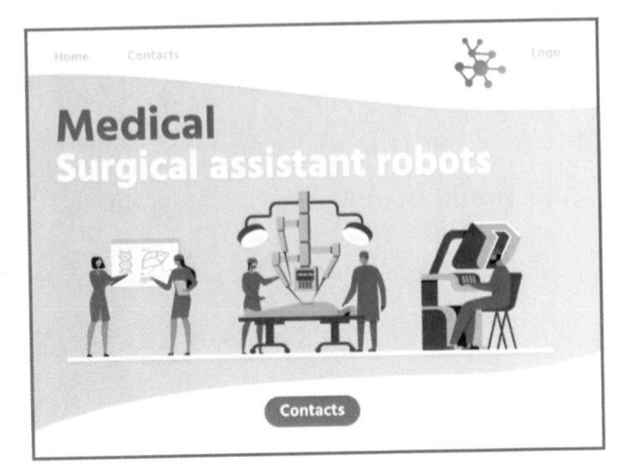

When I awoke, I was aware immediately that this surgery was major. Although the pain hadn't hit me, I felt as though probes were in my abdomen. My stomach was bloated with gas and pressing on the incisions. I had not seen the pictures above and wasn't sure what to expect. Sometimes it is best not to look on the internet for information, especially when the word cancer is associated. You can get lost and depressed almost beyond repair. It wasn't necessary in this case. I was having the surgery and would deal with it when it happened. And it was happening.

Nila was the first to look at my incisions. The expression on her face was telling.

"Nothing you say is going to sugarcoat that look!"

She said, "Oh my God. I had no idea. I wasn't expecting this."

"Take a picture!" I asked her. Or told her.

Then she said, "Uh, there's something you should know. You have a catheter."

What? A catheter? Like in my penis? No one said anything about a catheter.

"What goes in must come out," I thought. "I dread when that day comes. What the hell! How did they even get that in? I hope they put me to sleep to pull it out!"

I was rolled to my room and then transferred to my bed. Even with the leftover drugs in my system, the transfer was enormously painful.

I thought back to 1973. My friends and I crashed the pool at the Holiday Inn in Dalton, Georgia, like we did often. We swam for thirty to forty-five minutes. Back then there were still diving boards at hotel pools. I ran, bounced, jumped, and positioned myself for my famous cannonball. As soon as I hit the water, I was met with excruciating pain in my side, back, and abdomen. The pain paralyzed me, making swimming impossible; I thought I might drown in this pool because I didn't think I could make my arms and legs move. I let my momentum carry me to the bottom of the pool, where I was able to push off enough to reach the surface.

Back in my hospital bed, for a moment it was like my recurring nightmare where I could see the surface of the water, but pain numbed my body into inaction, and I was never able to reach air and life. But this was no dream. I remembered back to that pool many years ago, when it was imperative that I reach the surface. If I had inhaled, it wouldn't have ended in me waking up with a tremendous gasp!

When I was in that hotel pool, once I surfaced, someone noticed I was in trouble. The pain was so intense. An ambulance was called, and I was transported to the hospital. Shortly after arriving, I was being prepped and headed to surgery. I awoke with an incision about four to six inches in length, running horizontally on my front right side. Beneath it, my appendix no longer resided.

My friends and visitors wanted to cheer me up, but laughing was so painful. I kept a pillow across the incision and applied light pressure whenever I had to cough or laugh. That experience made me acutely aware that almost every movement of the body uses the abdominal muscles. If there is an incision, and body parts are removed, lying still is the thing to do. That is until you must move.

No sooner had the nurses gotten everything hooked up to the many machines in my room after my prostatectomy, than I was told that walking as soon as possible was important. I felt like I was going to need some medication before attempting that. Once the room had cleared, I looked at the picture Nila had taken. I had a long, curvy incision starting inside my belly button and heading north. It was much like the curvy road where I sped away from Nila on my CBR600RR in August 2009, not realizing back then that the curvy path was leading me straight to pain.

On my left side was a drain tube with a pump. I wondered how far the tube ran down inside my body. I didn't know at the moment, but I would find out the answer in three days. There were two small incisions, one on each side of the belly button and slightly above. Each was made at approximately the same distance from the center.

Higher up on my right side, even with the top of the long, curvy incision, was a slightly wider incision. Later I will explain why this incision was likely the most wicked of them all. My stomach was swollen and full of gas. The pressure could be felt at every incision and deep inside where the prostate and two lymph nodes had been a few hours prior but were now removed and the empty spaces forced to heal out of sight. And then there was the catheter, the revolting tube connected to a bag to hold my urine. It was at that moment that the gravity of the surgery set in.

"No time for self-pity, Sagittarius," I thought. "It is time to get mentally tough and prepared for what is surely going to be a painful recovery."

I began by telling Nila to get my phone and start making some calls and texts. Of course, she was already ahead of me. Then I asked her to look at my emails. She wasn't a fan of this request. I'm sure it felt similar to me ordering her to "Take off my PowerTrip jacket" before calling 911. But I needed the distraction. I needed to let work know I was all right and available. I asked her to read through the new email titles. The ones that sounded important were to be opened, and the body read to me.

"The tables have turned, and Nila is reading to me now," I thought. "It's awesome, but this is all required reading, not entertainment."

I had her type a couple of responses or comments that would suffice on Friday the 13th. The plants closed early, and I would now have the weekend to heal.

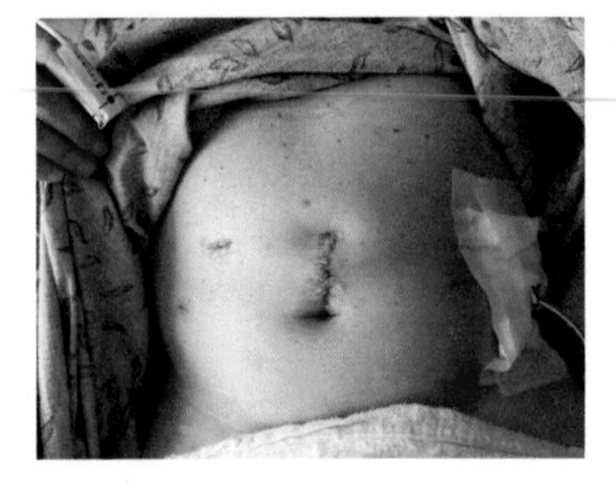

My abdomen immediately following surgery

Shortly afterward, I was able to get out of bed with a lot of assistance. Looking back, I can see how this must have been hard on Nila. I could deal with the pain much more easily than if I had to watch her suffer through it. But that was what she did. Our children, except Alanna, were strewn about the nation. Our brothers, sisters, and other relatives. were several hours away. Our friends were few in our new town. In the end, they were absent. Nila would spend every moment with me in the hospital. Our only visitor was Alanna. Though Alanna tried, Nila was determined not to leave my side.

Getting out of bed and walking was dreadful. The pain oscillated between an eight and a ten, depending on my movement. It lessened to some degree after several steps, but my pain tolerance was being overtaxed. This wasn't like the Tin Man from the *Wizard of Oz,* who is suddenly caught in a rain shower and rusts up. A few squirts of oil, and he gradually begins to break the rust loose, little by little freeing himself up to walk again.

Each time I lay in the bed and went through the process of getting up to walk, it was more like *Groundhog Day*. In the movie, Bill Murray wakes up to it being the same day, every day. For me, each time was like the first time following surgery all over again. I didn't feel progress. I felt the same pain and soreness over and over. I had to make sure I was mentally prepared each time for the pain that came with each walk.

That evening I met the night nurse. He was overly jovial and talkative for my first day. He was happy to explain my medication options after a short introduction. He knew better than I how important this conversation was. "You can have Vicodin, generically known as hydrocodone, every four hours. You can also have morphine every four hours. However, you can't have both at the same time."

Vicodin contains a combination of acetaminophen and hydrocodone. Hydrocodone is an opioid pain medication. An opioid is sometimes called a narcotic. Acetaminophen is a less potent pain reliever that increases the effects of hydrocodone. Vicodin tablets are used for the relief of moderate to moderately severe pain. Morphine is an opioid medication. Morphine is used to treat moderate to severe pain. Short-acting formulations are taken as needed for pain. The extended-release form of morphine is for around-the-clock treatment of pain.

Night #1 definitely felt like what one would imagine from a major surgery on Friday the 13th. I made the wrong choice of medications to start the night, going with the Vicodin. It began to wear off in three hours. The bloating was worse and caused increased pressure. I was thankful that the nurse understood my situation and volunteered some much-needed options.

"If you stagger the morphine and Vicodin, it will hold you through better," he said.

I got it! I didn't realize I could do both, just not at the same time. From that point, I took one of the medications, and two hours later, I took the other. Although this allowed me to rest a bit more, the pain was still in the red. By 5:00 a.m., I was literally yelling in pain. My pantry of tolerance was empty. I had tried walking two times during the night. Was I overdoing it? It's what I was instructed to do. I was a good patient, and I followed my orders completely. Something was seriously wrong.

The nurse finally gave in and called the doctor. The doctor ordered double the morphine. It took thirty minutes, and I was thrashing and writhing in pain. Once administered, I still had to wait for it to take effect. To my dismay, the impact was hardly noticeable.

After more than two and a half hours, the nurse returned with additional medication. I pleaded with him to do something else. Something was obviously wrong.

"Did I tear something loose deep inside? The wounds where my prostate and lymph nodes once resided are surely torn open. I may be bleeding, and no one would know because no one can see."

He left and returned with two more pills. It was basically Gasex. It gives relief for abdominal distension, intestinal gas, belching, flatulence, and indigestion. Of course! The bloating was gas, and the gas was putting pressure on everything that had been invaded by the robot. I looked pregnant and thought it was swelling. Nila went to work on Google and found the explanation.

Post-op gas pain can occur after any type of surgery but is most common after abdominal and pelvic surgery. Open surgery with longer incisions and laparoscopic surgery in the abdominal cavity can leave the bowels (intestines) "stunned." Anesthesia (general, as well as epidural and spinal) can slow down the bowels, preventing the passage of gas and stool. Pain medications (narcotic) add to and contribute to this effect. As a result, patients frequently report constipation and gas buildup after surgery. During laparoscopic surgery, multiple ports are inserted into the abdomen through small incisions. Then carbon dioxide is blown into the abdomen to make room for the surgeon to operate.

They didn't want to give me something to eliminate the gas bubbles. They wanted me to walk and do leg exercises. I did all of those. I didn't do the minimal requirement. I went above and beyond. No one would expect less from a Sagittarius, after all.

Alanna arrived to visit later that morning and give Nila a break. Nila made it a mission to buy some Gasex and bring it back. It was a saving grace, and I was able to extend my rest time, partly due to relief and partly due to exhaustion.

Each day and each shift, I was asked if I had a bowel movement. The answer was always the same. "No." Each time I was reminded that before I would be allowed to go home, I *must* have a bowel movement. I wasn't eating, so I wasn't sure how that would happen. I thought of an episode of *Shameless.* Frank had sold some Vicodin to someone.

He said, "Remember to stay well hydrated when you're taking the hydros if you don't want to die on the toilet like Elvis."

Who would ever have believed that I would get something educational out of an episode of *Shameless*?

By day three, I was walking every couple of hours. The pain was always there waiting. Each time I walked further. It was a well-laid-out plan. Walk to the nurses' station first. Then, two doors past. Each time you had to beat your previous record until you completed a full lap. Then, work on two laps. I had only found out the day after surgery that two lymph nodes were removed during the procedure. This incited new panic. I thought I was out of danger when the CT scan showed my bones and organs were clear. Now I knew they were concerned it had spread into some of the nearby lymph nodes.

"No need to work so hard breaking records and consuming pain. If the cancer is in your lymph nodes, it will all be for nothing."

But I paid no mind to the morbid thoughts and continued breaking records. On the third day, I was asked again about a bowel movement. This time my answer was "Yes." Not because I heeded Frank Gallagher's advice and made sure I was well hydrated. And not because my bowels were no longer stunned from the laparoscopic procedure, but because it was a lie. I was ready to trade in the compressed hospital bed for my recliner. I was ready to dispense with the nurses and let Nila help me to heal. The nurses showed up later that morning and began the process of unplugging me. It was a welcome sight when I was disconnected. My arm was bruised and sore.

Then, last but not least (by far), it was time to remove the drain on my left side. It was more of a terrible sensation than pain. Still, there was pain. The nurse placed her hand on my side above where the tube entered. Then a single long pull, and I caught myself being loud. But it wasn't over. A second long pull. The pain and sensation weren't just in my head. It was as bad as the first. I could feel the tube snaking up from deep in my pelvis. I imagined it coiled somewhere deep in there, where blood and fluids puddled in the wounds where once a prostate and two lymph nodes existed.

I looked down to see the tube still hadn't exited. I felt lightheaded and took a breath as she made one last, long pull. I felt the tube slither out, and exhaustion immediately overcame me. So, on Monday, October 16, 2017, my new nurse drove me home.

The ride certainly had its moments. Nila was so careful, but she couldn't control the lack of attention from whoever was responsible for the conditions of roads between the hospital and Olgia Lane. We'd purchased new recliners (electric) just for this moment. I couldn't walk downstairs, so the longer path around the house was taken. The short trip home was still lengthy enough for me to rust up. The last record-breaking walk at the hospital had me prepared for the long walk. Finally, I was in the basement and in my new recliner. It was always cool in the basement, and the large-screen TV with surround sound provided entertainment.

Once settled, my first order of business was to take a stool softener that Nila had picked up with the Gasex. It was important that I get things functioning, and I prescribed this for myself to help. Next order of business was to call each plant and catch up on what was going on. Of course, adequate pain meds were needed ahead of time. Nurse Nila issued them, always within guidelines.

Shortly after, I joined in on a conference call. I mostly listened, but made it a point to contribute and show I was paying attention. This was an important call. My boss was one of the participants. He never said it, but I knew there was concern for my future and my ability to continue leading. It was a fair concern, one that occupied my thoughts more than the cancer itself. One that I intended to put to rest.

Next was a well-deserved nap. When the pain woke me, Nila was ready, as always. When the meds kicked in, it was time for a walk. The fall air was cool, breezy, and easy to breathe. The leaves were close to their most spectacular season of colors. Being home was good medicine, and the walk seemed more gratifying and less painful somehow. The animals welcomed me with love and attention. They were curious and seemed to understand my condition. They were so very gentle around me.

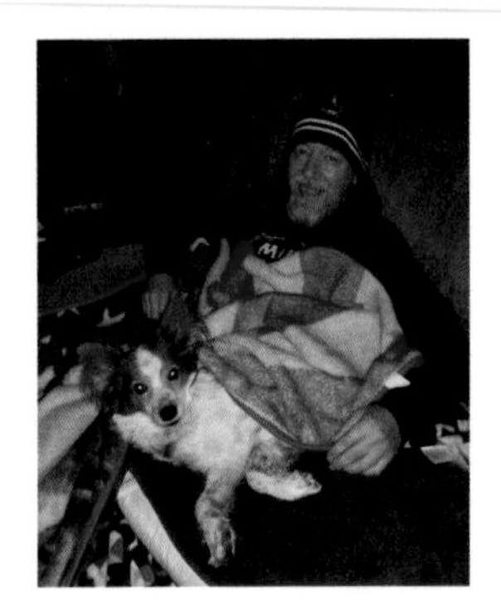

In the recliner with Sparky

Once back in the recliner, it was time for Nurse Nila to become Secretary Nila and go through my emails. After I caught up, my mind was freed from its to-do list. The pain was eased, and I could once again sleep. This became my routine. I soon took over the secretary functions, so Nila could focus on being a nurse and getting some well-deserved rest of her own.

The catheter was a menace to me. I was disgusted with emptying the bag. I had no clue when it was even filling. Whenever I went for my walk, it was a whole routine to change from the larger bag to the smaller-profile bag that was strapped to my leg. Just as I had done after my motorcycle wreck, I got Nila to take me to the plant as soon as I could handle it. I had to be able to walk and show how well I was doing. I knew there would be plenty of scrutiny. I was constantly aware of the urine bag strapped secretly to my leg.

"I'm making a good showing for the troops. Everyone is very welcoming and glad to see I am doing so well, so soon. I just hope there isn't a catheter malfunction, and I don't find myself drenched in urine. That would ruin it all."

On October 26, I went to see Dr. Hinder and hopefully get the catheter removed. I expected it to be uncomfortable. I had no idea what was really coming. The short visit with Dr. Hinder went well. He was happy with my progress. He also informed me the lymph nodes had tested negative for cancer.

"Thank God I didn't stop breaking those records!" I thought.

I was still thinking about the good news when he ran through some exercises I needed to do.

"Just act like you are urinating and cutting it off midstream. Repeat this over and over. It will strengthen your urethra," he said.

The doctor left, and Nila and I went into another room, similar to when I received my first Lupron shot. I was embarrassed to see Dr. Hinder's nurse come in to do the catheter removal. My penis looked dead and abused. I didn't recognize it as part of myself. She positioned herself with one hand on my lower abdomen and the other on the tube.

"Are you ready?" she asked.

Before I could answer, she pulled the tube. The sensation was that of a tube dragging along raw nerves. In an instant, the tube was out, and I found myself trying to disguise the discomfort and embarrassment. At that point, I was free to leave. Nila led. I followed. Down the hall and left at the nurse's station. Then down another hall and past the checkout window. I didn't have to stop, and Nila continued through the door into the large waiting area. I scanned the full room of mostly older gentlemen and their wives.

"I wonder how many of you have your catheter bag secretly strapped to your leg?"

I felt a strange sensation and looked down to find my pants were soaked. I had peed myself and didn't even know. I was shocked and embarrassed. How could I have done this? By the time I got home, I was drenched in urine down to my knees. No one told me I would not be able to control myself. Why didn't Dr. Hinder give me a Depends diaper? How did they expect me to make it home without this happening? Nila and I reviewed the visit and all of the instructions from pre-surgery to present. Nothing suggested that I bring a diaper to the catheter removal. Nila and I were furious.

Being the good patient, I did my exercises. Sleeping was nearly impossible through the entire recovery. My shoulder ached and minimized what options I had for positioning myself in the recliner. It seemed as though the shoulder pain I had neglected was worsening over time. In case there weren't enough things going on after surgery to challenge my ability to sleep, my shoulder pain limited the positions in which I could lie.

I was humbled and motivated by wearing the Depends. I remember starting to work my way up the stairs rather than the leisurely walk in the yard. I weaned myself off the medications early. This came at a cost, but I needed to see what my true progress was.

"I had better get off the narcotics. It would be a shame if the cancer is gone, but I die on the toilet."

I mentally celebrated starting to go into work. At first for a few hours, with Nurse Nila always with me. I was starting to sit in meetings when I would feel the sensation as I uncontrollably urinated into my Depends. No one knew, but I did. I was the one who had to show everyone that I was fine. I couldn't let Foam Products down. But my uncontrollable bladder didn't feel like I was fine. Meanwhile, I had noticeably more pain in the shoulder and significant loss in my range of motion (ROM). I tried to find a silver lining.

"Perhaps my golf game will be better. I will surely have that 'old man' swing."

In the back of my mind, I knew I had to work on the shoulder next. How would that be received at work? Another issue to keep me from being 100 percent? I knew there wasn't a choice in the matter. The pain and loss of ROM would make it a challenge to drive. I am predominantly left-handed, and this was my left shoulder.

As with anything that causes a person to endure a lot of pain over time, depression tries to seep in unnoticed. Add cancer to the mix, and the mental aspect of healing took work and focus. Still, I had Nila, and, for me, it was all I needed to exchange the depression for motivation. I couldn't hide it from her. But I didn't let it own me or get in my way.

If I could write the lyrics for a song that expressed how I felt (and still feel) about my wife, this would be the one. The lyrics to this song say it all for me.

WITHOUT YOU

Mötley Crüe 1989

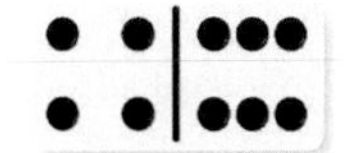

Chapter 10

VORSÄTZLICHE MANIPULATION!

The Sagittarius man is typically a natural scholar and loves both to learn and to teach, making conversations highly stimulating.

My fatigue was a roller-coaster ride, courtesy of my ricocheting health issues. In four months, I had undergone eighteen iron infusions to combat the anemia, a colonoscopy, an endoscopy of my esophagus, a prostate biopsy procedure, and a radical prostatectomy surgery. Although I was extremely tired, rest didn't come often or easy. My mind raced constantly, developing to-do lists or focusing on work that never ended. My shoulder had gotten progressively worse, and that meant more pain.

When I got a boost from the infusions, I worked even harder to be on top of the job that paid my bills. Plus, recovery from the prostatectomy was a struggle and tested my pain tolerance and patience. At this point, I had lost thirty-six pounds that my muscular frame could not afford to lose. Mr. Skeleton was becoming more apparent, and my appetite was lacking. Oh, yeah, then there was the cancer.

On November 14, 2017, I sat stiffly in Dr. Famoyin's office. I didn't know it yet, but it was on this day that our relationship would be transformed and become more personal.

I had researched Lupron treatments and prostate cancer.

I had educated myself thoroughly on anemia and the infusions.

I was determined there would be no more surprises like the day I had urinated on myself leaving Dr. Hinder's office.

When Dr. Famoyin walked in, I began to speak as though I were the doctor talking to my patient. He listened contentedly, and a smile began to appear as I recited medical terms and phrases. I was resolute on getting some answers, and that meant he needed to know I was a student of my own condition. When I finished, his first remark was a question

"And what is it you do for a living, Mr. Perry?" he said.

"I am a full-time Sagittarius if you are wondering why I did all of this research," was my initial thought. However, I answered his question by sharing my actual job title.

He replied, "So you have done a lot of homework and research similar to what you do in your professional work."

"Yes, sir. You are correct," I said.

Then, Dr. Famoyin said, "Now, let me tell you the rest of the story."

From that day forward, we have enjoyed a wonderful, honest, spiritual, and intellectual relationship.

Still to this day, he walks in and asks, "Mr. Perry, what is it you have learned that you wish to discuss today?" Regardless of my preparedness, he always tells me "the rest of the story."

On this particular visit in November 2017, only a few short weeks after my prostatectomy, we discussed Lupron reducing my testosterone and also the retreat of the psoriasis that had plagued me as a domino effect of the anemia. As usual, I told him about how I stayed tired, although having the iron infusions retarded the fatigue considerably, until my iron would once again drop. Dr. Famoyin understood.

In the summary reports under "Assessment," he always noted: "Adult failure to thrive."

"Perry, I notice here that you have begun taking a multivitamin?" he said, looking at the nurse's notes. "Tell me about that."

"Well, I've been trying to combat the fatigue, so I switched to something called Mega Men's 50," I said.

"You must stop immediately," he forcefully said. "I will check the ingredients, but because it says, 'Mega Men's,' and because it says 'fifty,' I believe this means it has testosterone boosters as a part of the ingredients," he paused here for emphasis and then went on.

"What you failed to uncover in your research is that prostate cancer feeds off testosterone. The Lupron shots are reducing your testosterone, so the cancer will starve," he finished.

"I've been feeding my cancer!" I thought, shocked at my own blunder. There is a good reason "doctor" is a part of his name prefix and not mine.

Because my shoulder pain was getting so bad, on November 17, 2017, just three days after learning that some vitamins can feed cancer, I met Dr. Wells. He was an orthopedic surgeon. Once I caught him up on my shoulder complaint and all of my health details, I was sent for an MRI (magnetic resonance imaging).

An MRI is a test that uses powerful magnets, radio waves, and a computer to make detailed pictures inside your body. The machine looks similar to the machine for a CT scan. However, unlike CT scans, MRIs do not use the damaging ionizing radiation of X-rays, and thus, there's no need to drink contrast.

Dr. Wells reviewed the results of my MRI. I had a 5 mm x 4 mm intratendinous-insertional tear that involved greater than 75 percent of the (rotator cuff) tendon thickness. I also had a 4 x 1 x 1 mm delaminating tear of the distal fibers of the infraspinatus muscle. There were signs of bursitis. Shoulder bursitis is an inflammation of the bursa in your shoulder. The bursa is a fluid-filled sac that acts as a cushion between a bone and a tendon.

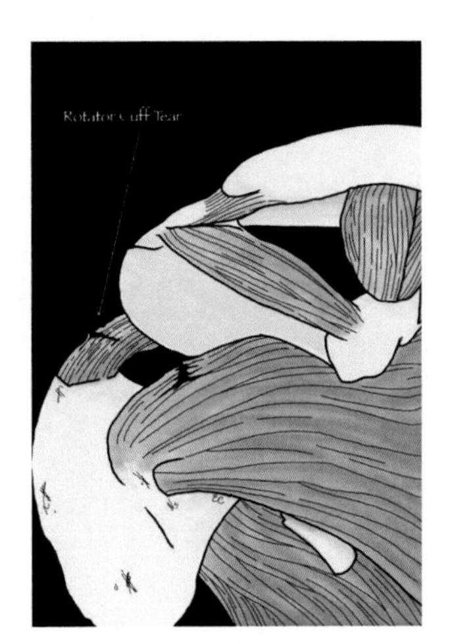

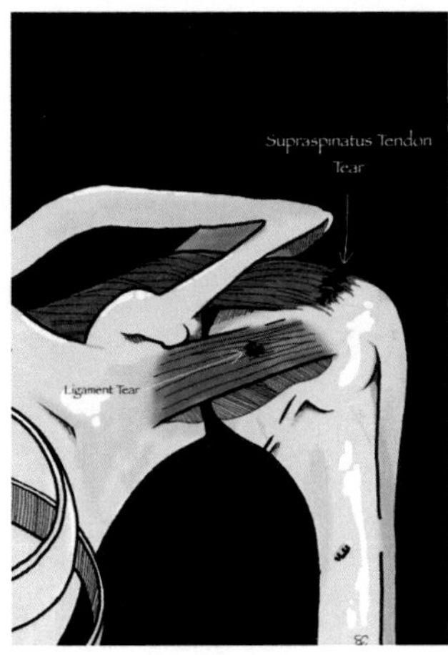

Shoulder drawings by Ezekial Cooper

It was also noted that there was labral fraying. The shoulder labrum is a piece of soft cartilage in the socket-shaped joint in your shoulder bone. It cups the ball-shaped joint at the top of your upper arm bone, connecting the two joints. The four muscles of the rotator cuff help the labrum keep the ball in the socket. This allows your upper arm to rotate.

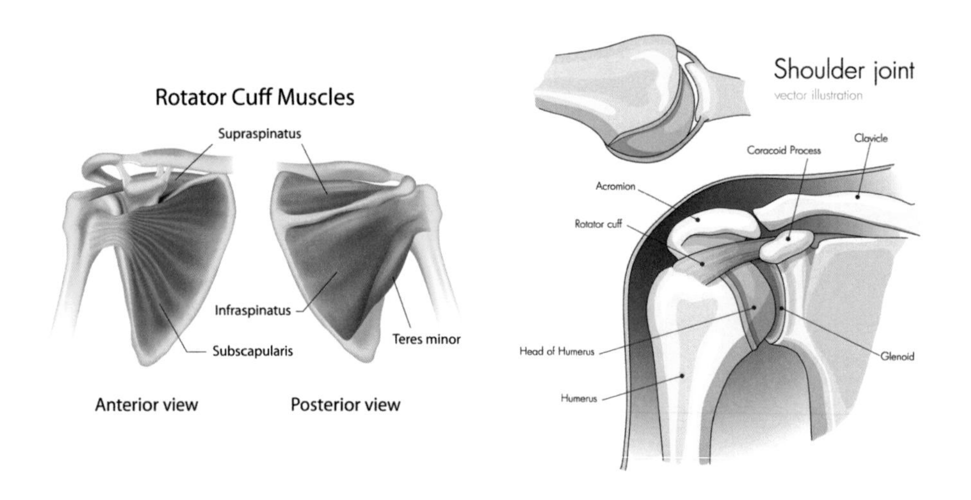

A section of the report referenced "Osseous / bone marrow." The report read, "Small subcortical cyst at the posterolateral aspect of the humeral head."

"Is a cyst the same thing as a tumor? If so, does this mean shoulder cancer?" I thought, walking to my car after the visit was over. I was reading the report because Dr. Wells had never mentioned cancer during the visit. Hmmm—more homework.

Subcortical or subchondral bone cysts (SBCs) are sacs filled with fluid that form inside of joints such as knees, hips, and shoulders. The sac is usually primarily filled with hyaluronic acid. Hyaluronic acid is a liquid in the joint fluid that lubricates the joint. SBCs aren't technically cysts. Instead, they are fluid-filled lesions surrounded by bone. Sometimes doctors call them geodes. SBCs are a sign of osteoarthritis (OA), a disorder in which the cartilage between joints wears away. These fluid-filled lesions are typically a response to an injury, such as a fracture, or conditions such as osteoarthritis.

Dr. Wells said that I desperately needed to have my shoulder repaired. I was already aware but wasn't going there yet on purpose. He then explained that a lot of time had elapsed since the injury. While I was dealing with all of my other medical problems, I had neglected my shoulder.

“You haven’t been using it because of the pain and discomfort,” Dr. Wells said. “Now you have a ‘frozen shoulder’ or adhesive capsulitis, and it must be addressed before we can repair the rotator cuff.”

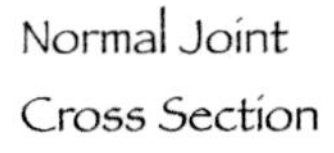

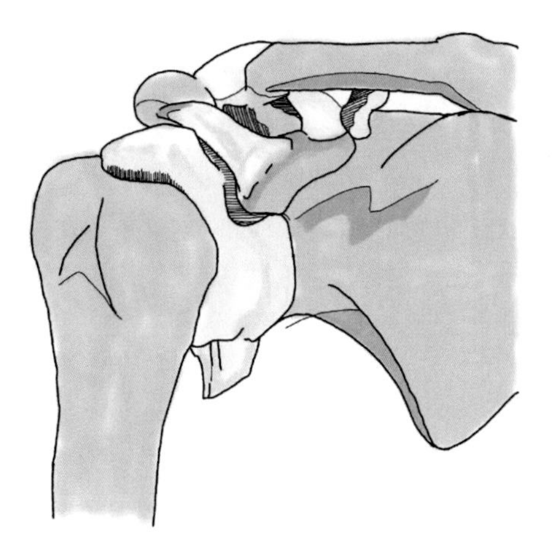

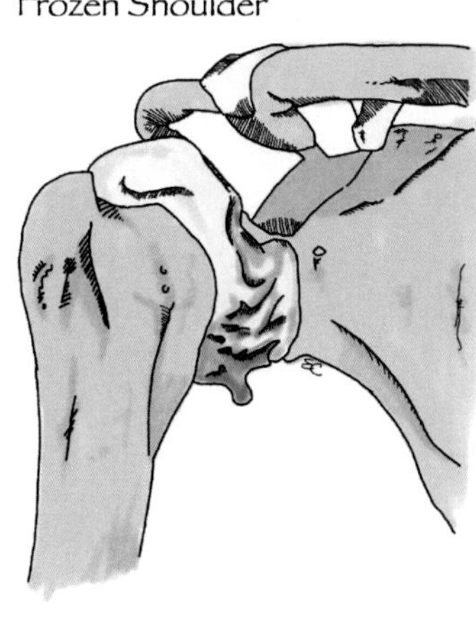

“So, how exactly do we address it, Doc?” I asked.

He said something about “intentional manipulation” surgery.

“I need to have surgery before I can have my surgery? I’m not fully recovered from the last surgery,” I thought.

Twenty-six days later, on December 12, 2017, I returned to the surgery center. This was the familiar place where, only two months prior, Dr. Fry had made me think of the sixties.

Vorsåtzliche is German for the word *intentional*. I have always thought the German language sounds forceful and sometimes angry. For example, the band Tool has a song named “Die Eier von Satan.” It is German. It begins with a word that appears to be “Die” in English. It has Satan in the title. But it is really not a song. There is a German fellow reciting the words (lyrics) over a loudspeaker in front of a huge crowd. He recites the words with strong emphasis. It is easy to visualize a German officer motivating his brigade of troops before battle. A strong point is made, and I imagine his fist slamming onto the podium. The troops erupt in support!

Of course, I had to know what was being said. All of the lyrics were in German. I bought the album in 1996. It was still two more years before the launch of the Google search engine. This meant I had to translate it the hard way.

Once translated, I was amused to find out the whole speech was a recipe. The title translated into "The Eggs of Satan." It was a recipe to make eyeball-sized pieces of dough, powdered and containing nuts. Hilarious.

But my manipulation surgery wouldn't be amusing. It would be forceful and done with great emphasis, like the fist slamming onto the podium. *Vorsåtzliche bearbeitung!*

Shoulder manipulation is a procedure to relieve shoulder stiffness and poor ROM. During the procedure, the doctor breaks away scar tissue that keeps your shoulder from moving properly. The scar tissue was responsible for the severe pain and stiffness in my shoulder. However, shoulder manipulation can also cause injuries to nerves and other parts of your shoulder. It may not fix the problem, and your shoulder could continue to be stiff and not stable. Shoulder manipulation may even cause a bone in your arm to break!

"Great, I could go in with a frozen shoulder and come out with a broken arm. Mr. Skeleton would not be happy with that outcome."

It was one week before my fifty-seventh birthday when I arrived for the intentional manipulation of my left shoulder. If my research was accurate, and it was, then it would not be a very happy birthday the following week.

After processing through the normal routine, the anesthesiologist administered the initial relaxation dose. Shortly after, I was rolled into the room where the procedure would occur. This time there were about half of the number of people working and prepping as were present for the prostate surgery. Understandably so—it was a much simpler procedure.

I was given the final dose to make me sleep. As I fought it, I once again enjoyed the feeling of alcoholic-like intemperance. I was lying flat on my back, and the surface angered my ribs. Just before slipping into a blissful sleep, I vaguely remember getting a shot in my neck. It alarmed me for only a couple of seconds, and I was out.

Dr. Wells moved my left arm up and out and then down and in. The goal was to break up the scar tissue holding my frozen shoulder in place. He made sure that my shoulder was moved through its entire ROM. Then, the movements were repeated. This continued until he felt as though the scar tissue was completely broken loose.

"I imagine the resistance that he must have felt at first, and then pushing my arm further until a crisp, crackling and popping sound was heard. Push in: crack, pop, and stop. Then out. Perhaps they turned up the music in the operating room to hide the sickening sounds coming from my shoulder. Perhaps a relaxing tune to aid the doctor in being gentle. Or perhaps 'Die Eier von Satan,' the troops cheering as the scar tissue shattered."

Nila was the first thing I remember seeing when I woke up in recovery, which was extremely comforting because I couldn't remember where I was or what had happened at first.

"How are you doing?" Nila asked.

"My shoulder," I gritted out through clenched teeth. "It's so bad...worse than ever."

"The nurse said to tell you that it's normal for it to feel worse at first. They already gave you some narcotic medication, but I will buzz someone," Nila said and pressed a button on the side of the bed.

A nurse breezed in within two minutes carrying a new black arm sling.

"Oh great, he's awake and doing so well! Look at that!" she said, oozing cheer. Then, she showed me and Nila the sling. Unlike previous slings, this one had a four-inch pad that, when I had it on, rested against my body. It forced my arm away from my body to hold my shoulder in the correct position.

"Any questions? Do you need anything?" the nurse asked.

"Why can't I feel my left arm or hand?" I said to her.

"The doctor gave you a shot in your neck that was a nerve blocker to deaden the feeling in your shoulder, arm, and hand," she said. "Eventually, it will wear off, but it will make your recovery easier." And she breezed out of my cubicle in recovery as quickly as she had breezed in.

It felt odd to touch my arm and not to feel the touch. It was like touching someone else. Other than being warm, it felt like touching a dead person. There was no response as I rubbed it or pinched it.

Dr. Wells came by after I had been awake for about an hour.

"Your procedure was a success, Perry! Everything went just great!" he said. Then, he turned to shake Nila's hand again and tell her some things I needed to do in the next several days, including some rules I needed to follow and some things I needed to do for the best recovery. Then, he turned to face both of us again to say, "He needs to be at physical therapy in an hour. It is located right next to the office."

"How can I do physical therapy in an hour with a dead arm?" I wondered.

But Nila dressed me and put on my stylish new black sling. We walked out, and she drove me to my first physical therapy appointment.

A favorite band of mine from the 1980s was Triumph. It was a three-person band out of Canada. After my cancer diagnosis, a particular song caught my attention on the radio one day. It was an old favorite called "Fight the Good Fight." It was released in 1981, the first year of my enlistment in the army. This unofficially became my mantra for my cancer battle.

When we arrived at the location for my physical therapy (PT), Nila helped me out of the car and into the building. I was still groggy from the anesthesia and likely appeared impaired walking through the front door. Even so, I was introduced to my therapist, David Lily.

Dave had me lie on my back on a table off in one corner of the room. Luckily, the pain meds were working, and my ribs were less concerned about the table I lay on. A round cylinder was placed under my knees, which further helped my ribs tolerate the table. As Dave was talking, he wrapped my shoulder in a heated pad. Although my shoulder was numb to the pad, the warmth radiated into my body and felt nice.

I lay there observing the activity in the room. There were many beds, or tables, and a lot of various therapy tools. There were stationary bikes, balls, resistance bands, and four therapists. I watched as people were given tasks by their therapists based on their personal needs. Then I saw something that shocked and surprised me. I wasn't sure at first and looked around at each of the therapists to confirm. They all wore T-shirts that had the company logo on the front left quadrant of the shirt. On the back read, "2 Timothy 4:7—I have fought the good fight. I have finished the race. I have kept the faith."

This epistle, written to Timothy, was Paul's last before his martyrdom. Earlier in this same epistle, Paul reminded Timothy to "endure hardship as a good soldier of Jesus Christ."

I had no doubt that this was a message to me. I was meant to be here and read this. It was uplifting, motivating, and far from coincidental.

I continued my PT schedule. Each visit began with a warm heating pad. Each ended with an ice compress, which was equally welcomed after the exercises. My first night home, Nurse Nila did a great job of massaging and exercising the numb hand, arm, and shoulder.

That first night, I was sitting beside her, watching a movie. Suddenly, something passed before me.

I jumped and yelled, “Hey!” It was unexpected and scared me.

Nila had picked up my arm and moved it across my body, in front of me. I had no clue. Nila had to pause for a good long laugh.

“I bet it wouldn’t be so funny if *you* saw a dead arm float in front of your face,” I thought as she laughed.

The numbness lingered for two days. While I was glad to get the feeling back, I was not so happy with the return of the pain. The exercise and therapy had obviously angered the shoulder.

“Careful about what you wish for. Maybe dead was best,” the little voice in my head whispered.

I came to love the ice compress as it provided relief.

At home, I spent my time downstairs in the recliner. My right hip became sore as I had to lie with my weight on it. It was a struggle to endure the pain between times to take my medication.

I resolved that I would not go through this again. I had a pulley installed above the door. Every couple of hours, I sat in a chair beneath the pulley. A rope ran through the pulley with hand grips attached to each end. I held the grips and pulled down with my right hand in order to raise my left arm skyward. It was an agonizing routine. But I was determined to fight the good fight and not let the shoulder freeze again. Exhausted, I would sit back in the recliner and begin my other exercises, the ones Dr. Hinder had assigned: “Just act like you are urinating and cutting it off midstream. Repeat this over and over.”

A week passed in this fashion, and my fifty-seventh birthday came. This Sagittarius was going to overcome the pain and incontinence to celebrate! I skipped my narcotics and had beer instead. It was just Nila and me, but I relished feeling well enough to revel. However, before I finished the second beer, I found myself soaked in urine again. Nila helped clean me up and get dressed. This time I took two sleeping pills and fell asleep.

Before seeing Dr. Wells, I had no idea about frozen shoulder or "adhesive capsulitis." I had created this domino effect as a result of my neglect or procrastination. As a result, rather than having three months to heal from my prostatectomy before radiation treatments began, I had six weeks to heal my shoulder through PT on top of having to teach myself how to hold my urine. The manipulation surgery wasn't intentional on my part. Nonetheless, it was compulsory.

I continued to go to work with Nila driving while I sported the black sling. I had to focus on leading and managing the two manufacturing plants that my boss had entrusted to me. I had a long way to go in the next six weeks. I had no idea what to expect from the upcoming radiation treatments. Every day I just hoped and prayed to be able to sleep, so I could keep up this pace.

I have loved this song since the first time I heard it in 1981. The lyrics are inspiring and so positively motivating. It is no wonder the lyrics made this my life's theme song after the cancer diagnosis.

FIGHT THE GOOD FIGHT

Triumph 1981

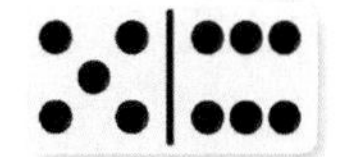

Chapter 11

BEAM ME UP!

Inspiring and spontaneous, Sagittarians can sometimes be seen as too aggressive or impatient by those who prefer a more subtle approach to life.

Halloween, Thanksgiving, my fifty-seventh birthday, and Christmas came and went in 2017 with a bitter pill of somber. In the past, Nila and I had had so much fun decorating and taking part in the festivities during the holiday season. We always dressed up like a couple of kids for Halloween. Since Nila lost her mom and dad, Thanksgiving had been hard on her; however, my mom and dad were in their mid-eighties, living alone in the house they built in the early seventies when my dad retired from the US Army. Thanksgiving and Christmas were the only two times each year that we got together as a family. However, in 2017, Nila and I would be absent from the holidays, compliments of my cancer.

At home, we even skipped all our holiday traditions even though Christmas had always been a huge deal for us. Our attic was primarily full of interior and exterior decorations. This included two trees. One was a five-foot-tall tree that we placed in the basement for us to enjoy when downstairs. The other was a seventeen-foot-tall tree that matched the height of the front window in our living room.

From October through December 2017, I spent the vast majority of my days and nights in the basement. That is, except for when I was at a doctor's office, a surgery center, PT, or being escorted by Nurse Nila to work.

Nila also dedicated time to decorating the five-foot tree, and she made it colorful and beautiful. She also set out an array of snowmen. This was her way of lifting my spirits. Truth be known, it was medicinal for us both. All in all, it gave me comfort and joy to see. I had fought feelings of depression because I knew I would not be able to help decorate. I knew we wouldn't be traveling back to Georgia to spend time with family and friends. I knew we would mostly be alone.

The seventeen-foot tree wouldn't even make it out of the attic, much less have ornaments or lights. Getting it down alone was a two-person job, not to mention the rest. But this year, Nila wasn't feeling the spirit of the holidays either. We celebrated Jesus's birthday with much less fanfare. We talked to God often and were sure He didn't miss the rest.

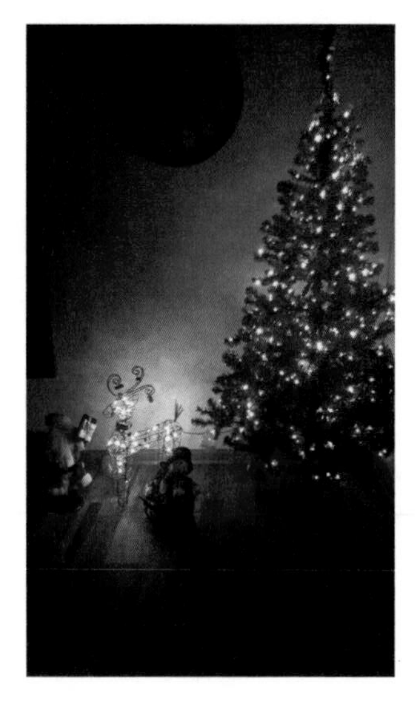

Five-foot Christmas tree downstairs

I was incredibly thankful for the holidays. I took a one-week vacation to add to the scheduled holidays at work. Christmas Eve and Christmas fell on a Saturday and Sunday. Therefore, my employer shut down on the Thursday and Friday prior. The Georgia facility was shut down completely the following week, and many took off at the Tennessee facility, as well. January 1, 2018, New Year's Day, was on a Monday, and the plants were down for the scheduled holiday. All in all, I had twelve days to mend. I needed to have a big comeback at work. On January 24, I would begin my thirty-eight radiation treatments.

Another side effect of my anemia was that I stayed cold, especially my extremities. As I said, we live in a mountainous area and in the forest. We had snow, which made our Saint Bernards happy. Nila kept a fire going in the wood-burning stove downstairs. She would even throw in the occasional foil pack that made the fire change colors. I knew it was her way of trying to lighten the mood and brighten my day. But I was constantly cold.

It was hard for me to be upbeat when my fingers and toes were like icicles. I spent my time at home wearing flannel pajama bottoms, knee-high socks, a sweatshirt, and a toboggan. Then, I would cover up with my heavy American flag blanket. I could always count on Sparky and Mr. Mitten to cozy up beside me for a little extra warmth.

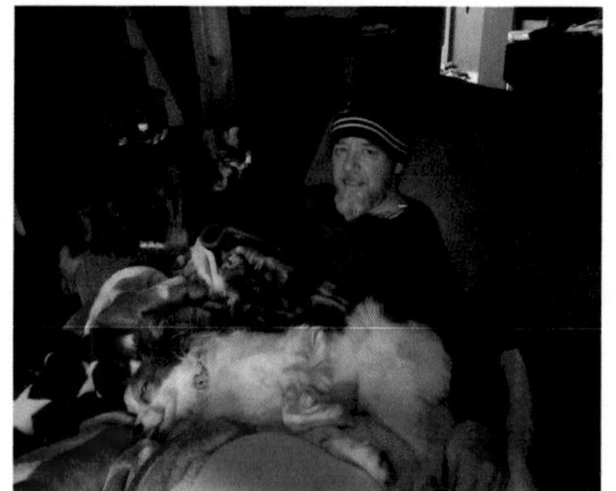

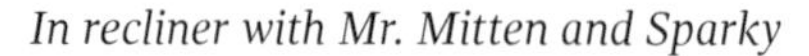

In recliner with Mr. Mitten and Sparky

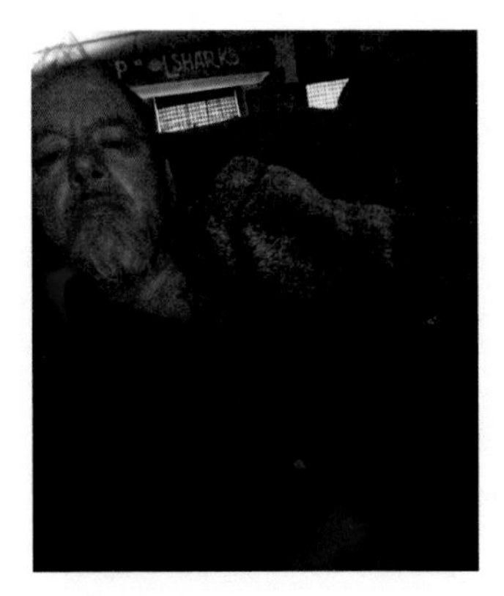

After shoulder manipulation surgery

On January 15, 2018, Nila surprised me with something wonderful.

She walked into the basement with colored hair! I looked at her hair and could not believe my eyes! Her hair had four different colors. It was red, green, blue, and purple. It was beautiful!

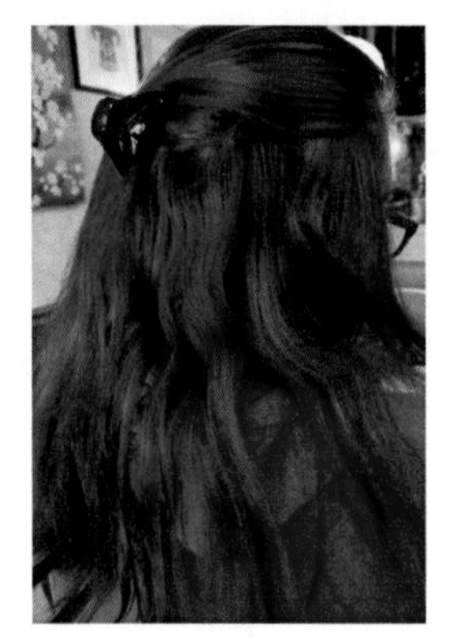

Nila with multicolored hair

I asked her, "Are you having a midlife crisis or what?"

Nila smiled at me and said, "No. I just wanted to brighten your day."

I teared up. Nila helped me uncover and grabbed my hand to lift me from the recliner. Then, I gave her a huge hug. Her hair did brighten my day. It also made my heart swell. I couldn't say anything for fear of crying. So, I just stood there and held her.

Two days later, I went to my appointment at a local medical radiation and oncology facility so that I could get new tattoos.

Most people would be surprised to learn I have tattoos because my tattoos are on my body in places where people can only see them if I allow it. All my tattoos have special meanings to me. Of course, me being a Sagittarius, none of them are small.

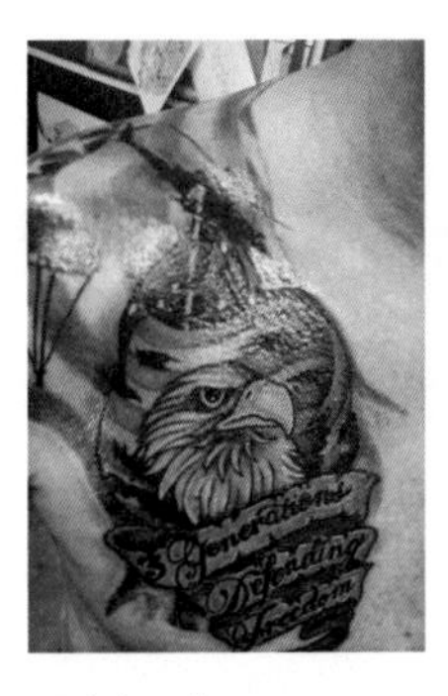

Right chest tattoo

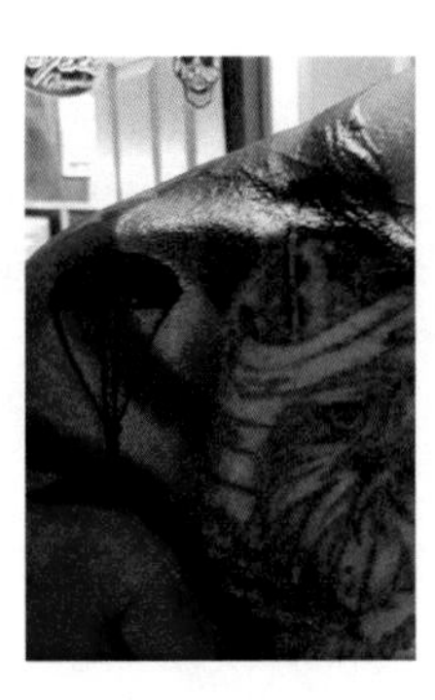

Right shoulder tattoo

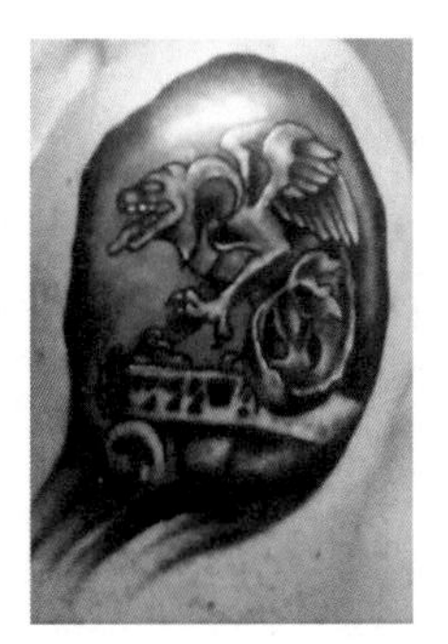

Right shoulder tattoo

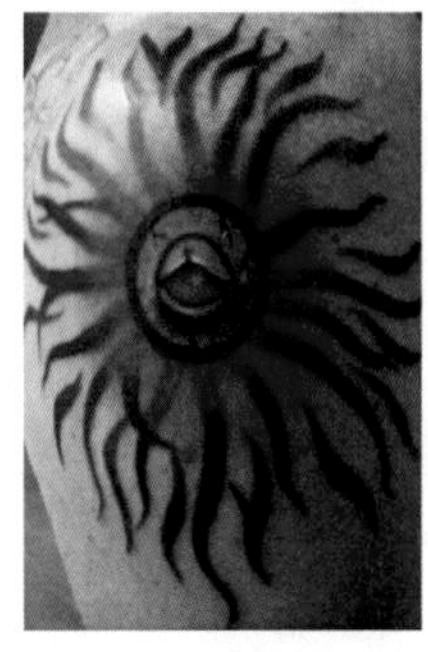

Left shoulder tattoo

But the tattoos I was getting on this day were going to have a very special meaning.

I walked into the radiation center.

"Hello, please sign in," said the nice lady at the front desk. Between now and my last treatment on March 19, we would come to know one another on a first-name basis. But for today, it was just the formal reciting of information and personal verification.

I sat in the large, empty waiting area until my name was called. That day I saw a younger radiology technician, whom I would see almost every weekday for the duration of my treatments. She gave me the nickel tour of the place.

There was an area with semi-private dressing rooms that had curtains in the place of doors. Past that was a small waiting room with a television. *Gunsmoke* was on. This made me flashback to my childhood years when we watched *Gunsmoke* routinely at home. There was one gentleman seated and watching the television. He and the technician exchanged pleasantries, and we moved on. I glanced at the clock. It read 2:15 p.m. That was the exact time of my appointment.

Across the hall was a long, rectangular room in which two technicians would operate the controls where the radiation equipment was located. On the wall was a radiation warning sign.

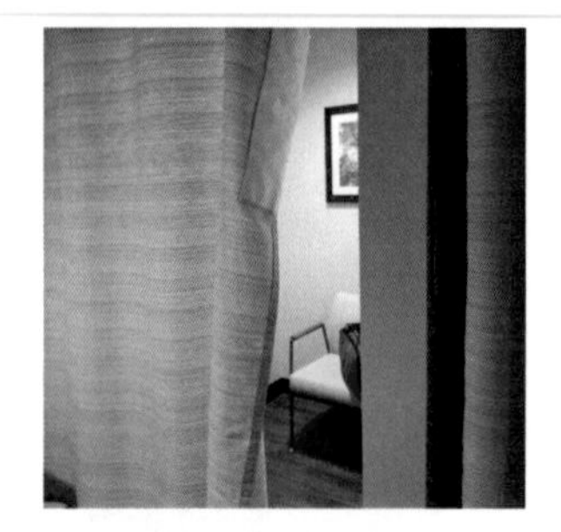

Dressing room

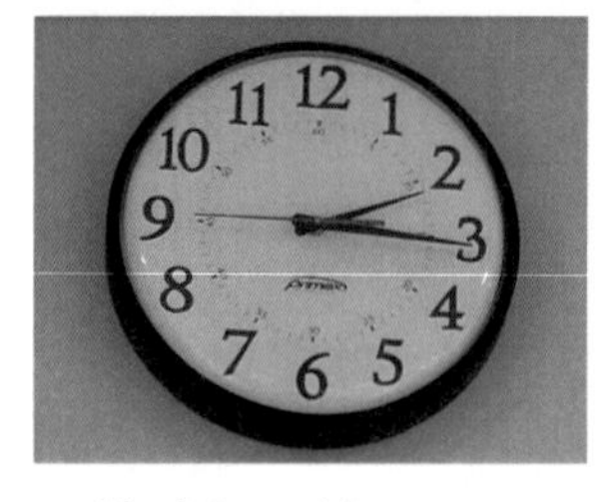

Clock in waiting room

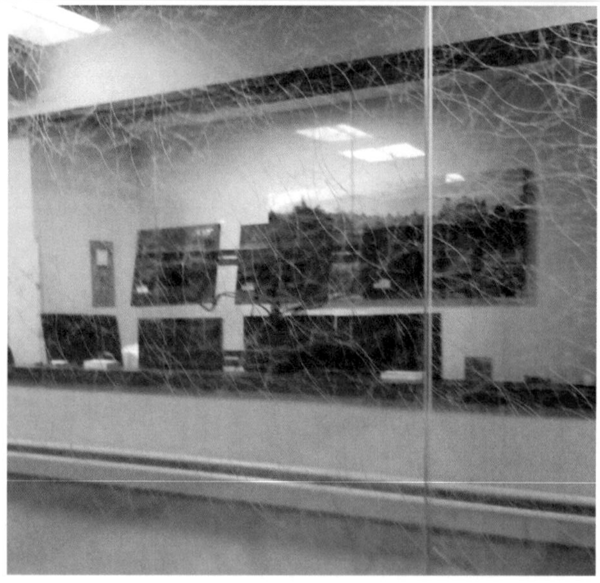

Control room

This was the second sign I had passed on my tour. The first sign simply read "Radiation Treatment LN231." The second sign was more graphic. It read, "CAUTION—VERY HIGH RADIATION AREA WHEN THE RADIATION BEAM IS ON."

My imagination kicked in, and I thought of technicians walking around the room with the attire of a post-apocalyptic era. They would have on full radiation suits and boots. They would be wearing masks, with large goggles for better vision, and a long hose extending from the front that connected to an oxygen bag on their side. I was sure they might be dressed like that, but not me. I would have on only my sweats, knee-high socks, and toboggan.

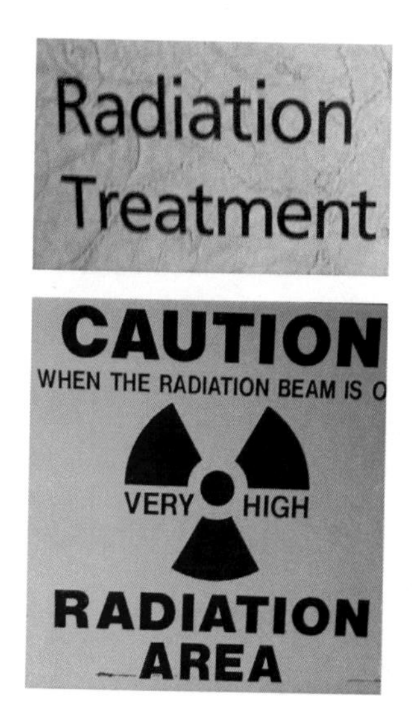

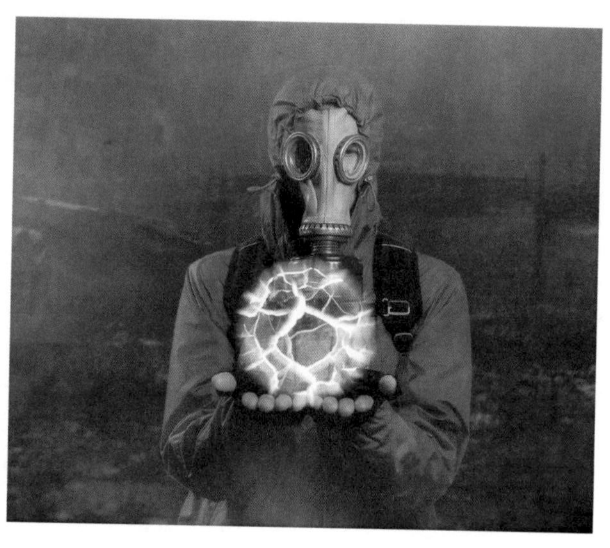

However, it did not look like a post-apocalyptic world behind the curtain. Everyone was dressed just as any other health professional would be. I was introduced to the other technician, and we all proceeded through a huge iron door.

Past the heavy door was the room where it would all happen.

I listened to the technician. She was droning while I looked at everything. A red light protruded from the wall. Beside it, the sign read, "Beam On."

"Lie on the table," the technician said, but I did not process the request at first. I was focused on the red light and the sign.

"Beam me up!" I thought, like on *Star Trek*.

"Mr. Muse," one of the techs repeated louder. "I need you to lie on the table, please."

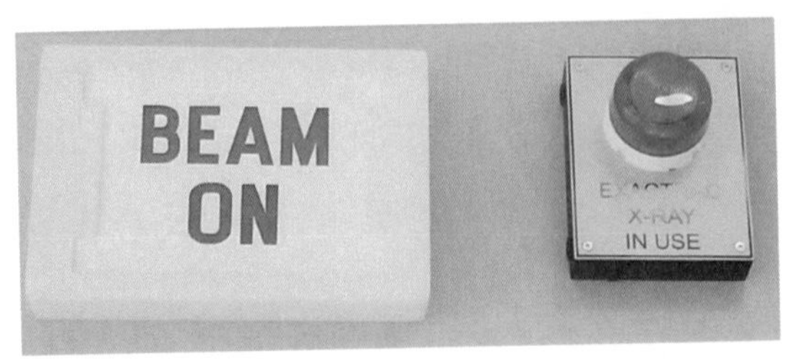

Beam On sign

I sat on the table, lifted my legs to the bottom, and rolled down.

"This table has a small amount of cushion," my thoughts registered, but, at this time in my life, it did not matter; it could be a bed, a recliner, or a table—they all caused me pain. I was immediately concerned about how I would get back up without embarrassment.

The taller technician covered me with a blanket from just below the waist and across my feet. I welcomed the blanket and wished it had been heavier, like the American flag blanket at home. I raised my sweatshirt and lowered my sweatpants to just above the crotch, as instructed. The technician took my hands to place them exactly in the correct position across my chest and gave me a blue device to hold. Little did I know how relevant the color blue would become.

Then she said, "Oh my. Your hands are frozen."

"If you think my hands are frozen, you should have seen my shoulder last month," passed through my mind.

In the form of small talk, she asked what kind of cancer I had.

"Prostate," I said. "I had a high PSA, and evidently it has spread outside of the prostate."

"What was your PSA, if you don't mind me asking?" she inquired.

"One seventy-nine," I responded.

There was a pause for a few seconds, and she replied, "Seventy-nine?" as if she hadn't heard me correctly, or I hadn't been correct in my initial answer. You know, my mistake or hers.

I corrected her, "No, you forgot the number one at the beginning."

The techs looked at one another as the one prepping me said to the other, "I have never heard of a PSA number that high, have you?"

"No," the short one said.

"Lie as still as possible," the tall one prepping me said.

My ribs were already screaming, "GET UP!" But I did lie still. I caught myself gripping the blue device so hard that my fingers began to go to sleep. I closed my eyes and reverted to something we were taught in the army to combat adrenaline. I focused all my attention on relaxation and convincing my heart to slow down.

The two techs were speaking to one another, and the alignment adjustments began.

Once the table on which I lay was placed in the exact spot targeted in the room, she repeated, "Really still, all right?"

I hesitated to answer, fearing I would move. Just like a master ventriloquist, I quietly replied, "Yes," not moving a muscle, including my lips.

They rolled a table over next to where I lay. I was focused on lying motionless. I was not able to see what was on the table. Straight above me was a large fixture with a glass cover. I tried to use the reflection on the glass to see what was on the table, but all I could see was my reflection.

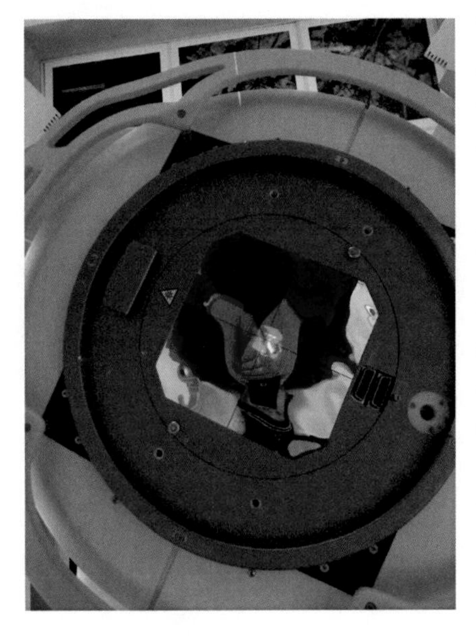

"Is this where the 'very high' radiation will come from to kill my cancer?" I wondered. "Unfortunately, this will not be the same as when I got fried at the surgery center."

A red laser light ran along the length of my body on each side, along with one down the middle. Another red light ran perpendicular across my abdomen. It was at the intersection of these red laser lights that my new tattoos would be placed.

Overhead radiation machine

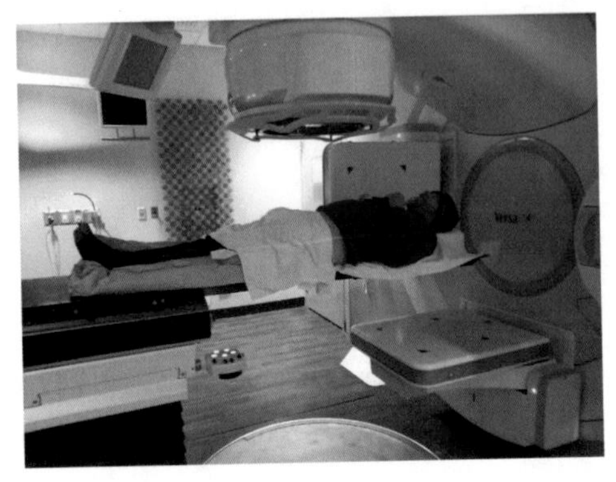

Positioned on radiation table with red laser lines

I felt a slight pressure as the technician worked on what would be three tattoos. This was nothing compared to the pain of my other tattoos, which made me lightheaded at times. Each design was the same. A single blue dot, with four lines, similar to the way a child would draw the sun. The preparation and alignment took about thirty minutes. The tattoos took only three.

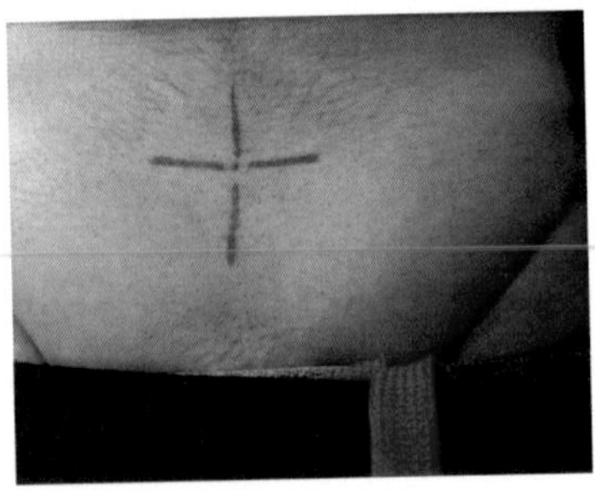

Tattoo center abdomen

"We're all done," announced the tech who gave me the new tattoos. "You can get up now." But it wasn't that easy. I strained and used my arms to try and lift my stiff body from the table. The effort made pain shoot through my back like electrical shock waves. Contrary to my best effort to be silent, a painful groan slipped out. My attempt to raise up was unsuccessful. I lacked the strength and pain tolerance to do it alone.

I remember thinking, "If only Nurse Nila were here to help me when the technicians were gone."

"Are you all right?" asked the techs in synchrony.

"Damn ribs," I replied with a grunt.

They immediately jumped in to help. All the work and mental preparation I had put into being able to appear normal was erased. It was obvious I was far from normal. The expressions of pity on their faces told me so.

As you may recall, my major at the University of West Georgia was jazz performance. I played the trumpet. My radiation treatments were scheduled to begin on January 24, 2018. When I want internet news, I use Bing, and I enjoy reading the daily news topics.

On January 23, 2018, one day before I began my treatments, one of the news topics caught my attention. Hugh Masekela, jazz trumpeter, had died. I clicked on the topic and read the following article from Billboard.com:

> *Legendary South African jazz musician Hugh Masekela has died at the age of 78 after a decade-long fight with cancer, according to a statement from his family on Tuesday (Jan. 23). Often called the "Father of South African jazz," Masekela died in Johannesburg after what his family said was a "protracted and courageous battle with prostate cancer."*
>
> *In October last year, Masekela issued a statement that he had been fighting prostate cancer since 2008 and would have to cancel his professional commitments to focus on his health. He said he started treatment after doctors found a "small speck" on his bladder and had surgery in March 2016 after the cancer spread.*
>
> *Hugh Masekela 1939–2018*

I was completely taken aback by the coincidence. It is still remarkable to think about it today.

The fact that it was a "decade-long battle" also got my attention. When I read about prostate cancer, if a person did not survive, it was often associated with a ten-year time frame. I didn't know why a decade was important, but I planned to find out.

"Is the goal to help me live ten more years? Perhaps that is why Dr. Famoyin's business is named Quality of Life. Are my treatments merely a way to improve my quality of life for a decade?"

I felt I had uncovered the ugly truth. The big idea the doctors didn't want to tell me so that I could live optimistically for a few more years until the truth was revealed on its own.

I returned to the medical center on January 24. I was driving to work each day and had all of my radiation appointments scheduled for 2:15 p.m. This way, I could go home afterward because the workday would be over.

I greeted the lady at the front desk. I was dressed as usual. I wore warm socks, sweatpants, a sweatshirt, and my toboggan. Each day of radiation was the same routine. Nila held my hand and walked me into the lobby. She gave me a loving hug and a kiss. I walked past the first radiation sign and into LN231. I walked past the dressing rooms and into the waiting area. *Gunsmoke* was just coming on. It was 2:00 p.m. A gentleman was sitting there, and I recognized him as the same person who was watching *Gunsmoke* the day I got my tattoos. He was wearing a medical mask on this day, as well. I would later find out why.

The familiar tech who had inscribed the tattoos came to the waiting area and asked me to follow her. We walked by the control room, and I greeted the other technician. We walked through the huge iron door, and I got onto the table. I laid back gingerly with the tech's help, offered without asking. I blushed with embarrassment, knowing she remembered the difficulty I'd displayed a little more than a week earlier. She handed me the familiar blue foam device to hold.

"Remember, you have to lie still," she said.

The other tech entered the room and walked over to a control panel. The first stood by me and made sure the new tattoos were visible. The red lasers reappeared, and she began manually adjusting the table. Once the manual adjustments were completed, the technician at the control panel began to call out numbers.

"Twelve back, fifty-nine left," she said.

The table was adjusted slightly according to the commands.

After the second set of numbers and corresponding table adjustment, the tech at the controls announced, "That's good. We will be right outside. Try to lie very still."

I did not answer this time. Sagittarius was trying to solve the mystery of the numbers and table alignment. Meanwhile, the sound of the enormous metal door closed. The sound reminded me of an old castle door, the hinges moaning from carrying the weight.

The view of the ceiling was very relaxing. It looked like a glass window with a dogwood tree in full bloom beyond it. The sky was a beautiful blue, with no clouds in sight. My grandmother was a devout Christian and the most influential person in my life. She was the reason for my faith and my motivation to be a better person. I lay there and remembered the story my grandmother told me about the dogwood tree.

If you ventured into the forests of Israel almost two thousand years ago, you would have seen plenty of sturdy oaks, lofty cedars, walnut trees, and more—all of which were fine and noble trees, loved and used by carpenters. However, one tree was prized above all others: the mighty dogwood. Back then, the dogwood lacked its distinct fruits and flowers, but it was still impressive, rising taller than any oak or cedar. Its wood was strong, hard, fine-grained, and easy to work with. It had no equal, and it was constantly in demand.

During this time, a simple carpenter was declared king of the Jews and was sentenced to death. The method of execution? Crucifixion. And the tree used to fashion the iconic wooden cross? A dogwood. According to the story my grandmother told, the dogwood felt great sorrow for the role it played in Jesus Christ's death. While on the cross, Jesus sensed the tree's anguish, and he decided to transform it so that it could never again be used in crucifixion.

From that point on, the dogwood was no longer a tall, stately forest tree. Rather, it became a small and shrub-like tree with thin and twisted limbs. Its four large petals represent the cross Jesus died upon, and each petal displays four red-tinged notches that are said to represent four nail holes. And in the center of each flower is a green cluster that is symbolic of Jesus's crown of thorns.

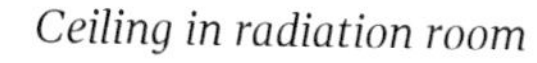
Ceiling in radiation room

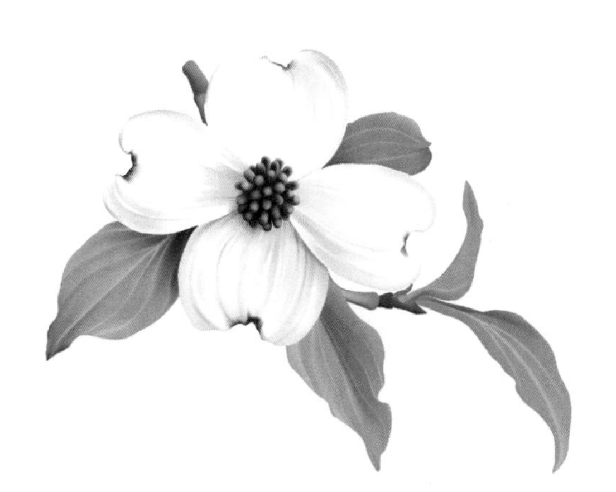

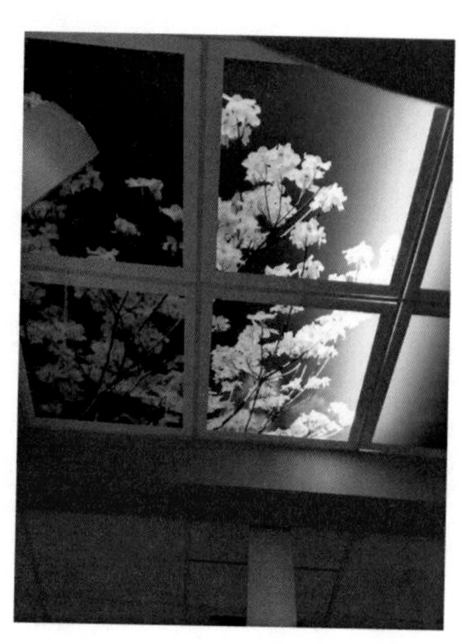

My thoughts were quickly brought back to the present as the red light came on with a loud click that echoed in the room. The sign lit up reading "BEAM ON," and treatment number one started.

I made myself relax and loosened my grip on the blue foam device. The light on the wall exuded its bright red light and constantly teased my peripheral vision. The large device above me had green lasers coming from it, surely sending very high radiation into a surgically accurate location inside of me. The device moved left to right at a slow, steady pace. Within a few minutes, the device stopped. The red light was extinguished, and the sign was turned off.

A voice came over the speaker. It was one of the technicians.

"You are all done, Mr. Muse," announced the voice.

I immediately began preparing to get up from the table. It was my goal to do so before they returned to the room, hopefully presenting them with a different opinion of my physical condition. The large iron door unlocked with an echoing *clack*! Then it creaked open. By the time the technician came into the room, I was sitting upright.

"Are you all right?" she asked.

"Spectacular," I responded. And I was because I had successfully cloaked how I truly felt.

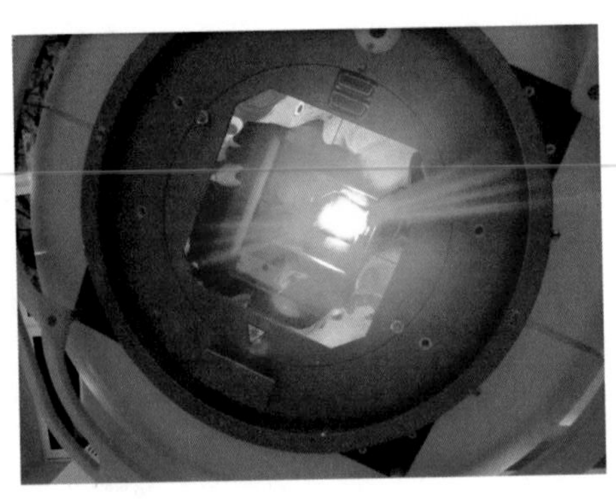

Radiation light beam

I left the room, subconsciously waiting for some type of pain or burning because of the treatment. It never came, and I was thankful. I walked into the large waiting area and was happy to see Nila. She immediately got up and delivered a loving hug.

I told her the details of the event as we rode home together. We talked about the numbers that were called out and the adjustments of the table. When we got home, she met me on the passenger side of the car to make sure I was fine getting out and into the house, just as any great nurse would do.

Once inside, I went downstairs and got into my recliner. Sparky met me at the door and followed me downstairs. Nila covered me with my American flag blanket, and I fell fast asleep. One down, thirty-seven to go. As soon as I woke up, I located a dry-erase board that was stored away. I used a red marker and drew the red light and wrote the words "Beam On Radiation." I put the first of thirty-eight hash marks, representing a completed treatment.

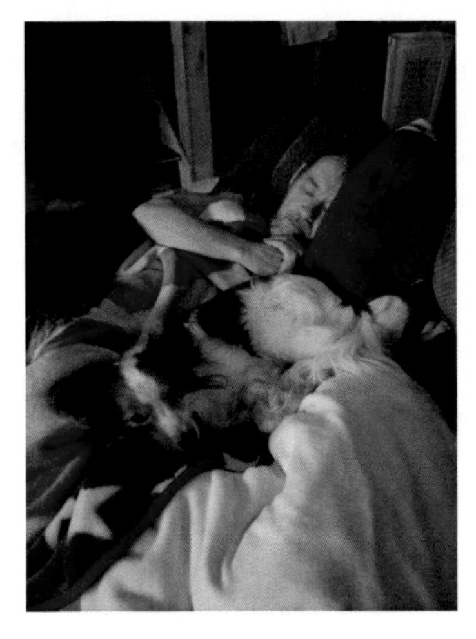

In recliner with Sparky and Mr. Mitten after treatment

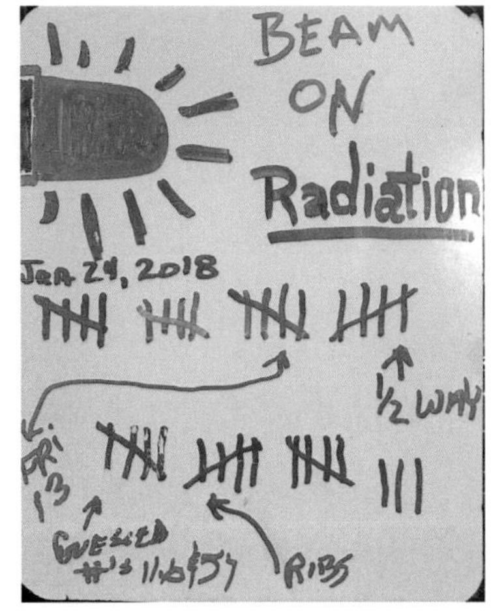

Dry-erase board

The days passed, and I added more red hash marks to my dry-erase board. I remember February 13, 2018.

"Maybe I should skip my treatment today. It seems like an omen that my thirteenth radiation treatment is on the thirteenth. If something is going to go wrong with the 'very high radiation,' it will likely be today. I don't need anything unexpected getting fried," I thought.

But I did not skip out. Other than the coincidence with the thirteens, it was a typical day. I got up, went to work, skipped lunch, went to my treatment, went home, added a red hash mark, notated the date, curled up with Nila and Sparky, and fell fast asleep.

During this time, every time I went to a doctor and got my vital signs taken, I tried to guess my numbers. This included my weight, temperature, and blood pressure. I got very good at it over time. In statistics, we say repetition leads to predictability. There was no shortage of repetition for me in the medical arena. So, every day when I lay on the table, holding the blue foam device, I listened intently to the numbers communicated between the technicians. I began to guess the numbers. They found humor in the game and joined in.

On my twenty-first treatment, I got both of them right! Eleven back and fifty-seven left. I couldn't believe it. Nor could they. I am still amazed when I look at the dry-erase board and remember that day.

On my twenty-sixth treatment day, my ribs were especially painful. I had popped some out of place sleeping and forced them back in more often than usual. They hurt so badly I could hardly tolerate leaning back in a chair.

"How am I going to be able to handle lying on the table?" I wondered.

I wore the TENS unit all day. I loaded up on anti-inflammatory medication. Then, about an hour before my treatment, I resorted to taking a leftover hydrocodone from my most recent surgery. Even with all of that, I could not bear the pain of the table.

By this time in my treatments, the technicians and I had become well acquainted. They knew the story of my motorcycle wreck and the one hundred and ninety-two-foot trip down the pavement. So, they understood about my ribs and allowed me a few extra minutes to get into a position that was tolerable.

Once the red light went off and the treatment was over, I found myself unable to get up. Both ladies came in and helped me to sit up. The pain took my breath, and I paused before getting off the table. This day was unusually painful and difficult, even with the medications and TENS unit. Without them, I would not have been able to lie on the table. This warranted a special note on my board.

The treatments were going well. I was able to continue working each day, and the effects of radiation were only minimal at this point. Nila and I managed to maintain optimism, which made it possible to enjoy every second together.

Every few weeks, we would go back to a small room beyond "Radiation Treatment LN231." We sat in the small room, waiting for Dr. Channeler to appear and review where things stood.

On the day of my thirty-fifth treatment, he came in and greeted us as normal.

"How have your side effects been? And your fatigue?" Dr. Channeler asked in his stiff, formal way.

"Other than a little more fatigue and some upset stomach, I feel fine," I said.

"An upset stomach is normal," he said. "You can consider diet changes if it seems like something you are eating is not agreeing with you."

"I understand," I said.

"Is there anything we can do about the fatigue?" Nila asked.

"The fatigue is normal. You have four more treatments left. You have come a long way."

"Should we follow up with Perry's oncologist?" Nila asked.

"Yes, this will be our last visit together," said Dr. Channeler. "Are there any other questions before I leave?"

I did have a question that haunted me. It centered around my cancer research and how it often referenced ten-year segments. I kept thinking of Hugh Masekela and his ten-year bout with prostate cancer. I explained all of this to Dr. Channeler.

"What I really need to know is...Is there a reason for looking at prostate cancer in ten-year segments?" I said to sum up my ramble. In truth, I felt my life hanging on his next words.

Yet, his answer was short and to the point.

Dr. Channeler simply said, "Yes, we typically look at this type of cancer in ten-year increments."

I persisted.

"Do you mean this type of cancer, meaning prostate cancer?"

The doctor nodded a full long second before stating, "Prostate cancer that has spread beyond the prostate gland, especially with a PSA of one seventy-nine."

"I see," I said, letting him know that I understood the specifics he was sharing.

"So, what is next for me?" I ask. I wish he had told me that each case is different and unpredictable. It would have been much better than what he chose to say.

Without hesitation or expression, Dr. Channeler laid out his prediction in detail. "*Once you have completed your radiation treatments, there will be some really mean microscopic cancer cells that will have proven to be immune to the Lupron and radiation treatments. Over time, your testosterone will begin to come back up. At that time, those really mean cells will start to multiply and spread. Prostate cancer and breast cancer tend to spread to the bones. We really don't know exactly why.*

"At that time, you will begin to experience pain in your bones. Slight at first and then increasing with time. You may even find that you start fracturing easily. You will then have prostate cancer in your bones. You will not be able to have any additional radiation, but that won't matter because those really mean cells will have already proven immunity. So, chemotherapy will be the last option. Cancer in your bones is not curable."

I was dazed and confused.

This was not what I was hoping to hear.

Then I asked the million-dollar question, "And so, Doc, with all of your years of experience, what do you feel are my chances of making it ten more years?"

I thought it was a valid question. Looking back, perhaps it was unfair. Again, he could have told me it was impossible to answer such a question. But instead, he answered without hesitation.

"Thirty-five percent. I will give you a 35 percent chance of living ten years," he said. "Until then it is a matter of providing you with the best quality of life possible based on the circumstances."

Nila and I were speechless. Dr. Channeler stood up and walked away. If he said goodbye, we do not recall it.

"If I have a 35 percent chance, does that equal three and a half years? Maybe not. Maybe it is like when the weather app says 65 percent chance of thunderstorms. In that case, there is only a 35 percent chance the area will not get the thunderstorm. With a one seventy-nine PSA, I know I am in the 65 percent chance of rain area."

I completed my radiation and received a certificate, which everyone from radiology had signed. Everyone except Dr. Channeler.

"It doesn't matter that he didn't take the time to sign my certificate," I thought. "I am in the 65 percent chance of rain region and will likely never see him again anyway."

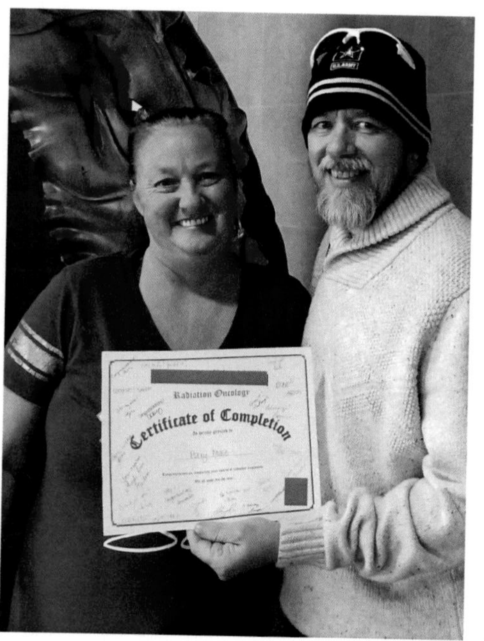

The signed certificate was a nice gesture, but it felt symbolic of something terrible. A reminder each time I looked at it of the final visit with Dr. Channeler. That visit was devastating to our morale and optimism. It created a hole that I am still trying to crawl from. Even today, when I get an ache or pain, I wonder if it is cancer. I worry about Mr. Skeleton daily, just as I worry about Mr. Mitten and my dogs. I know they will leave me one day, and Mr. Skeleton will, as well.

The visit with Dr. Channeler on March 14, 2018, impacted my life forever.

Me and Nila after radiation graduation

My battle was taking a toll on me, mentally and emotionally. The events were starting to make me think more about what the end of life really meant. The lyrics to this song turned the negative, fearful thoughts into something more positive. Coincidentally, it was released in 2013. I will explain the significance of that year later.

ACID RAIN

Avenged Sevenfold 2013

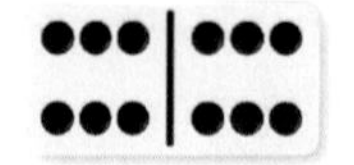

Chapter 12

REACH FOR THE SKY... MAYBE, MAYBE NOT

The Sagittarius man craves to obtain as much knowledge about diverse things as he can during his lifetime. However, he won't want to learn in a boring traditional classroom.

Nila and I came to an agreement a very long time ago that we would not celebrate Valentine's Day. Instead, we celebrate being in love all year long. However, just by sheer coincidence, we both secretly got gifts for one another this year.

It was the weekend following graduation from radiation and, with my feeling of impending doom, I started organizing pictures from my phone and computer. One folder was named PLM NVM, which is both our initials. It took me hours to go through all of them.

Nila was downstairs, and I decided to sit in the computer room and watch a slideshow of the folder named with our initials. There were pictures ranging from before we married up to this week. I watched the pictures scroll by in random order and began to weep...no, cry. Tears were not in short supply. I began to struggle with the current state of things.

"I am supposed to be here and take care of her until the end. If I live ten years (which the doctor said I will not), she will only be sixty years old. How horrible will it be to live with me for those years as I slowly "die on the vine"? Then what? She lives in this big house...her days and nights alone? How many countless rainy, gloomy days did I call her when I was at work because I knew depression would be getting the best of her here at home alone?"

"What about the anniversaries of the deaths of her family members? Those are days she needs me to be there. It is not fair to her. I was supposed to be there forever to love her, comfort her, care for her. I haven't even been able to make love to her in months. Now I am going to slowly die in front of my wife and leave her alone."

I knew it would be best if she found someone after me. I knew that was true. Yet, that thought also broke my heart.

"What if she doesn't want to be buried beside me when she passes one day? What if she wants to be beside my replacement?"

That felt so very selfish on my part. I knew it was selfish. Clearly, I was trying to come to terms with what was best for her. Why in the hell would I want her to live twenty or more years in this big house alone? I would not and do not want that.

If I could only figure out how not to die, yet nobody knows that except for God.

Radiation was over. My last treatment was March 19, 2018. It was Tuesday the twentieth and, fittingly, the first day of spring. A new season, and with it should come a new chapter in life. I was healed from the prostate surgery and much better from the shoulder manipulation. Radiation was behind me and the future before me. But I did not feel like the first day of spring. I felt like winter: cold and dreary.

I could not stop thinking about what Dr. Channeler had said with his icy tone and blank expression. However, some things needed to change. I had to step up my game at work, and my naps in the basement needed to come to an end. The radiation had stolen energy from me that I did not have to spare. So, I stocked up on 5-Hour Energy shots.

After radiation, there was a noticeable difference in my digestive system. It was a slow change enacted upon my internal body parts by the very high radiation. I became intolerant of dairy. Plus, anything fried made me blow up with gas like a helium balloon. Furthermore, my anemia was still up and down, but now it was difficult to determine the difference in radiation fatigue and low iron. I never knew what was going to make me sick when I ate, so I just did not eat often. Even when I did eat, it was a few bites and done. And there was depression. Nila and I together had plenty to go around. We were mostly alone, and there was an abundance of morbid thoughts these days.

"I need to find a burial plot close to home," I thought. "Then Nila can visit me. But we do not live close to any friends or family, except Alanna. That means me spending most days and nights alone buried in the ground. Maybe I should just be cremated. Then I could stay in the house with Nila. It's cold in the graveyard. But would that be weird for the person who replaces me if I am sitting on the shelf?"

We had a rock patio and firepit built in the yard and were hanging out on a Sunday afternoon. The mountain air in spring was slightly chilled, so we built a fire. It was a place filled with happy memories of playing corn hole with friends and uncountable nights of Nila and me playing Angry Birds and getting lost dancing.

Nila had gone to the house to get something. A large mound of dirt was piled nearby, and as I sat on the patio, petting Sebastian, I stared at the mound of dirt when a thought came to mind.

"Perhaps I could be buried here. It is out of the way, and I could be closer to Nila. However, it is unfortunate that friends, family, and my eventual replacement would ask why she was starting a cemetery in her backyard."

Other than the psychological effects I was dealing with, there were still physical problems. It was highly disappointing that I still needed help getting out of bed or even out of the recliner if I sat too long. I kept telling myself that it was just a matter of time to finish the healing process, and then I would start an exercise regimen to build back my core strength.

My body had been through a lot.

Patience is not the Sagittarian's forte. But my shoulder still required surgery. I stopped going to see Dave at the PT clinic, and I was struggling to "fight the good fight." Insurance only allows a set number of PT visits each year. I needed to save some visits for the real surgery and not burn them up from the manipulation. As any true Sagittarian would do, I observed all of what was going on in the PT room and learned what I needed to become my own therapist. But progress had slowed, or halted, with my shoulder. I was unable to get the ROM back to normal, regardless of my efforts. Each day I sat beneath the homemade pulley mounted above the door. Each day I lowered the right side as my left arm reached for the sky. Each time I was limited by the sheer pain that kept progress from being obtained.

"Perhaps the manipulation was only a temporary fix. Perhaps I needed the real surgery to move past the stalemate," I thought. But I was not so sure about having the surgery. I was back to the same dispiriting mental place again, wondering if I would live long enough for it to be worth the pain and struggle.

"There is a 35 percent chance I may get to throw a ball again, to shoot basketball or to go to the gym and get back in shape. Come on, Sagittarius, reach for the sky!" I thought as I unsuccessfully tried to raise my arm to be perpendicular to the floor. "Will I ever be able to reach for the sky again? Maybe, maybe not."

Every day I would lie on the floor with a blue cylinder beneath my shoulders. I would cross my arms and push with my feet to roll my body across the cylinder. Each time, various ribs would pop back into place. It was a painful routine that delivered immediate relief. But fifteen minutes later, I needed to be prepared for the ribs to be angry. Each week I made my way into Ballard and Kind Chiropractic. Both of these doctors became special people in our lives. I can never figure out how to repay them for everything they have meant to us.

After a few days of "woe is me," I changed my focus. I was watching television, and a commercial came on. I hate commercials, but this one caught my attention before I could fast forward past. It was advertising a specialty cancer center (SCC). I hit pause and called the number on the screen.

There was a lengthy discussion with the friendly voice on the other end. He had a ton of questions and made it a point to let me know he was a cancer survivor and a patient of SCC. That was uplifting to hear. By the time the call was over, I had an appointment at one of several locations across America. It was chosen because it specializes in my type of cancer, among others.

This motivated me enough to go downstairs and do my PT. It had been a couple of days since I had the willingness to do so. I didn't want my shoulder to freeze up again. Who knows, I might even want to get that surgery after all.

My appointment at SCC was scheduled for April 2, 2018, only a couple of weeks away. I wanted to go tomorrow. But it was time for my appointment with Dr. Famoyin at Quality of Life. When I pulled into the parking lot, the reason for the name of his business struck me as obvious for the first time. I had decided to fire my urologist and radiologist. Their plan of waiting for the cancer to spread to my bones was unacceptable. I looked forward to the upcoming conversation with Dr. Famoyin. I knew he would be forthcoming and candid.

Dr. Famoyin walked in, and we exchanged pleasant regards.

"So, Mr. Perry, how are you doing these days?" questioned the doctor.

"Well, Doc," I replied, "Physical therapy on my shoulder sucks. I wake up tired every day; my digestive system seems to have turned on me since the radiation; and my radiologist said I was likely to die a slow and painful death."

There was a moment of pause before Dr. Famoyin responded, "This doesn't sound like the Perry Muse I have come to know. Let us take this one thing at a time," he suggested.

Dr. Famoyin continued, "Your body has been through a great deal in a short amount of time. You also must realize that with a PSA of one seventy-nine, your body has likely been dealing with cancer for five years. Let us not forget that we are not the young men we once were. Recovery is slower and requires more effort. It all starts with a positive attitude, which you have shown since coming here."

"It is difficult to wake up with that positive attitude each day when the fatigue makes it hard to wake up," I replied.

"Do you feel like your iron is low again?" Dr. Famoyin asked.

"Yes. Absolutely," I said immediately.

Dr. Famoyin assured me we would get the blood lab and line up more infusions if needed.

"Why are you still having to do PT?" he asked.

I explained how my ROM was still lacking and about my fear that the shoulder would freeze up again.

Nila jumped in and told Dr. Famoyin that she was still having to help me from the bed and from sitting. He reviewed my inflammation markers, which are sedimentation (SED) rate, C-reactive protein (CRP), and rheumatoid factor (RF).

Our final topic of discussion for the day was about "dying a slow, painful death," although the doctor phrased his question with elegance and professionalism.

"What's this about dying?" ask Dr. Famoyin.

I clarified my initial remarks by recounting the conversation we had with Dr. Channeler about the "ten-year" prostate cancer.

"*He said what?*" Dr. Famoyin asked loudly and with an uncharacteristically stern tone. Then, returning to a normal tone but very serious, he continued, "Let me explain something; no one can answer the question you asked of him. He should not have even tried. Only God knows what our future holds, and we are not promised tomorrow."

Then he continued his lesson.

"You make an appointment each time you leave. I always say I will see you in six weeks. But I am assuming you will still be here, and you are assuming I will still be here. Do you understand?" I did understand. It was absolutely the truth and made me realize a new outlook.

"I don't know whether to quit worrying about when cancer will kill me or start worrying about everything else that may do the job sooner," whispered the dark shadow sitting on my shoulder.

I smiled and thanked Dr. Famoyin for the wise, uplifting remarks. We left the room, and he escorted me to the lab for my blood draw. Along the way we chatted, and he casually continued to inspire me back to a more optimistic mood.

The next time I saw Dr. Famoyin was fifteen minutes later, and he held my lab results.

The lab results revealed several problems. My red blood cell count (RBC), hemoglobin, hematocrit, platelets, mean platelet volume (MPV), and iron were all low.

A red blood cell count is a blood test that is used to find out how many red blood cells (RBCs) you have. The test is important because RBCs contain hemoglobin, which carries oxygen to your body's tissues. The number of RBCs you have can affect how much oxygen your tissues receive. Your tissues need oxygen to function.

A low RBC count can cause fatigue and shortness of breath, among other things. I was experiencing both. I had assumed the shortness of breath was just being out of shape.

The hematocrit (HCT) is expressed as a percentage by volume of blood. It is the proportion of blood that consists of packed red blood cells. The term "hematocrit" was coined in 1903 and comes from the Greek roots hemat, blood, krites, and judge, meaning to judge or gauge the blood.

Platelets are tiny fragments of cells that are essential for normal blood clotting. They are formed from very large cells in the bone marrow and are released into the blood to circulate. The platelet count is a test that determines the number of platelets in your sample of blood, and the platelets play a role in preventing excessive bleeding. People with low blood platelets do not typically display symptoms but may be at risk for serious bleeding during and following trauma or surgery.

Hemoglobin (Hb or Hgb) is a protein in red blood cells that carries oxygen throughout the body. A low hemoglobin count, only slightly below normal, does not affect how you feel. If it gets more severe and causes symptoms, your low hemoglobin count may indicate you have anemia. Mine was listed as abnormally low.

Iron deficiency is an abnormally low level of iron in the body. Iron is an essential mineral found in red meat and certain fruits and vegetables. In the body, iron is needed to form myoglobin, a protein in muscle cells, and it is essential for certain enzymes that drive the body's chemical reactions. In the bone marrow, iron is used to make hemoglobin, the oxygen-carrying chemical inside the body's red blood cells. If iron levels fall too low, it causes iron deficiency anemia.

All these results indicated I again needed iron infusions. However, my ferritin level was normal this time. Ferritin tests can tell if you have an iron deficiency or an iron overload. Keep in mind that ferritin is not the same thing as iron in your body. Instead, it is a protein that stores iron, releasing it when it is time to make more red blood cells. You can think of it as a pantry for storing your iron.

It was perplexing to Dr. Famoyin and me as to why I had all the symptoms of low iron, yet my pantry was full. We agreed the iron infusions were the right move, and I would start the first one immediately. The mystery of my ferritin level would be left unsolved for today.

Next were my inflammation markers. My last lab from Deanna had been shared with Dr. Famoyin. I was unaware of the results.

My SED rate, CRP, and RF were all high. The results of my SED rate were ninety-six. This was more than six times above the high limit of fifteen. My CRP was sixty. This was twelve times above the high limit of five. And my RF was two hundred. This was fourteen times above the high limit of fourteen. The inflammation in my body was through the roof.

"Have those really mean cells already found their way into Mr. Skeleton undetected? Why else would my inflammation be so high? Perhaps 35 percent was a generous number after all."

I now understood why I needed Nila's assistance getting up, why I was so stiff, and why I was taking naproxen (an anti-inflammatory OTC drug) every day. Because of the super high rheumatoid number, I began to think back on the motorcycle accident. I recalled the doctor telling me to "expect to have some arthritis as a result of the damage you have done to your body."

"I need to find a rheumatologist," I thought.

I went back to the infusion room and was greeted by the nurses who worked there. The room was lined on three sides by blue-colored recliners, most of them filled with patients. Everyone was hooked up to an IV. Many of the hanging bags were different in color. It was similar to scanning the patrons' drinks while sitting at the local bar. Yet here the mood was melancholic and not celebratory. Most of the patients lay sleeping and covered in blankets. They looked very ill with gaunt, pale, or ashy faces and cracked lips. One patient wore a mask, just like the man I saw watching *Gunsmoke* in LN231. This was where I learned he had esophageal cancer.

The IV needle was inserted into my arm, and the nurse asked if I wanted a blanket. Of course, I did.

"No Benadryl in my drip, please," I said.

"Okay," the nurse said as she tucked the blanket around me and helped me recline the chair.

I lay there in silence beneath my blanket. It was very somber, watching the seemingly lifeless bodies that filled the room.

Nila refused to leave me and found a place on a couch at the end of the room, near the back exit, and laid down. She would lie there for the next three hours as my liquid concoction dripped slowly into my arm. I carefully scanned the room and took note of each individual.

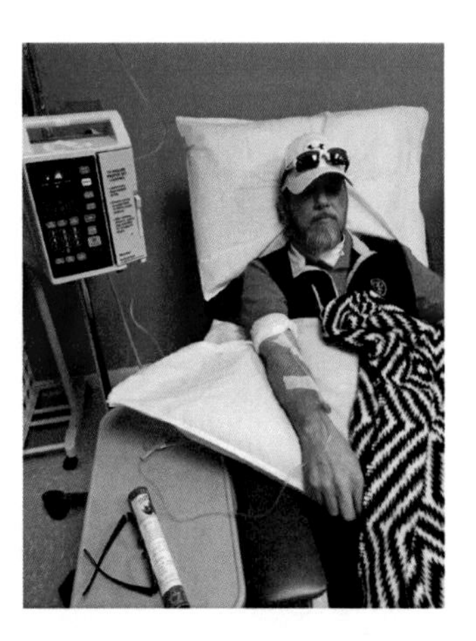

Sitting in infusion room

"This is what it looks like to slowly die on the vine like grapes hanging on far too long," I thought.

Once the IV bag was emptied, the nurses removed the needle. I was able to catch up on all work emails while sitting there. Nila helped me up. It was very difficult to get moving, like all my joints had rusted. We slowly made our way to the front and scheduled my next five infusions.

Once in the car, Nila took us home. There was a lot of silence as we both processed the news.

"On the bright side," I began, "I know my energy will be back after a few more of these." The inflammation was worrisome, but we did not talk about it. Other than my conversation with Dr. Famoyin, the environment surrounding my visit was depressing. Once home, we went downstairs and fell asleep.

Over the next couple of weeks, I completed the remaining five infusions. I needed to make a trip to the plant in Georgia. Although I was in constant contact, nothing replaced being there live. We planned a trip that would coincide with my visit to SCC. It made sense because the plant was along the same route. My energy had returned and, along with it, my optimistic attitude.

Before heading south, I received a call from my orthopedic office. I was informed that my shoulder surgery was scheduled for May 1, only four weeks away. It seemed like everything was heading in the right direction.

SCC was, and remains, top class in the field in terms of medical facilities. Their special rate with the nearby hotels was $25/night. You can take the free shuttle or take advantage of the free valet parking. There was a road en route called Celebration of Life Drive. It reminded me of the celebration of life I had planned when I lost at Family Feud. It felt more than coincidental that my journey led me here.

"I see by the street name that they are already working on improving my psychological quality of life," I said to myself.

My first impression was how vast the hall was. We were met at the doorway.

"Please don't hesitate to ask if you need any help, and welcome to Specialty Cancer Centers," was the greeting.

My attention was drawn immediately to a huge metal tree on the wall. It was beautiful. It reminded me of a two-hundred-year-old oak with bare limbs except for several individual leaves. They reminded me of fall. As I got closer, it was obvious the leaves were bronze, silver, and gold. We walked right up to the beautiful art and realized the leaves were individually engraved. Above the tree were the words "Tree of Life."

Every leaf had a person's name engraved on it. Below the name was a number and the word "years." Bronze said five. Silver ten. And gold was twenty years. These were cancer survivors' names and how long they were cancer free.

I turned to Nila and said, "I want to be a leaf on this tree."

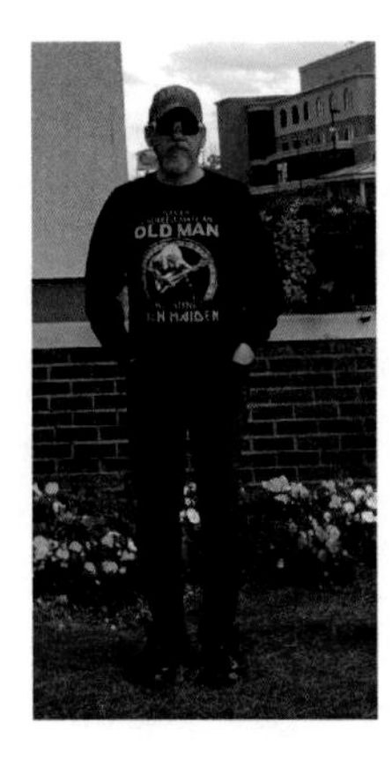

Before entering SCC

We continued walking and reading the printed schedule that had been emailed to me a few days earlier. Nila and I stood in the middle of the immense hall, searching for "Maple." A custodial worker was emptying a trash can about twenty-five feet from us. The hallway was bustling with people. He stopped working and made his way over.

"Can I help you folks?" asked the gentleman. "It's a big place and can be confusing at first," he continued.

"Thank you," Nila and I replied in unison. "We are looking for Maple."

The kind man pointed out the maple tree on the wall further down on the left.

"You were almost there," the man said and bid us a good day.

I checked in at Maple and got my new bracelet after confirming my name and birth date. I was sent across the hall for a blood draw.

The next scheduled stop was a small chapel. A Doctor of Divinity greeted us and asked that we sit down. He explained that services were held two times daily, and we were welcome to attend as many as we cared to. He also let us know that pastoral support was available twenty-four-seven.

Afterward, we had a break in the schedule. The cafeteria was down the hall from Maple, adjacent to the area I had been in for my blood draw. There was a wide variety of foods and drinks. A large salad and soup bar sat in the center. To the left there was a line formed where two cooks prepared food to order from the menu behind them. The food was incredibly inexpensive and delicious. Of course, all of the ingredients were organic and lacked all of the bad things that we eat daily.

Next stop was a trip to another floor. There we would meet the nutritionist who would change my eating habits forever. We sat and listened as she gave us a class on Nutrition 101. Some of the more notable suggestions were to limit red meat to once every four days. The most surprising suggestion involved my favorite color and the color of my 1972 Chevelle, the color orange.

"Eat anything orange as often as possible," she suggested. "Have a sweet potato instead of a white potato. Eat carrots, cooked or raw. Orange fights cancer."

From there we went to the end of the large room and waited for our next visit. It was with a naturopathic expert. I was somewhat skeptical of this visit. I dabbled in supplements, but I wasn't sure how this visit would impact me.

"Maybe she will have a cancer-killing mushroom for me," I thought.

But she was a spectacular person and extremely knowledgeable. I learned a lot and still use all of the supplements prescribed on that initial visit.

- Vitamin C helps absorb iron, boosts the immune system, and reduces the risk of chronic disease.
- Theracurmin is the concentrated ingredient in curcumin for inflammation and cancer fighting.
- Turkey tail is a mushroom that boosts the immune system and is cancer fighting.
- Zinc is for the immune system and cancer fighting.
- Vitamin D3 is for Mr. Skeleton.
- Calcium helps the D3 to absorb.
- Green tea is for inflammation and cancer fighting.

I was blown away and wondered how all of this nutritional and naturopathic information had not been a part of my plan all along. Downstairs was a pharmacy. This was where I picked up all the natural supplements that were prescribed. I was assured that, unlike many supplements sold, these were the highest quality anywhere. If they were out of anything, it would be shipped, free of charge, to our home.

My last stop was oncology. This was where I met Dr. Taha. I had finally found another great person to help me fight the good fight.

"Perry, your PSA has dropped to .9," Dr. Taha said.

It sounded great, but I was disappointed. I wanted to hear zero.

"So, the mean cells that were immune to the very high radiation are still hiding in there," I thought.

Dr. Taha explained that my testosterone was still elevated, and we would see a further drop in PSA as the testosterone was reduced. He said that my Lupron shots were not being given in the most effective manner and could be contributing to the PSA.

"What do you mean by the most effective manner?" I asked.

Dr. Taha explained, "Scientific research shows that a one-month Lupron dose lasts greater than one month. A three-month dose of Lupron lasts greater than three months. But a six-month Lupron shot is only effective for four to six months. The effectiveness starts to wear off by the four-month mark. You should be on the three-month dose, not the six-month dose."

"I suppose the six-month dose Dr. Hinder prescribed is wearing off early, and the testosterone has continued feeding my cancer until the next shot," I thought.

Dr. Taha and I talked for twenty-five minutes before he departed. From there I went back to where my blood had been drawn earlier. This was where I received my first quarterly Lupron shot.

Last stop was back to the second floor, where I was taken to a private room. An IV was put into my arm. This wasn't for iron. It was strictly for Mr. Skeleton. I sat in the dimly lit room and pondered the reason for the IV.

Upon leaving, I received an email with my hotel reservation and schedule for the next visit. We were very encouraged as we left the facility. In the grassy area across from the entrance was the statue of a boy playing with a toy plane. It took me back to my childhood. I reminisced about the small wooden planes I loved to play with. The wing slipped into a slot through the body. I would spin the propeller, which was attached to a rubber band. Then, I launched it into flight and imagined what it would feel like to fly.

On the drive back, I stopped over to work at the Georgia plant for a couple of days. My shoulder surgery was fast approaching, and I had to make the most of the time I had.

When we got back home to the mountains of Northeast Tennessee, I went into my patient portal to read the lab results and clinical summary from my first visit to SCC.

The lab results were similar to those Dr. Famoyin had shared the week prior. My iron level was improved from the infusions, but still in the lower quadrant. It was the clinical summary that piqued my interest.

The parts that caught my attention were where Dr. Taha stated, "... *high-risk* Gleason 8 adenocarcinoma..." and "Radical prostatectomy with *unfortunate* disease progression."

"Dr. Taha nailed it! It was definitely unfortunate for me," I thought.

I spent the following three weeks trying to get everything possible in place at work, preparing for my downtime. Each passing day I submerged myself in my work, thanks to my daily dose of 5-Hour Energy. This allowed me to avoid the morbid thoughts and depression. Although upbeat, I couldn't lie down to sleep at night without contemplative thought about Dr. Channeler's prediction of there being a 35 percent chance that I would live ten more years.

On Tuesday, May 1, 2018, I showed up at the familiar surgery center I had become accustomed to visiting for my recent surgeries. The routine was the same as before.

Nila came back to give me a loving kiss and to say, "I will see you shortly, hunny bunny."

When in the operating room, I noticed the same busy atmosphere. Just as before, the blower hose under the edge of my blanket provided welcome warmth.

I was fully prepared for the injection into my IV port. A mask providing oxygen was placed over my nose and mouth. Slowly, I became lightheaded. The conversations were becoming muffled. I could no longer make out the words to the song playing through the speakers. I caught a glimpse of Dr. Wells.

I felt the urge to sing out the lyrics from Pink Floyd's album The Wall, "*Your lips move, but I can't hear what you're saying. I-I-I-I-I have become comfortably numb.*"

I woke up in recovery with Nurse Nila at my side.

My first words were, "I bet you're getting tired of us coming to this room."

My arm was firmly secured in place. Dr. Wells explained what all he had done during the operation.

"The rotator cuff tear was worse than originally thought," he said. "We used a fabric to sew into the rotator cuff for added support and strength. I performed what is called subacromial decompression."

But he did not explain what any of that really meant, so I had to look it up later.

A subacromial decompression is an operation performed to treat shoulder impingement that occurs when soft tissues in the shoulder repeatedly rub against bone, causing pain and inflammation, particularly when you raise your arm. *The aim of shoulder impingement surgery is to regain full, pain-free range of movement.*

"Last," said Dr. Wells, "I performed an extensive glenohumeral debridement."

Extensive fraying cartilage is debrided using a debridement tool and suction. Debridement typically is performed in the anterior and posterior shoulder. Cartilage, but no soft tissue, is removed.

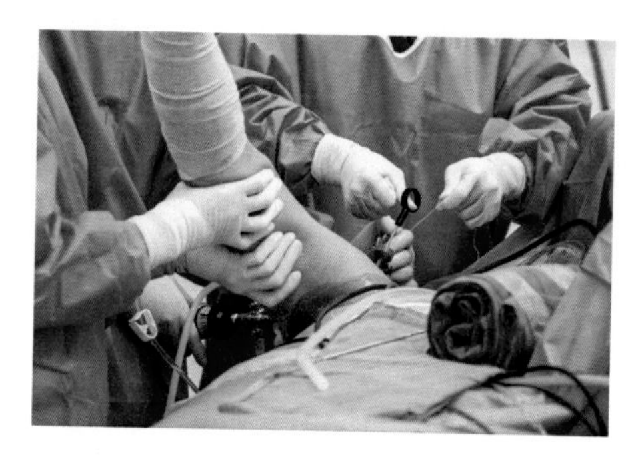

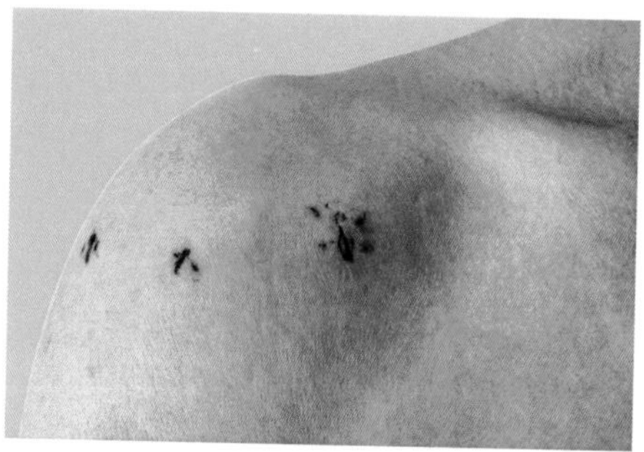

The healing and recovery process was similar to the manipulation. I wore my familiar black arm sling. However, the pain and discomfort were many times worse. Nurse Nila helped me with emails and phone calls. She knew I would not rest without knowing I was keeping up with my responsibilities to Foam Products. She made sure I had my medication on time throughout the day and night. She drove me to PT and sat patiently in the waiting room until I returned.

I did not see Dave this time during my PT. I was sent to a new location. The therapist was very upbeat and motivational. It was a six-week recovery period. I worked at home, as well as at the PT facility, using the pulley and resistance bands. The Sagittarius in me was focused on shortening those six weeks as much as possible.

While I made progress each visit, one area struggled to improve. Actually, I never achieved the goal during the six weeks or for weeks after. When I lay on my back with my arm bent at the elbow, my hand was perpendicular to horizontal. My therapist would sit beside me and place his hand on my shoulder. Then, he would pull my hand toward him. Sometimes it was so painful I would let out a short yell or turn my body toward him to force relief. Over the six weeks of PT, his tone became more discouraged.

"I just don't understand why I can't get your arm to come on over further," he would say.

"It's not your fault," I thought. "My RF is thirteen times too high. I probably have some really mean cancer cells in Mr. Skeleton. I doubt *manipulation vorsätzliche* could even move it!"

Early in my recovery, I noticed it was getting more difficult to breathe. Sometimes I felt it was just the position I was lying in. Other times I thought it was just where I was so out of shape that I got winded a lot easier. Either way, as time passed, it became more obvious. It was especially noticeable, lying on my right side. This was a common position while my left shoulder healed.

"I hope the cancer hasn't spread to my lungs. I need to see Deanna again."

I'm sure many people start to think of how they can change for the better when faced with a possible terminal condition. I was no different. One day, as I ponder such things, this song played, and the lyrics perfectly described what I was doing with a lot of my time.

SOUL SEARCHIN'

Glenn Frey 1988

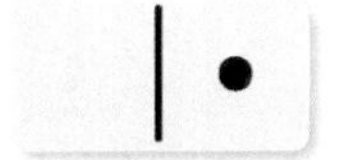
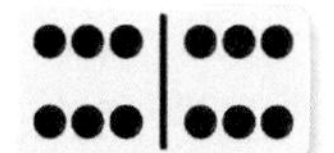

Chapter 13

BECOMING A WOMAN

Sagittarians in a relationship are very attentive and generously plan special things to make their loved ones happy.

Women have always played a significant role in my life. You see, I have been heavily influenced by women since I was born.

My mother and her mother were the first most influential people that I recall. No one needs to explain how significant their mother is to their life, yet I have always felt mine is exemplary in every way. She is a Christian woman who took on the responsibility of caring for three children for the twenty-four years my father was in the army. All while bouncing around from location to location.

During those early years, when my father was away fighting some horrific war, some other women were involved in my life too.

My mom had two sisters. One of the aunts had a daughter who was very close to my sister Gail.

I fondly remember visiting with my family. We would travel to Cleveland, Tennessee, to visit one of my aunts, which was always quite fun. My grandmother's house was right next door. It was very old and still had an outhouse in the backyard. I loved the mimosa trees across the front yard. The pink blooms were like feathers with long seed pods that reminded me of green beans.

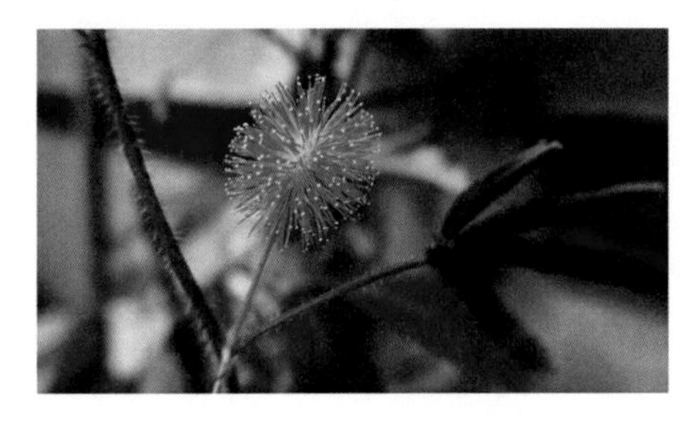
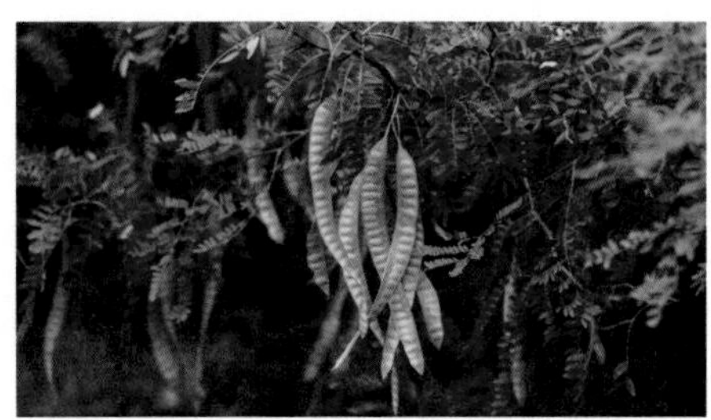

My aunt also had a piano that she would tolerate me experimenting on—at least for a little while! But the one thing I could always be assured of was the vanilla ice cream in the freezer.

At that time, I was surrounded by mostly women. There is a saying: "It takes a village to raise a child." In fact, in 1996, another woman, Hillary Clinton, wrote a book titled *It Takes a Village*. My village was composed mainly of women, which I never realized until later in life. It probably explains why I had so many female friends throughout school. They weren't "girlfriends"; they were just female friends.

My sister is seven years my senior. The relationship we have is not typical for a brother and sister. Because of the age difference, I always looked up to her. I know I was a pest of a little brother. I am quite sure there were times when she wanted to lock me in my bedroom just to have some peace. But instead, she positively influenced my life in many ways. She never judged me. She just provided support, mentoring, and even a place to live in my teen years. Looking back, I wish I could have been to my younger brother David what Gail was to me.

David is a brilliant, wonderful person. For the life of me, I don't know why I was such a bad brother to him. I have spent my life wishing I could go back and be to him what my sister was to me.

And then there is my grandmother (Granny to me). My mom's mother was the only living grandparent I had in my life. She was soft-spoken and deeply religious. I think I am correct in saying she never cut her hair. She always wore it in a bun.

Granny took time staying with each of her daughters in the later years of her life. She is the number one person who positively impacted my life.

Granny never said, "Don't be selfish," or "Don't talk that way," or even "There's no reason to be angry." By being with her, you wanted to be like her and earn her pride and respect—she never needed to tell her grandchildren what to do because her actions spoke louder than words ever could. And she *never* raised her voice.

For a long time, the daily routine was the same. I got off the bus, and, when I came into the house, Granny had the checkerboard set up. Remember, I am a Sagittarius and an athlete. My character is competitive, and my ego is larger than life. But every day, I walked in and sat down with Granny and played checkers. Every day I lost. Each and every day, I walked in more determined to win. I was pretty good at chess, and I just knew I could win at checkers. Every time I lost.

I never won a single game of checkers against my grandmother. It was humbling. I would get twisted up and rant about losing. Granny would just sit and laugh at my childish behavior.

In her last years, it became difficult for Granny to get out of bed. One particular Mother's Day, I recall the struggle of my mom and dad to get her out of bed, bathed, hair washed and put up in a bun, and dressed in a beautiful dress. Mom and Dad finally got her into the den and sat her down. The waiting began.

I remember my granny sitting there all day, waiting for her children to come. Of course, her daughters didn't forget her. However, none of her five sons came. No call, no card in the mail (I checked the mailbox myself), and no visit. Even at my young age of thirteen, I knew how difficult it must have been for her to sit there.

By the end of the day, I was full of anger. I wanted to call all of my uncles and let out my hostility.

"Don't you know how hard it was for your mother to get up and ready today?" is how I would have started the conversation.

"How inconsiderate could you possibly be of the woman who brought you into this world and raised you?" is how I would have continued.

I would have ended by saying something like, "When I get old enough, I am coming to your house to whoop your ass." Then I would slam the receiver down onto its holder.

Before taking Granny back to bed, I walked over and talked to her.

"I am so sorry, Granny," I started. "I don't understand how your own boys can be so inconsiderate. I am so mad and wish I were old enough to drive. I would go find each of them and bring them here."

I wasn't finished telling Granny exactly how I felt before she interrupted me with laughter. I was completely caught off guard.

"It's not funny," I said sternly.

Granny replied, "I'm laughing at your behavior." She paused, and then she continued, "It's all right, Perry. Everyone has their own family now. They have mothers in their families and children. And it's a long drive, too. I had a wonderful day sitting with you all. That's all I need."

I was stunned and speechless. How could she not be mad? How could she not be on my side? But that is the woman she was. Always. She was always kind and forgiving. She inspired me to be a better person without ever quoting scripture, although she knew the Bible intimately.

My dad picked me up from high school one day. Granny was in the hospital and was in a coma. Dad said she had asked for me.

When I got to the room, I wasn't sure what to expect. I walked over and took her hand beside the bed. A few minutes later, her eyes opened, and her head turned toward me. I felt life in her hand—it twitched in mine like a brief squeeze—and I began to get excited about the prospect of her healing.

She looked at me and said, "You know, Perry, it doesn't hurt anymore." Her lips turned up; it was a brief smile—then, she died.

To this day, I believe that Granny is my guardian angel, watching over me, protecting me from myself, and guiding me through life.

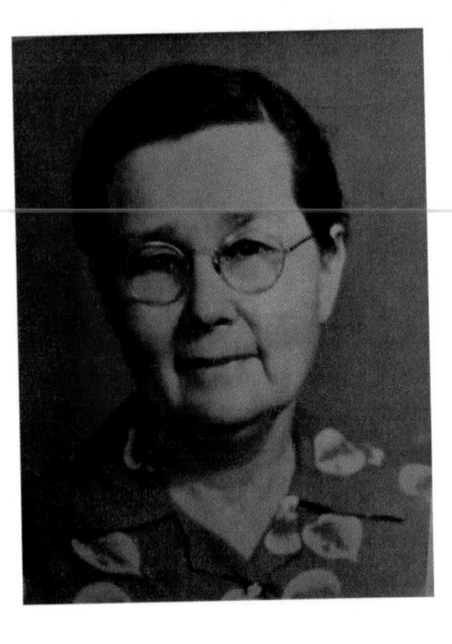

My grandmother, Lily Henderson

Another saying is, "The apple doesn't fall far from the tree." This certainly applies to my mother. My mother is very much like my granny.

I am grateful to still have my mother. She is in her late eighties and still lives at home with my dad.

One of my favorite memories is from December 19. This is my birth date, and every year that I can remember, my mom has sung to me.

The telephone rings, and I see the caller ID. It reads "Mom." I answer, "Hi, Mom." The first thing I hear is my mom singing, "Happy birthday to you. Happy birthday to you."

No matter my whereabouts, or whether I have gotten myself in trouble, Mom always sings to me on December 19.

My sister Gail was somewhere between a sister, a mom, and a great friend to me. She, too, inspired me and mentored me. Just like my mom and Granny, she has set an example for me to follow. Without speaking a word, she helps me to realize my faults and see how to be a better person.

I would be remiss if I didn't mention Nila. She is the strongest woman I have ever known. Underneath that layer of strength is a caring, loving, passionate woman. I can't begin to list all I have learned from her, but the list is quite long.

The list goes on and on of women who have touched my life and motivated me to aspire to be smarter and better. My daughter, my daughters-in-law, to name a few more. Even the female teachers that made my life better are a long list.

Ms. Thompson was my third-grade teacher. She was beautiful, and I fell in love with her. "I'm going to marry Ms. Thompson when I grow up," I would tell my buddies.

But Ms. Thompson didn't get the memo. One day she came to class and announced she was getting married and moving away. Ms. Thompson was my favorite teacher, and I excelled at learning from her. There were more great teachers that followed her.

It was only when I got older that I realized I had been surrounded mostly by women growing up. I began to notice how others mistreated women or spoke disrespectfully to or about women. I didn't understand those views. I also noticed how television shamelessly exploited women.

I even noticed as I progressed through life, working various jobs, that men were predominantly at the top of the food chain. And in these jobs, women were spoken to disrespectfully. It was confusing to see women treated like second-class citizens.

While I was in school, I learned that, throughout history, traditional gender roles have often defined and limited women's activities and opportunities. Even many religious doctrines stipulate certain rules for women. I learned that during the twentieth century, restrictions began loosening in many societies. Women began to have greater access to careers, outside of being homemakers, and got the ability to pursue higher education.

Yet, unfortunately, there is a long history of violence against women at home and within their communities. This violence is primarily committed by men.

In some societies, women are even denied reproductive rights.

As a man surrounded by women, I have always been in awe of what it takes to be a woman. In addition to the aforementioned atrocities, a woman's life is incredibly tough by design.

Puberty hits boys and girls, but when a girl's body starts to change, it is often the boys at school who make the girls objects of ridicule.

As exciting as it is to begin the change into adulthood for boys and girls alike, it is the female that is introduced to menstruation. I have watched the women in my life struggle with painful cramps and more. Their emotions are affected, and I have seen them struggling to understand why they are suddenly sad. This goes on for decades. It just doesn't seem fair.

Pregnancy is a miracle I couldn't handle. I think in amazement about having a child grow and develop inside of me. There is no greater responsibility than that. I would probably just stay home and surround myself with pillows to make sure the baby was protected.

But women don't think that way. An aforementioned, remarkable woman in my life, Nila, worked a job in a factory until the week she gave birth...to another wonderful female, my daughter, Alanna.

As though all of these things aren't enough, women still have more to contend with: menopause.

Menopause occurs when a woman reaches her forties or fifties, but the average age is fifty-one in the United States. Menopause is a natural biological process. But there are physical symptoms to contend with, such as hot flashes and emotional symptoms that may disrupt sleep, lower energy, or affect emotional health in general.

It just doesn't seem fair. After decades of having monthly menstruation, it finally ends with menopause and the side effects that come with it.

When I began having my Lupron shots, I remember Dr. Hinder saying, "Once your testosterone drops, it will be like a woman going through menopause. You will experience hot flashes, night sweats, and mood swings."

As time progressed, it was easy to see the doctor was correct in his prediction. I began having hot flashes routinely, about every two to three hours. I would wake up throughout the night feeling as though the room temperature was elevated. Then, I would break out into sweat, similar to when a fever breaks.

My emotions were definitely impacted. I am an eternally optimistic person, but sadness would show up without warning. It might only take a commercial or just something kind spoken to me by Nila.

Perhaps the feelings can best be described by a picture from a movie.

It was Christmas time, and I was watching *National Lampoon's Christmas Vacation*, starring Chevy Chase. In the movie, he had locked himself in the attic. It was cold, so he rummaged through some containers to find articles of clothing to put on. He also ran across some home movies and set up the projector to watch them.

In the scene, Clark (Chevy Chase) finds himself sitting in the attic, wearing women's clothing, watching home movies, and crying.

Throughout my life, I remember hearing phrases like "Crying like a little girl," or "You hit like a girl." That was meant to make us boys dry it up or hit harder. I often felt it was derogatory for someone to say, "You fight like a girl" to another person. But driving one day, I saw this in the back window of the car in front of me.

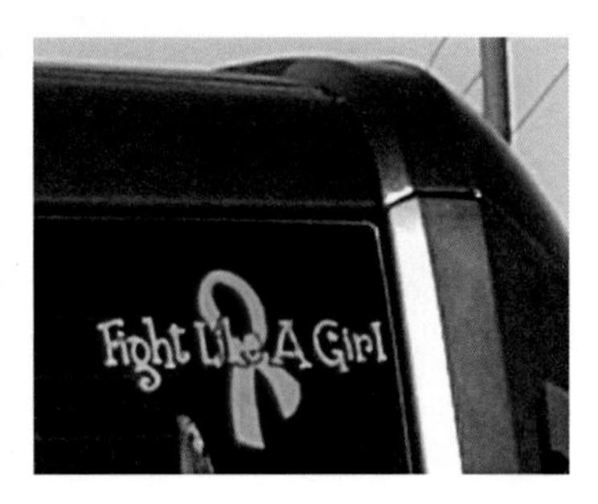

Back window of a random car

The effects of Lupron lowering my testosterone were in full force. Hot flashes, night sweats, and suddenly sad. My muscles shriveled away, and I was a weaker version of myself. Nothing about my manhood worked anymore. Nila and I often jokingly told people we were lesbians now.

On September 17, 2019, Mr. Mitten passed away after seventeen years of being with us. From the day I was diagnosed with cancer, he never left my side. He shared my food, my recliner, and my pillow. Still today, I think of him and cry like a little girl.

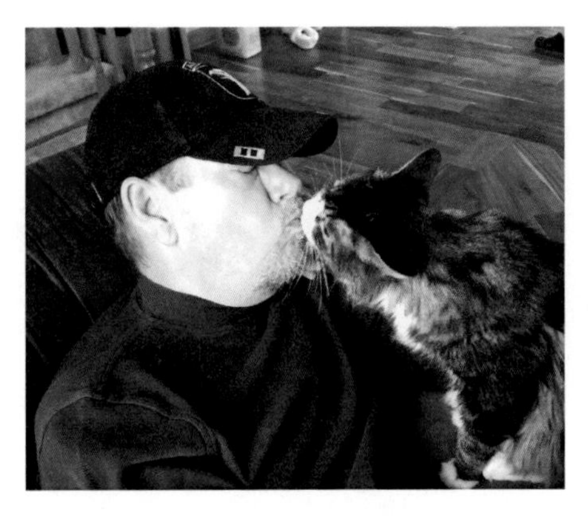

Kisses from Mr. Mitten

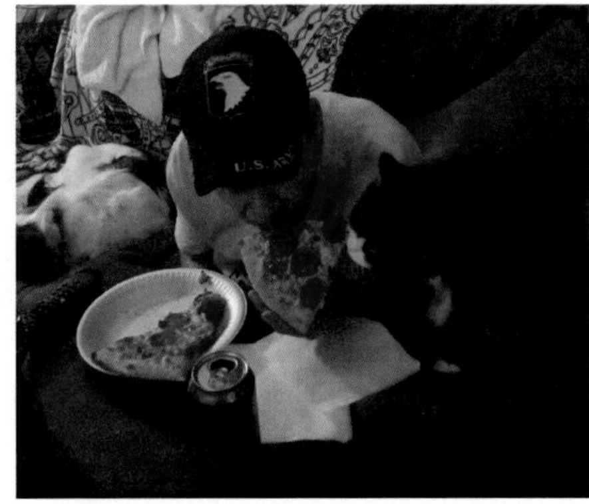

Mr. Mitten sharing my pizza

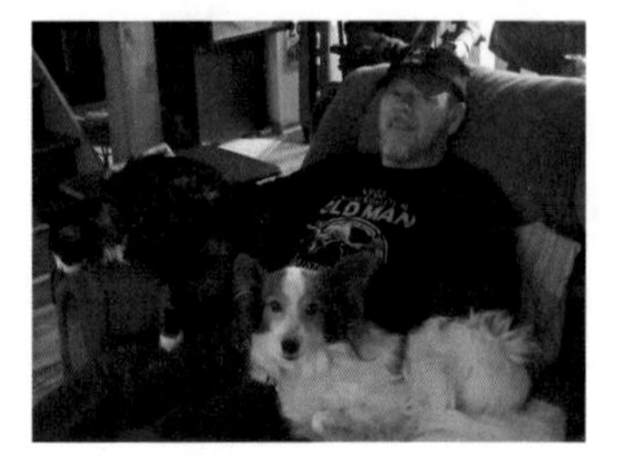

Mr. Mitten and Sparky in a familiar place

Women have made great strides in establishing themselves in top-tier careers. Another woman I have a great deal of respect for is the female doctor who invented a new fusion rocket thruster concept, which could power humans to Mars and beyond.

She is a physicist who works for the US Department of Energy and designed a rocket that will use magnetic fields to shoot plasma particles—electrically charged gas—into the vacuum of space.

According to Newton's second and third laws of motion, the conservation of momentum would mean the rocket was propelled forward—and at speeds ten times faster than comparable devices.

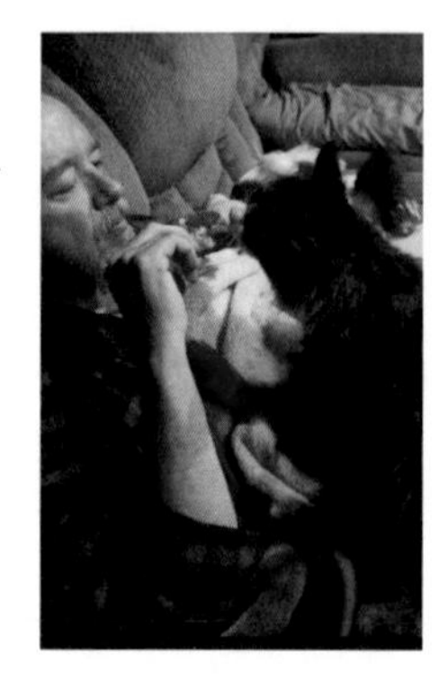

Mr. Mitten sharing pizza again

Currently, space-proven plasma propulsion engines use electric fields to propel the plasma particles. But the doctor's new rocket design will accelerate them using magnetic reconnection.

Magnetic reconnection is found throughout the universe. The most well-known observation is found on the surface of the sun. When magnetic field lines converge there, they produce an enormous amount of energy.

It's just rocket science!!

Thanks to cancer, I felt like I was becoming a woman. But being a woman is something to have great pride in.

Having menopause symptoms was new for me as a man. I had no idea the degree of hot flashes and other symptoms, although my wife had told me on many occasions. One day I took the opportunity to watch the musical, Menopause. *The lyrics to this song made me laugh out loud. I could definitely relate.*

HEAT WAVE LYRICS

Menopause the Musical 2001

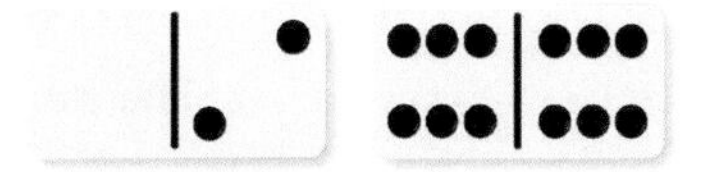

Chapter 14

CANCER BOUGHT ME A FENCE

A Sagittarius is an adventurous, courageous, and immensely social man. Optimism is his favorite word.

Sometime during my radiation treatments and through the weeks prior, I began having an odd catch in my right thumb. At first, I dismissed it as just one of those things that happen as you get older. I would bend my thumb, and it would click occasionally when I straightened it back out. It was weird, but in no way did it impede my ability to use it.

Besides, I told myself, my right hand *was* the part of my body that had been through more than the collective rest. Let me explain.

Let's go back to the 1970s when I was playing "pony league" baseball. I loved baseball and never minded practice. Unlike basketball, we didn't do the endless wind sprints and laps to get into shape. Running bored me. (Today, I would love to experience the boredom of running a few laps.)

In baseball, I once played for a team named the Roadrunners. I was usually assigned to the lead-off batting position. In order to obtain this position in the batting order, the coaches must have confidence in your ability to get on base more often than not. Secondly, you need to have speed to steal bases or to gain extra bases in the event a subsequent batter gets a base hit.

As I mentioned before, I was a small guy. In fact, I was below average size for my age. This made me a smaller target for the opposing pitcher, and, therefore, I led the team in walks. Small also usually equates to speed. The big bullies on the playground couldn't catch this undersized speedster. I didn't get bored running fast, just running without an obvious purpose.

One particular season, while playing for the Roadrunners, I mastered a new form of trickery to get on base and gain an advantage. I started by crouching a little more than normal to further reduce the targeted strike zone. Then, I crowded the plate. This was a psychological ploy. I wanted the pitcher to be conscious of not hitting me. Not that he cared if I was hit by a baseball, but it would automatically award me a walk.

On more than one occasion during this season, I had earned a walk. Most often it was due to accumulating four called balls. I had a routine. I would casually toss my bat aside and begin to trot down the first base line. I would carefully study the pitcher's demeanor. I knew that if I saw frustration and distraction from giving up the walk, I should check to see what the second baseman was doing.

Oftentimes, the pitcher's demeanor was contagious, and the second baseman would be distracted. He might be kicking the dirt or adjusting his glove between batters. I would then watch for him to walk away from second base toward his position for the next batter. As soon as all of these boxes were checked off, I would step on first base and kick it into turbo! I would run as though the big bully on the playground was hot on my heels.

The opposing players were always caught off guard. They would begin yelling to get the attention of the pitcher, who was holding the ball. His first instinct was to look at first base. But I wasn't there any longer. The second baseman would turn and run to his base. Sometimes I would pass him. Sometimes it was a tie. However, he and the baseball together never made it there before me.

In the last game of the season, we were playing for the championship. I pulled the same stunt. I didn't always get a walk. I actually had a pretty good batting average. Sometimes I was lucky enough that my speed was able to beat out an infield grounder. The word was out about my tricky talent, so I had to be extra cautious and extra sneaky.

As I crowded the plate, I tuned everything else out. I stared hard at the pitcher and gripped the bat with two sweaty hands.

"Ball!" the umpire yelled as the second ball missed my strike zone.

I stepped back from the plate and swung my bat around to ease some of the tension in my back. Then, I moved up to the plate again, hunching over and getting low, ready for the pitcher's next throw.

The pitcher stared hard at my stance and then peeled his arm back and let one fly in my direction—straight into my left shoulder.

Written by Perry Muse

I dropped the bat and made out like the ball had been a cannon shot. My coach came out and checked me over.

"Can you go on?" he asked.

I held my shoulder and nodded my head bravely, putting on a strong front.

The trot to first was slower than normal as I held my shoulder where the ball had struck me.

"Don't worry about me; I'm too hurt to pull anything today," I thought hard at the pitcher as I hung my head lower and cut my eyes in his direction to see if my ploy was working. He was rolling his shoulders and looking toward home.

My foot hit the first base, and I geared into turbo time.

I guess the pitcher wasn't completely surprised. He spun and threw the ball toward second before anyone was even there. I could see that the second baseman was going to beat me to the bag, and I was going to need to slide. However, before I slid, I saw the ball fly well over the second baseman's head and into right center field. Adrenaline had gotten the best of the pitcher's ball control.

I touched second base and never slowed, heading for third. My third-base coach was jumping and waving for me to stop. But I rounded third and looked for the ball. I could always stop and go back. The ball was in the air with the catcher standing over the plate at home, waiting. I never let up. I saw the ball bounce several feet in front of him, and I dove headfirst toward the catcher's feet. It was him or me. My eyes were fixated on the open area of the home plate—I knew I could slip by him, touch there, and be safe. I slid with both arms outstretched before me. My right hand touched just before the catcher reached down and tagged me with the glove that was now holding the ball.

"SAFE!!!" yelled the umpire.

I had just turned a walk into a home run.

My teammates greeted me with an enthusiastic "way to go" and "all rights," plus hearty slaps on the back. I felt like I could fly.

I needed to catch my breath, so I went into the dugout. We were undefeated, and this last game of the season was a nailbiter, but my home run had pushed us into the lead.

Rather suddenly, I realized that my hand was wet. When I looked down, my right hand was bleeding profusely. Between my pinky and third finger was a huge gash. How had I missed that? All I could see was dirt, blood, and white tissue.

What could have happened? I thought back over the last couple of minutes...when I dove into home, my hand slid across the plate, but my pinky finger must have found its way under the edge. As I slid across, the rubber edge of the home plate had to have carved through my hand.

I was immediately taken from the game and to the local hospital, where I received stitches and the first of many scars on my right hand. I always revered the scar as my personal trophy, for it was a forever reminder of the day I turned a walk into a home run.

Later in life, I began to add to the scars on my right hand. I developed Dupuytren's disease. Guillaume Dupuytren was a famous military surgeon and French anatomist. He is best known for treating Napoleon Bonaparte's hemorrhoids and originally describing Dupuytren's contracture.

Dupuytren's disease, also called Dupuytren's contracture, is an abnormal thickening and tightening of the normally loose and flexible tissue beneath the skin of the palm and fingers, called fascia. The pinky and ring fingers are most often affected.

The fascia contains strands of fibers, like cords, that run from the palm upward into the fingers. In Dupuytren's disease, these cords tighten or contract, causing the fingers to curl forward. In severe cases, it can lead to crippling hand deformities.

The signs of Dupuytren's disease show up in three phases. The first sign is the development of nodules. These lumps under the skin in the palm of the hand are the first symptoms for many people. The lump may feel tender and sore at first, but this discomfort eventually goes away.

Second are cords. The nodules cause these tough bands of tissue to form under the skin in the palm. These inflexible bands cause the fingers to bend, or "curl," forward toward the wrist.

The last development is contracture. As the curling gets worse, it becomes difficult, if not impossible, to straighten the fingers. People with Dupuytren's disease often have a hard time picking up large objects, or placing their hands into their pockets, something you might do every day to retrieve coins, cash, or your ID card. If you have this condition, you may also find it difficult to place your hand flat on the table, wear gloves, or shake hands, among other things.

In order to treat Dupuytren's contracture, I underwent four surgeries on my right hand less than a year before my cancer diagnosis. I have been fortunate to not have any on my left. I am the only such case my orthopedic hand surgeon has ever seen.

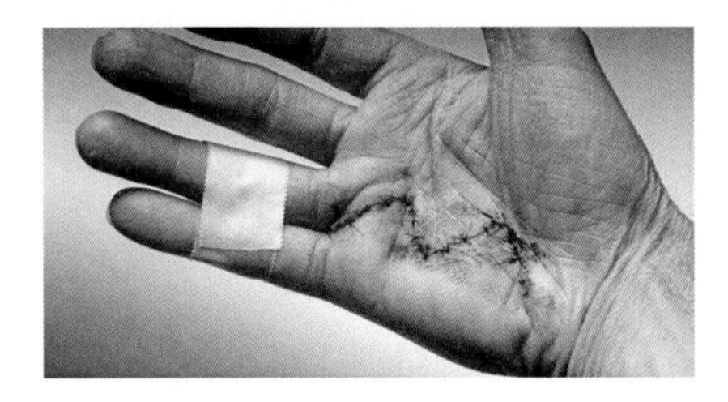

The surgery is usually a long, zigzag incision. The skin is folded back to allow the surgeon vast access. This is so they can remove any newly forming nodules. It also allows them to unwind the bands and, hopefully, avoid nerve damage.

Scars on my right hand

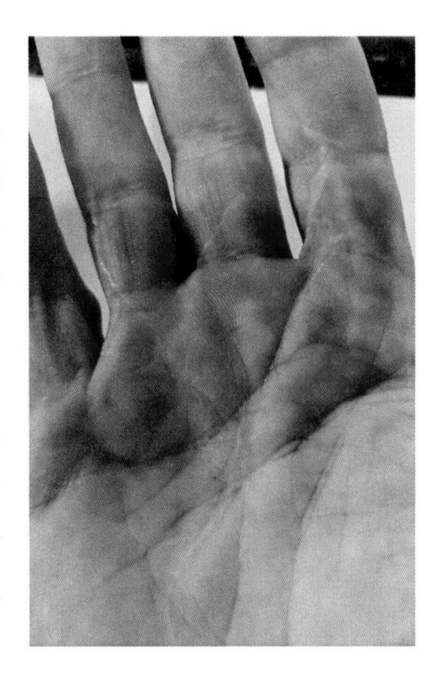

During the recovery period for my shoulder surgery, the thumb worsened. It began to lock in place. During the time leading up to the surgery, I took an opportunity to discuss my condition with Dr. Wells. He brought in a coworker who specialized in the hand. The coworker was Dr. Lord.

Dr. Lord explained that I had a condition called trigger finger. My initial treatment was a shot of cortisone into the bend of the thumb at the palm. It worked for a few weeks, and I was relieved, thinking the problem was solved. I was wrong.

My second shot of cortisone lasted only two days. The thumb locking was more of a problem because I could not use my left hand due to the shoulder surgery. Now I was limited as to what I could do with my right hand. So, twenty-seven days after wanting to sing a Pink Floyd song to Dr. Wells, I went to a different surgery center so Dr. Lord could fix my thumb.

The surgery went well and was low on the pain scale. Each day Nila took a vitamin E gel cap and punctured it with a needle. She would then squeeze the contents onto my incision. This is a practice we followed for all of my surgeries. It accelerated the healing and minimized the scarring.

By the time I was scheduled to have the stitches removed, I was busy working in Georgia. The time away while healing from the rotator cuff surgery concerned me. I needed to make an appearance and a contribution. I needed to make up for lost time. So, I skipped my appointment. Then I skipped the rescheduled appointment. Before I realized it, I was two weeks overdue for getting the stitches removed.

Nila and I finally made it to the rescheduled appointment. One of Dr. Lord's female nurses came in to take the sutures out.

"Mr. Muse, there is a problem here with your stitches," the nurse said.

"Okay," I said, waiting to hear the problem. I hated to hear I had a problem and then get a long pause. You could state the problem in the same breath.

"It seems your skin has grown over the sutures," she said. "I can give you a local numbing agent, but it will still likely hurt to remove these today."

"Gee, thanks, accelerated healing," I thought.

"Well, if you had not postponed your appointment, maybe this would not have happened," replied the little voice in my head, not to be outdone.

"Can we leave them in?" I asked, thinking she had implied we didn't need to take them out.

"No."

"Okay, let's go," I said. "It's better to get bad, painful things over and done with," I thought.

I lay on my back and the nurse sprayed something on my hand to numb it, but I would not have the urge to sing, nor would I be comfortably numb. The pain was immediate and intense. In fact, it was far more intense than recovery from the surgery itself. I held off making any noises as long as possible, until I couldn't bear the pain any longer.

I yelled, "OH SHIT!" and farted.

That's right.

It hurt, then I cussed and farted loudly from the strain as the nurse tried to do her job. Which promptly made her stop.

After an awkward moment, I apologized.

"I hope she only heard me cuss and didn't hear the fart," I thought, embarrassed.

She kindly replied, "It's all right. We all fart."

I reached a point where the pain and tenderness were more than I could bear. It seemed as though she was trying unsuccessfully to peel the skin off my hands.

"Not another second," I said. "Get me a scalpel, please, and I'll cut the stitches out for you. Peeling off the outer skin to get the stitches is not working. Please get me the scalpel."

Without another word, she left the room to talk to the doctor. After privately consulting with Dr. Lord (I assume), she returned and brought a magnifying glass, a pair of tweezers, and a surgical scalpel and laid them on a table across the room. Without a word, she turned and left.

"Grab them before they come back," said Nila.

I understood the issue; they couldn't give me permission, so they gave me time and tools. I grabbed the utensils and went to work. I can't say for sure that was their intention. Nevertheless, I took advantage of the situation.

Immediately I could see why the nurse had literally been peeling my skin off. It was a conundrum. The stitches were tied in multiple places. All but one of them were out of sight beneath the skin. I began to slice my skin, however, certainly not with the skill and precision of Dr. Lord.

The newly grown skin was incredibly sensitive. I had to be careful not to cut the stitches, or more slicing would be needed. Nila held the magnifying glass in one hand and held the single visible stitch with the tweezers using her other. As I sliced away at the skin's surface, blood began to pool, making it increasingly difficult to see.

The nurse peeked in, and we froze. I'm sure we looked like a couple of children being caught by Mom doing something bad.

She said, "I will be back in a few. We are having difficulty with another patient."

The door closed, and I began working with the scalpel again. We hoped that was code for "I will give you more time to finish."

The pain never let up. Actually, it intensified. But I had to get to the buried sutures. There was no way I was letting the nurse have another go at it. Finally, I whittled my way down to the final small knot and cut it free. Nila pulled it out slowly, and the feeling of relief was intoxicating.

The foundation for the sixth scar on my right hand was complete. It was the smallest of all. But, just as the first one will always remind me of that special baseball game in the seventies, this one will always remind me of a cuss, a fart, and the scalpel left on the table.

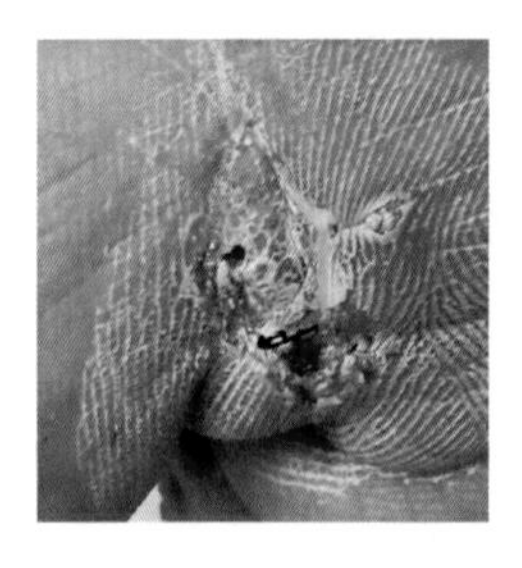

Thumb before stitches were removed

It was now June 2018 and already time for another trip to SCC. My outlook was optimistic after a year of what felt like falling apart at the seams. The fact that I had cancer never left my thoughts for long. As the time for my second appointment approached, the reality and anxiety were augmented. I needed my PSA to be lower. I needed to know that I was continuing my journey to a zero PSA and being cancer free.

My breathing continued to be an issue. I was through with all of the surgeries (as far as I was aware at that time) and had begun to ramp up my physical activity. I became acutely aware of the loss in strength and muscle mass. It was never more apparent than when I tried to do menial tasks, like putting dishes up into the kitchen cabinet. There were three shelves, but I could only reach the second one now. If I had too many plates or bowls, I was unable to even reach the second shelf.

I lost a total of thirty-six pounds. I weighed one hundred and seventy-eight pounds before cancer. To lose thirty-six pounds meant losing 20 percent of my overall weight. Most of the weight loss was muscle, and I could tell.

"Mr. Skeleton can't even lift a few plates above his head. He needs some muscles. Too bad he is way too tired and stiff to work out. I wonder what cancer does with all of that energy it steals."

Nila and I made the trip to SCC. We knew what to expect this time. It felt more upbeat on the drive down, unlike trips to most of the other appointments. We checked into our hotel room, had a nice dinner, and turned in.

The next morning, we headed down Celebration of Life Drive to SCC. We walked into a familiar greeting and headed straight to Maple. From there we went across the hall to get blood drawn.

"Take your time," I said to the nurse, "I need some really good numbers today."

The nurse smiled and replied, "I'm gonna do my level best to get you those good numbers."

We went into the main entrance area. There was a large round table with a beautiful flower arrangement there. I asked the person greeting everyone if they would take a picture, and they happily agreed. This became a routine from that day forth.

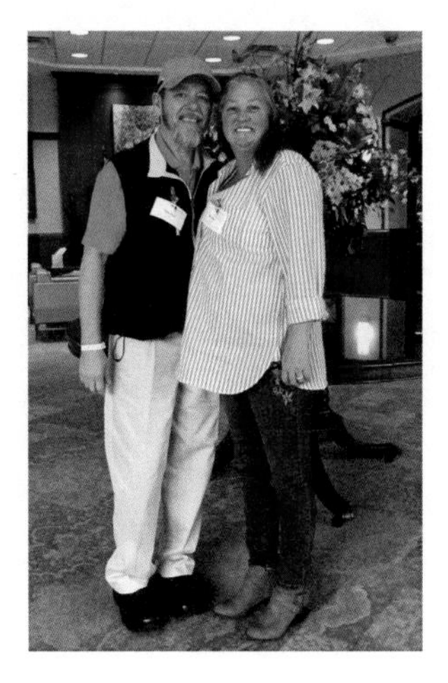

Nila and I at SCC

We had lunch and headed to see Dr. Taha. Once I was checked in, we anxiously awaited to be called back.

Finally, it was my turn.

Once settled in the room, the nurse ran through the typical line of questions. "Have you been to the hospital since your last visit? Are you still taking A, B, C, D, E, F medications? How are you feeling in general?"

"Yes, of course I am still taking all of my medications. Most of them are cancer fighting! Yes, I have been to the hospital twice. The first time I tried to sing. The last time I cussed, farted, and got my scalpel self-service license..." all ran through my mind.

But I answered honestly and patiently, although I really wanted to get to the part where Dr. Taha told me my PSA.

The time came. Dr. Taha walked in with a small entourage of folks he was mentoring. We had a little chitchat, and he opened my file. I did not see any change of expression. I couldn't read anything that hinted at what the news was for today. At this point the emotion was like that of a child waiting his turn to sit on Santa's lap.

"Your numbers look pretty good," he began with a tone as though he were pleased.

"Your PSA is .9..."

I didn't hear what came after the number. My PSA was unchanged.

"That is the same as the last time," I interrupted.

He immediately replied, "Yes, but that is still really good compared to one seventy-nine."

He then went on to say more.

In my mind, I thought, "That's not good enough. It's not progress if the number is unchanged. It's not zero because I still have cancer, but no one wants to screw up my quality of life and tell me. No one except Dr. Channeler, and I fired him."

I don't recall most of the remaining conversation. I do recall Dr. Taha suggesting I take a shot. I agreed and didn't even ask what it was for.

"Don't you remember—you wanted a picture with Dr. Taha for your book?" Nila reminded me as we stood up to leave.

I had forgotten and no longer cared, but it was too late to call it off. I unfairly felt Dr. Taha was being less than fully transparent. Dr. Taha stood beside me to pose. The next day I cropped myself from the picture. It was symbolic to me. Dr. Taha was exceptional to me, and my anger was unfairly directed toward him. I was really angry with the cancer.

We walked out and proceeded to the lab for my shot.

While the nurse prepped me, I asked, "And what is this for?"

She replied, "Your bones."

"I see the doctor is concerned for Mr. Skeleton. I know why. I am too," I thought.

To me, the news was very concerning. I researched all I could but never found any medical explanations about having a PSA number without a prostate that didn't point to cancer.

"Surgical procedures aren't perfect. Surgeons aren't perfect. Sometimes when the prostate is removed, there are fragments left behind. If these fragments contain cancer cells, your PSA will continue to show" is a quote from an article on WebMD, a reputable medical publication. It concurred with other explanations I found during my research. I did see where it could take several months after radiation for the PSA to fully drop. That was my only hope. I had to wait and see. My next appointment was in three months. I was already anxious about the results that would be reported on September 5, 2018, at the end of Celebration of Life Drive.

Meanwhile, I turned my focus to continued work on my ROM and getting into better shape. At the end of June, I stood on the scales in my bathroom. I had avoided this since the last SCC visit. I didn't want to see a further decline in weight. I stepped on the scale, looked down at the digital readout, and saw one forty-seven. I had gained five pounds back.

"That cancer may be hiding in there somewhere, but I'm getting my weight and strength back," was my first thought.

I was really motivated to work hard on my strength and ROM. But by the end of a workday, there wasn't much left in the tank. I couldn't do cardio because I struggled to breathe.

"Man, this cancer has kicked my ass. I haven't ever been so out of shape," I thought.

I made an appointment to see Dr. Famoyin. It felt like time for some iron infusion IVs and some intellectual conversation.

The dogs had become a real issue at home. Sparky would be let out and make a speedy run through the woods out back and across a field to a distant neighborhood. As the crow flies, it wasn't that far. But to drive was a good five miles. Then he didn't want to get into the car and go home, knowing it would mean the end of his freedom.

Thor was in love with the neighbors' Great Dane, Sangria, and would slip off to their house whenever the opportunity presented itself. We lived on Olgia Lane, which turned off South Greenwood, a very busy main road. Cars and trucks raced by on Greenwood. We were always panicky about the dogs making it all of the way to the main road.

At 3:00 a.m. one morning, Alanna was coming home from work. This was when she still lived with us. She topped the hill and rounded the curve just prior to Olgia Lane. Standing in the middle of Greenwood, with a "deer in the headlights" look, was Sebastian.

After that incident, we kept Sebastian, and eventually Thor when he came to us, on runners. I had several runners, so I could mix it up and give them new, interesting places to hang out. We set up temperature control in the garage and locked them inside at night. We hated them not having freedom, but not as much as we hated the thought of them standing in the middle of Greenwood.

At work one day, I was told the Aflac representative was there whenever I could make time to see him. I had Aflac starting in 2012 but had never used it. I had thought often about cancelling it to save money.

I went in for my visit with the Aflac representative and asked him to tell me what I was paying for. I really didn't even remember. One of the items on the list he recited was a cancer policy.

"Wait a minute. I have a cancer policy?" I asked.

He explained the policy, and I explained what I had been through thus far with cancer. It turned out I qualified for several benefits. The representative explained how to file the claims, and suddenly, I felt the need to take notes.

"Finally, something positive related to cancer," I said to him.

I gathered all of the required documents to file my claims. I already had them printed off and filed away to use as reference material for my book.

I went home and told Nila the great news. This was a chance to have some extra cash. Maybe we could take a vacation. No, I had missed enough work. Besides, the relaxing downtime would just lend itself to additional morbid thoughts.

In the end, the check came, and we were thrilled. We installed a beautiful black chain-link fence around the entire property. We had multiple gates placed at various locations. For the driveway, we had a solar-powered electric gate installed. I also ordered a beautifully crafted metal "M" to go on each of the two electric gates.

In turn, this allowed me to be able to cross off another box on my cancer to-do list. If I wasn't going to be around for Nila, I wanted her to be safe and secure. The fence provided that security. I just needed a few more security cameras. Then I could have peace of mind, knowing she would feel safer without me.

We were able to turn the dogs loose without fear of them running off. Instead of giving ourselves a vacation, we gave them freedom.

The first time we turned them loose, I looked at Nila and said, "Well, Nila, at least cancer bought us a fence."

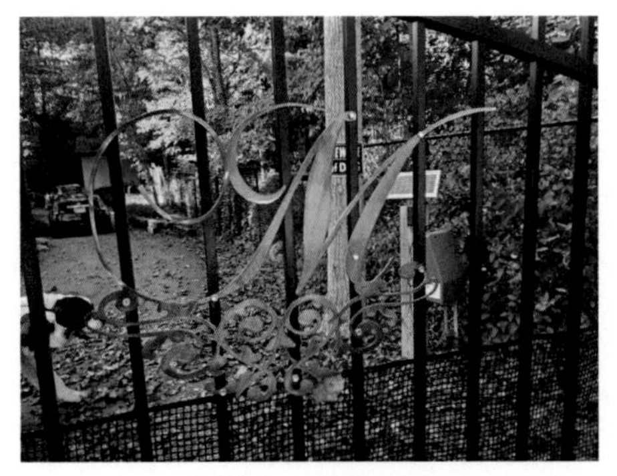

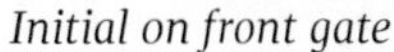

Initial on front gate

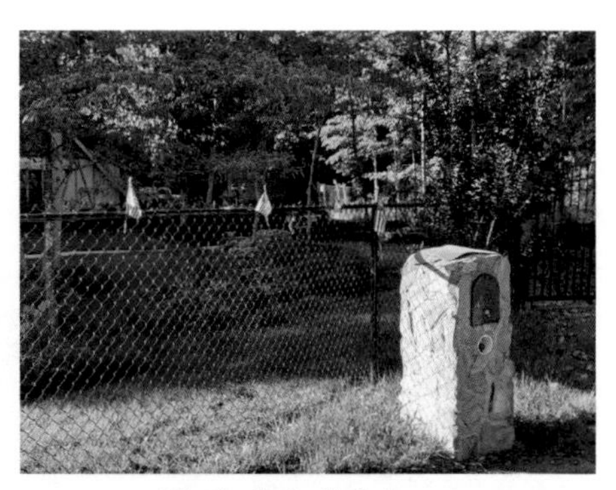

Black chain-link fence

WARNING
PROPERTY PROTECTED BY:
★GUNS
★KNIVES
★CAMERAS
★& DOGS
ENTER AT YOUR OWN PERIL

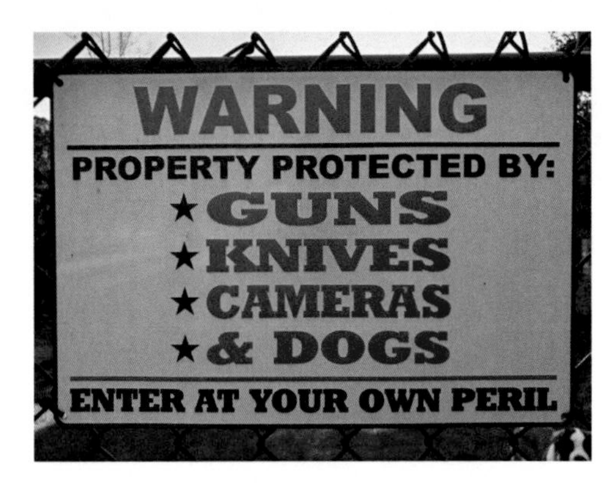

Signs I installed for added deterrence

I was a lifelong Neil Young fan. My iPod was set on Neil Young radio one day. After my surprise with the Aflac policy, and my ongoing cancer battle, I found the lyrics to this song to have a new meaning.

"HEY HEY, MY MY" (INTO THE BLACK)

Neil Young 1979

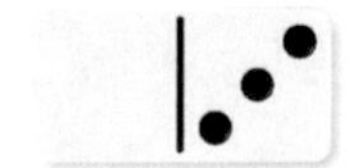 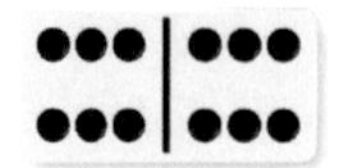

Chapter 15

TAKING MY BREATH AWAY PART I

Big-spirited and open-hearted Sagittarians are natural-born leaders who go after what they want, regardless of what other people think of them.

Few things will grab your attention like losing your breath.

My first experience happened when I was a child, and my dad was serving what would be his last tour of duty in Vietnam.

My mom, sister, and brother lived in an apartment complex in Dalton, Georgia. There were three to four apartments per building structure, and the complex covered many streets and blocks. This was a vividly memorable place for me. The apartments were small and made of concrete blocks; it was government housing, called the Dalton Housing Authority, but I remember it as Bluff Hill, the street on which our apartment was located. It was obviously low-income housing, which is strange to me after having served in the army myself. Low-income housing for those who pay a high price to serve. But I made tons of memories there.

I remember Mom working with me on my homework in the dimly lit and modest living room. Truth be known, I would never have been able to slide all the way through high school with A's and B's without her mentoring.

This was a place where neighborhood kids gathered and played wiffle ball. At least that was what we called baseball when we used a plastic bat and a plastic ball that had holes in it.

The backyard had a concrete wall that separated our space from the neighbors' space on the other end. Close to the wall was a metal fixture shaped like a T. There was another fixture several feet away, and wires that connected the two. This was where Mom hung our laundry to dry. But I used it for something totally different. The top of the T was the perfect height from the top of the wall if you were a superhero.

On days when there was no laundry hanging and blowing in the breeze, I would grab my favorite towel and tie it around my neck. If you were to ask my sister, she would say I tied a towel around my neck and played for years. Actually, I was still playing with a towel around my neck when I was in the army!

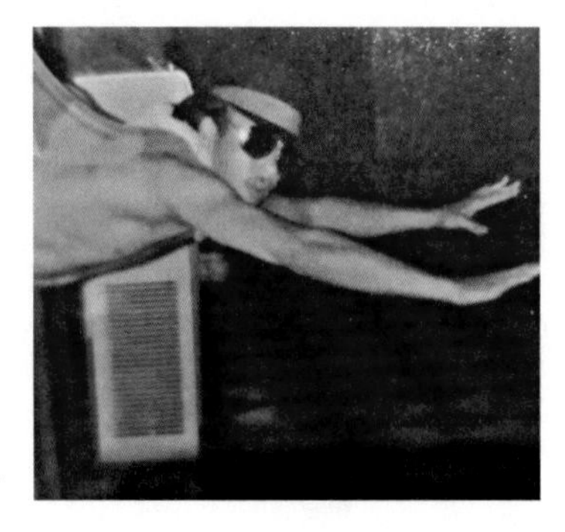

Pretending to fly in the barracks with towel

Once my cape was secured, I would position myself along the top of the concrete wall divider and place my hands on my hips. Just as any superhero would do, I scanned the city below for villains. Once spotted, I jumped into flight, my cape waving as I flew. To continue my imaginary flight, I grabbed the horizontal tube that made the top of the T-shape.

The T-tubing was painted gray. Little did I know, on my maiden flight, that the sun had oxidized the paint. It was more like powder than paint. On this day, when I first grabbed it, there was not any grip.

I tried to swing one-handed on the structure, likely kicking or swinging at the villains who had spotted me and came to entertain combat. But just as quickly as I grabbed the structure, my hand slipped off.

I was almost horizontal when gravity eventually sucked me to the ground. I hit with a dull thud, and all the air in my lungs raced away.

"I stopped breathing. I'm going to die," I immediately thought. Panic set in, and I jumped to my feet. I mustered all the strength I had, and after what felt like minutes, I inhaled.

There were other times in my life that I got the wind knocked out of me, and even though I knew each time what was going on, the panic was always there.

"What if I'm not so lucky this time? What if I can't force the air to return?" I often thought.

Richard Pryor once did a comedy standup and talked about Jim Brown of Cleveland Browns' fame hitting him.

Richard said, "Air just left my lungs, like F this. I'm outta here."

In eighth-grade football practice, it happened again. As I said before, I was undersized. I wore the smallest jersey available, and half of my number was tucked in my pants.

I was on defense, playing cornerback. I never played defense much and was just filling a spot while the offense worked on a new running sweep to their left.

The coach kept running the same play to the other side of the field, so I got bored and drifted off into imagination land. This was a dangerous place to go during football practice.

Vernon was a big strong country boy. In eighth grade he was five eight and probably weighed a hundred and sixty pounds. That was a hundred and sixty pounds of lean country boy.

Vernon didn't care that the play was running to the opposite side of the field. He was on offense, on my side of the formation. His objective was to block or hit someone with all of his overgrown might. Making physical contact was encouraged in football, and Vernon excelled at it.

I think Vernon must have gotten bored not being able to have any contact or being able to hit anyone since he was also on the opposite side of the offense that the play was running on. I later found out that the coach yelled at him for just standing around instead of engaging.

So, on the fifth or so time that the coach ran the same play, and at the very same time I took a break to go to imagination land, I snapped out of my daydream just in time to see Vernon running full speed toward me. He was about five feet from me, and the look on his face was that of anger and ill intentions. Vernon then proceeded to knock me on my ass.

I woke up on the ground to see Vernon standing over me, his feet on each side of my body. He was bent over, staring intently at me. The fact that his top front teeth were missing gave him an even more ominous appearance. I quickly realized that my breath had abandoned me again.

"I think he's dead, Coach. He ain't breathing!" shouted Vernon with his authentic Southern accent. For me, it was decidedly more difficult to summon my lungs to work again while lying on my back and wearing shoulder pads. For a split second, I wondered if Vernon would have to blow the air back into my lungs for me. I did not care, just so long as I could breathe again. Fortunately, that was not necessary.

Middle school football picture

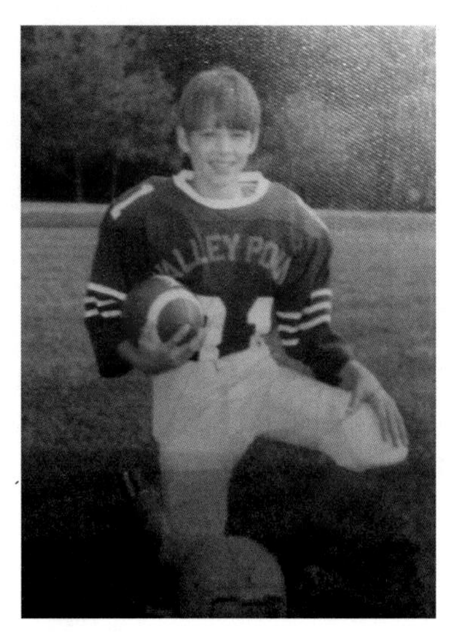

It isn't just getting the wind knocked out of you that is scary though. Anything that impedes your ability to breathe becomes concerning.

After my dad retired, he had a house built, and we moved to Ben Putnam Rd. My mom and dad are eighty-eight and still live there today.

After we moved, Dad had a load of chicken litter dumped in the yard. It was my job to take a shovel and spread it. It was fertilizer: stinky, nasty, disgusting fertilizer.

Chicken litter is the sawdust that is cleaned out of a chicken house. It absorbs all the urine and feces from the chickens. The aroma could be smelled for miles. The ammonia was so strong it made my eyes water.

After hours of spreading the litter, I started having difficulty breathing. My chest was tight, and the more time that passed, the more labored my breathing became.

By the next day, my labored breathing became congested breathing. I felt hazy, and it was likely due to my hundred-and-four-degree temperature. My parents took me to the emergency room.

After arriving, I was taken back to the treatment area, and the staff began working on me. I don't recall most of what occurred, except for one part. I was placed in a tub, and then it was filled with ice. I remember how wonderful the ice felt on my body.

It turned out that I had double pneumonia, and my temperature was out of control. The soothing ice was the last thing I recalled about the visit.

Pneumonia is caused by inhaling infected particles or aspiration. Aspiration is basically the equivalent of swallowing into the lungs.

Obviously, I made it through and recovered. However, since that incident back in 1975, it is not uncommon that I battle with pneumonia or bronchitis. It has been many years since I have dealt with pneumonia, but any time I get a head cold, it goes straight into my chest and eventually turns into bronchitis.

Bronchitis is an inflammation of the lining of your bronchial tubes, which carry air to and from your lungs. Often it develops from a cold or other respiratory infection. Acute bronchitis is quite common. Chronic bronchitis, a more serious condition, is a constant irritation or inflammation of the lining of the bronchial tubes, often due to smoking. I have experienced both.

Congestion and inflammation in the lungs or bronchial tubes restrict breathing. Maybe not to the degree of getting knocked on your ass by Vernon, or Superman being grounded by an archvillain. But enough to get your attention.

On July 25, 2018, I had an appointment to see Deanna. I was always touched by her sincere caring. The world would be a better place if we had a lot more like her. I'd finished my most recent series of iron infusions on May 3. My recent follow-up with Dr. Famoyin showed my iron levels to be good. I could feel the difference and was living in the time space where fatigue didn't dominate my life, thanks to my iron being in the normal range.

After catching up on all things cancer, we talked about my breathing. I explained how it had been a problem for months and said how I had written it off as me being out of shape or constantly recovering. I also talked about anxiety.

I shared with her how I have dealt with nightmares my whole life. It is something that has been handed down to me, my sister, and my daughter. I'm sure there are others in the family as well. I wish I had written all my nightmares down. They would have rivaled a book of Stephen King's short stories.

I previously mentioned the dreams of me being underwater and struggling to get to the surface. But I have other dreams where breathing was a struggle. One recurring dream is where I have food or tobacco in my mouth. It starts to slip down my throat, and I immediately stand, bend over, and start spitting it out. I spit and dig into my mouth, pulling out whatever it happens to be, but it keeps multiplying, filling my mouth and slipping further into my throat until I am finally suffocating. I am often surrounded by people, but no one notices, and I can't speak to get their attention. I mentally tell myself to relax and remain calm in order not to further complicate the dire situation. Finally, I wake up gasping, with my heart racing.

Sometimes I dream of having a hair in my mouth. I begin to pull it out, but there isn't an end to it. A single hair multiplies, and I can feel them sliding up through my throat as I frantically pull. Again, I wake up gasping, heart racing.

The nightmares aren't always about suffocating. Many times, they are about someone trying to kill me. A masked-faced man in overalls throws saw blades at me as I hide behind trees. Between throws, I try to run. My legs won't cooperate, and I resort to grabbing handfuls of grass and helping pull myself along.

There are many different scenarios where I have a gun. I load the gun as I am hiding from the stalking killer. Once loaded, I spring into the open, catching the assailant by surprise, and fire repeatedly at him, but the gun doesn't fire. Click, click, click, but no bang.

When my youngest son had a nightmare once, I got him to tell me about it. The dream involved a large green rat with a mohawk. As he described the star of his nightmare, I drew it. Once finished, he was no longer afraid.

At a young age, my daughter discovered the curse. So, at night, before she went to sleep, I tried planting thoughts in her mind. "Remember, Alanna, in dreams we can have whatever superpower we want. We just realize it is a dream and conjure the superpower needed to defeat evil," I would say.

I often drew our bad dreams. Until writing this book, I never realized it was the only art I didn't date.

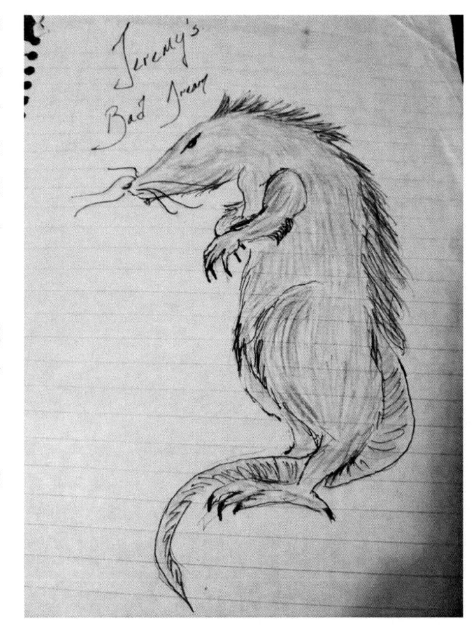

Drawing of rat with a green mohawk

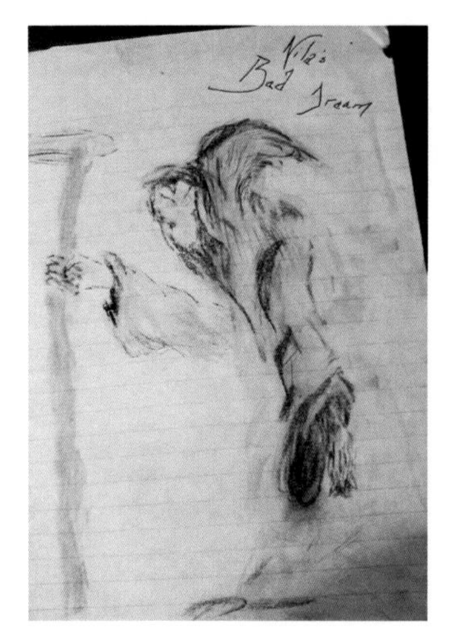

Drawing of grim reaper

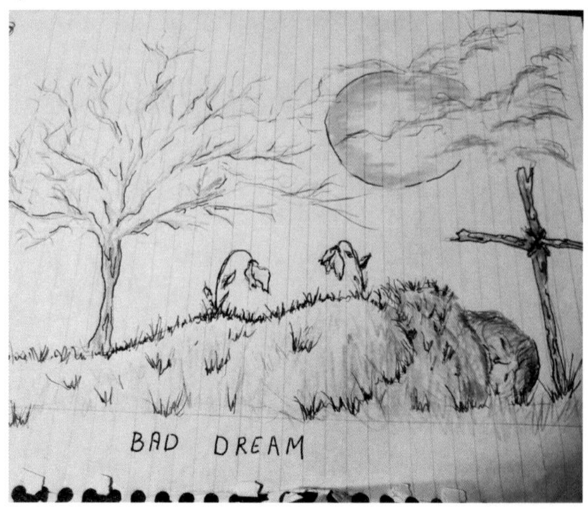

Drawing of person sleeping in grave under the turf

Since my cancer diagnosis, the nightmares had come more often. Some of the dreams were about not being able to breathe, but more of them were about wicked people doing wicked things and turning their attention to me.

After hearing some of my stories, Deanna said she was going to prescribe me .5 mg of Xanax to be taken at bedtime. I was willing to try anything. I had no idea that was even an option. I had just accepted my night terrors as a curse.

Next, Deanna sent me to X-ray. “Let’s see what is going on that is causing you to struggle with breathing,” she said.

I took the elevator down to the radiology floor of the medical facility and had my chest X-ray taken. Then, it was time to wait again.

When we were told the results, it was another unforeseen shock.

The report line that was of most consequence was titled “lung parenchyma,” which is the medical term for lung function. This line read: “*There is a partial collapse of the right lower lung with secondary elevation of the right hemidiaphragm. There is no visible central airway.*”

“Partial collapse? Secondary elevation of the diaphragm? No visible airway? My nightmares of suffocating may be coming to life,” I fearfully thought.

I was referred to a pulmonary specialist, which is a doctor who specializes in treating diseases of the lungs, such as lung cancer, chronic obstructive pulmonary disease (COPD), and tuberculosis. Nila and I would have to wait twenty-six days before my appointment with Dr. Ebeo.

Once again, Nila and I left a doctor's office astounded and in disbelief. How could this happen? Why would my diaphragm be elevated, collapsing more than half of my lung? How could this be fixed?

As the questions spiraled around in the car's cab on our way home, I was able to make sense of some of my struggles.

"My struggle to breathe wasn't from being out of shape or from my perpetual state of recovery. It was my elevated diaphragm preventing my lung from fully expanding. But why? How could cancer have done this? If it is the cancer, it likely can't be fixed," I thought wildly, consumed by thoughts I could not answer.

"Really?" Nila said repeatedly. "You haven't been through enough s**t without this happening? You can't get a damn break."

As soon as we arrived home, I started on my new homework assignment. I wanted to be prepared for my visit with Dr. Ebeo. But more importantly, I needed to understand how this could happen and what the possibilities were for treatment.

My research was very revealing and pointed me to the phrenic nerve.

The phrenic nerve is an extremely important nerve in the body, which controls the diaphragm and assists an individual in breathing on his or her own accord. This nerve is divided into two parts, although it begins as a single nerve from the neck, between C3–C5. The phrenic nerve also allows an individual to hold his or her breath and facilitates taking a deep breath whenever required.

This ability of an individual to control his or her breath is lost in cases of phrenic nerve damage, as the phrenic nerve is no longer able to send signals to the brain to control the diaphragm. This nerve begins in the brain and traverses down through the cervical spine, where it then gets divided into two parts. These two nerves now traverse down each side of the body and course in close proximity to the heart and lungs and meet at the diaphragm.

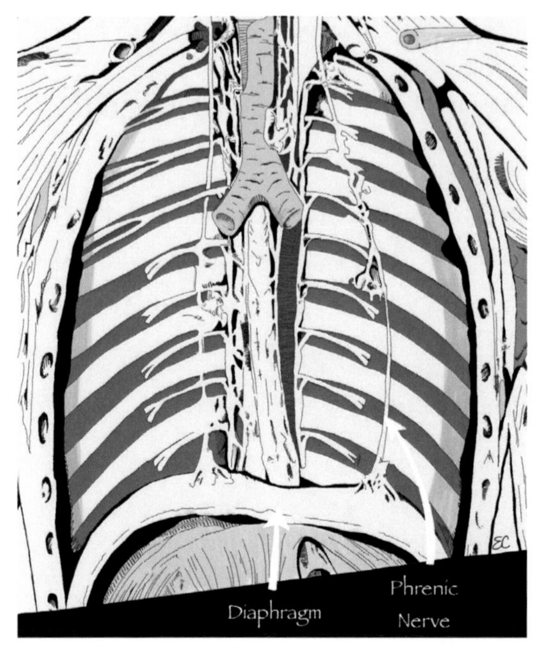

Drawing of phrenic nerve / diaphragm by Ezekial Cooper

Phrenic nerve damage is commonly caused by spinal cord injury (especially to the upper cervical spine); physical trauma like a motor vehicle accident or physical assault, especially to the abdomen; neck injury during a motor vehicle accident; and trauma from a surgical procedure (most typically from cardiac or abdominal surgeries).

After doing my research, my first thought was that my issues must have been caused by the physical trauma of my motorcycle wreck. But I did not have an abdominal, neck, or chest injury. Plus, the accident was nine years prior. I certainly would have known if my breathing had been affected for this long. But what about abdominal surgeries? I had had one of those just ten months earlier.

I went to my appointment with Dr. Ebeo on August 20, 2018, just over a year after my cancer diagnosis. Dr. Ebeo wanted to confirm the X-ray results to identify the exact symptoms and root cause.

The official medical term for my complaint is dyspnea or shortness of breath. It is often described as an intense tightening in the chest, air hunger, difficulty breathing, breathlessness or a feeling of suffocation.

I was given an exercise test, and my vitals were recorded. The doctor used a stethoscope to listen to each of my lungs. The exercise consisted of walking five hundred and eighty feet at an accelerated pace.

I was scheduled for a CT scan, with contrast, in order to perform a fluoroscopy.

Fluoroscopy is an imaging technique that uses X-rays to obtain real-time moving images of the interior of an object, such as the lungs. In its primary application of medical imaging, a fluoroscope allows a physician to see the internal structure and function of a patient, so that the pumping action of the heart or the motion of swallowing, or breathing, for example, can be watched.

I was also scheduled for a series of pulmonary function tests (PFTs). Spirometry (meaning the measuring of breath) is the most common of the PFTs. It measures lung function, specifically the amount (volume) and/or speed (flow) of air that can be inhaled and exhaled. Spirometry is helpful in assessing breathing patterns that identify conditions such as asthma, pulmonary fibrosis, cystic fibrosis, and COPD. It is also helpful as part of a system of health surveillance, in which breathing patterns are measured over time.

Both tests were scheduled for September 13, 2018.

"Again, on the 13th?" I thought. "This is becoming my unlucky number."

The appointment for my test was twenty-four days away, and fifty days since my appointment with Deanna. After prolonged anxiety, I arrived on time and, as usual, had followed my instructions exactly.

The nurse took my vitals and prepped me for the IV that would deliver the contrast. I made sure I was well hydrated to improve the odds of her hitting the vein on the first try. This was a small but important detail. The number of misses was starting to add up. The initial attempt to hit the vein was never bad. It was sliding it out and in while redirecting the needle, blindly trying to penetrate the evasive vein. That was the uncomfortable part. It often resulted in a sore spot that would be bruised.

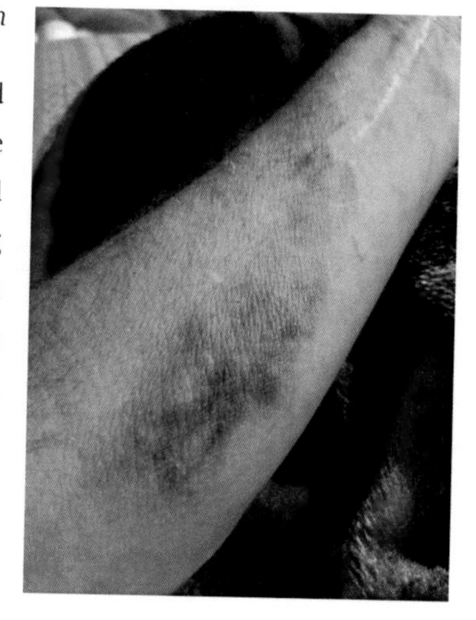

Bruised arm

I was taken to a familiar-looking room that was cold and dimly lit. The recognizable hard-surfaced table protruded from the entrance of the large donut, and it immediately reminded me of how painful lying on it had been in the past. I had taken naproxen an hour before arriving and used the TENS unit as an additional measure to reduce the inflammation and minimize the pain of lying on the hard table. Regardless of my efforts, when I laid back, the pain was intense and made me wonder if I could tolerate it for the duration of the test.

I closed my eyes and tried to relax and listen to the conversant sounds of the machine. In short order, the test was complete, and I was ejected from the donut ring. I couldn't raise myself from the table of my own accord. It was just too painful. My ribs and back muscles were angry and defiant. I was helped up by the nurse, and I started preparing myself to leave, trying to hide the embarrassment.

It was another eighteen days, sixty-eight total, until I returned to Dr. Ebeo for my results. After more than two months of mental acquisitiveness and angst, it was finally time to hear the report.

The clinical summary for my exercise test and office evaluation read as follows:

"The patient is a fifty-seven-year-old male who presents today for evaluation of dyspnea. The symptoms began months ago. The onset has been gradual. The symptoms are getting worse. The NYHA functional classification is II. Associated features include fatigue, but not cough or edema. Precipitating factors include exertion. The dyspnea is relieved by rest. The dyspnea is aggravated by a change in position (lying flat and on his right side)."

The New York Heart Association (NYHA) Functional Classification provides a simple way of classifying the extent of heart failure. It places patients in one of four categories based on how much they are limited during physical activity; the limitations/symptoms are in regard to normal breathing and varying degrees in shortness of breath and/or angina (a type of chest pain caused by reduced blood flow to the heart).

According to the clinical summary, my NYHA functional classification was II. This is defined as: "*Class II (Mild) Patients with cardiac disease resulting in slight limitation of physical activity. They are comfortable at rest. Ordinary physical activity results in fatigue, palpitation, dyspnea, or anginal pain.*

"This whole time I thought he was evaluating my lungs. Instead, he is focused on cardiac disease. So now I have heart disease? How can I go from perfectly healthy a year and a half ago to this? My body is failing me fast."

But the test wasn't about my heart after all. It was a test used by pulmonary doctors to evaluate and confirm my symptoms.

This was followed by the clinical impression from my fluoroscopy. The impression read: "*The spirometry was suggestive of severe restrictive airway disease with an FVC of 26 percent.*"

Forced vital capacity (FVC) is the amount of air that can be forcibly exhaled from your lungs after taking the deepest breath possible, as measured by spirometry. This test might help distinguish obstructive lung diseases. According to the test, I was only able to exhale 26 percent of my lungs' capacity when I took my deepest breath.

The report continued: "*There was no significant bronchodilator response. The lung volume studies were consistent with restrictive airway disease with total lung capacity of 52 percent and impairment of 67 percent.*"

The CT exam revealed no issues with my heart. "*No pulmonary emboli are identified. No coronary calcifications are seen. No adenopathy in the chest, and thyroid aorta is normal in appearance. No definite pneumonia or pleural effusions are seen, and no definite mass identified.*"

So, the heart was all right after all. Everything pointed to the elevated diaphragm. But no indication how it happened or why.

Then, I saw a solitary statement under the clinical impression from the CT scan. For me, this statement was like the kids on *Scooby-Doo* finding a clue that would eventually lead to solving the mystery.

The lone statement read: "*CT chest showed elevated right diaphragm with atelectasis. <u>This was not present with his chest X-ray done last 7/2017</u>.*"

I had totally forgotten about the prior X-ray. I was having severe chest pain and thought I was having a heart attack. Nila took me to the emergency room, where I was hooked up to an EKG and also taken for a chest X-ray. The final diagnosis on that day was pleurisy.

Pleurisy is inflammation of the pleurae, which impairs their lubricating function and causes pain when breathing. Pleurisy can be associated with an accumulation of fluid in the space between the lungs and chest wall (called a pleural effusion).

The excess fluid may be either protein-poor (transudative) or protein-rich (exudative). Mine was determined to be the latter. Exudative (protein-rich fluid) pleural effusions are most commonly caused by pneumonia, cancer, pulmonary embolism, kidney disease, or inflammatory disease.

It was extremely painful and felt like I would imagine the onset of a heart attack feeling.

Based on the fact that my diaphragm appeared normal on my previous X-ray, my elevated diaphragm was the result of something that happened after July 2017. While that narrowed the timeline, I had four surgeries and radiation in that time frame.

This newfound development appeared to be just another domino effect of the medical nightmare in which I was living. The Scooby mystery wasn't solved yet. I had more work to do.

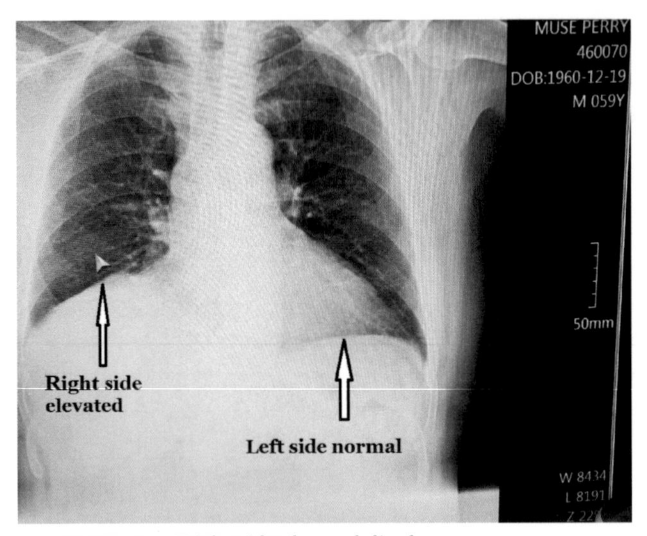

Right side elevated diaphragm
Left side normal diaphragm

Meanwhile, Dr. Ebeo discussed all of the results with us in detail. I asked questions about the phrenic nerve and why it might have stopped working. My primary question was, "Could my phrenic nerve have been severed during my radical prostatectomy?" Dr. Ebeo immediately responded with, "The prostate is far below the phrenic nerve on your right side. I think that would not be a possibility."

I had more questions than answers when it was over. It appeared I would also be welcoming a new doctor to my team. Dr. Ebeo referred me to a prominent University Medical Center to see Dr. Nesbitt.

The University Medical Center (UMC) is a renowned medical facility located several hours from home. We made the trip on October 9, 2018, and stayed overnight nearby. It was also an opportunity for me and Nila to have some time together and enjoy new scenery and restaurants. It was a long and challenging drive that took about seven hours.

The first half of the trip was even more challenging, considering we drove through a major city in the pouring rain.

After departing this major city, we headed west. The interstate took us through mountains with more than typical twists and turns for an interstate. The truck traffic was heavy and added to the poor vision during the trouncing downpour.

Once we arrived at our destination, we checked into our hotel room and then ventured out to sightsee and find tomorrow morning's appointment location.

The medical center complex was massive and spread across many vast locations. Thanks to our planning the day before, our arrival the following morning was on time.

Dr. Nesbitt entered the room, and my first impression was his serious tone and demeanor. He wore a brown tweed jacket and tie. His white hair helped us to better estimate his age range. He looked professional, all business, and experienced. I wouldn't have expected less from such a reputable organization.

This was another situation where the information came quickly and with unexpected content. As much as I had coached myself to pay attention and ask questions, the recommended option that Dr. Nesbitt offered was nothing I had prepared for.

"I have reviewed the findings to date and reevaluated the CT scan, sniff test, and all other data. I agree with the conclusions. I want to share my thoughts and concerns," he began.

"Although there are some limited alternatives for treatment, none will give you all the results you desire, which is to increase your lung capacity to normal by relieving the elevated diaphragm," he explained.

Dr. Nesbitt then continued, "I am proposing robotic diaphragmatic plication."

I didn't need to ask any questions yet. Dr. Nesbitt was like a robot. He stood straight and still, not changing in tone or facial expression throughout the counseling.

"This is a procedure where we use the da Vinci robotic surgical equipment to penetrate your chest cavity. I will fold the paralyzed diaphragm, similar to folding a curtain. Once in place, I will use reinforced strap material and sew the diaphragm in place. This will be done by sewing into the diaphragm muscle and fabric in a series of U patterns. It will then be sewn to the inside of your rib cage to hold it in place. This should allow your lung to expand and improve your ability to breathe," he continued.

"He said it should, not it will," I thought.

The picture he painted in my head was one of pain and irrevocability.

My first question was more about the conclusiveness of the surgery. "So, I will never be able to use my diaphragm again," I said.

Dr. Nesbitt didn't hesitate in his response, telling me, "You will never be able to use your diaphragm again, regardless. Once the phrenic nerve becomes inoperative, there is no way to find the location of the damage, much less repair it."

He continued, "The diaphragm is the primary muscle used for aspiration, but not the only one. Once your diaphragm has been lowered, your lung can expand, and the auxiliary muscles will aid in aspiration and improved breathing. Remember, a person can actually live with only half of a lung. Many people live with only one lung."

"I'm sure that is medically true. But with what quality of life? Panting after a few stairs. No more basketball, I'm sure. And what if the other phrenic nerve stops working?" I pondered.

Then it was time to make my decision. It was easy enough. I needed to be able to breathe more. My lack of breathing wasn't conducive to avoiding nightmares of suffocating or trying to clear my airway while everyone around me was oblivious.

I said, "Let's do this, Doc."

Dr. Nesbitt warned that this was going to be "a very tough surgery and recovery." He then ran through all of the typical risks and potential complications. Bleeding, infection, and pneumonia were just a few.

The holidays were looking to be a bust again this year. We left UMC and decided to stay over another night to soak in what we were just told. Nila and I found a quaint pizza place on the second floor that had a nice view from the outdoor seating of the busy street below. There weren't many people there at that time, which afforded us some privacy. I ordered a double chilled shot of Crown Royal and a beer. I had no idea what I might want to eat, only what I wanted to drink.

It wasn't the "very tough surgery" that occupied my thoughts as I sipped my Crown. It was realizing the termination of many things that I loved in life. Running, playing basketball, and more. I thought back on my years playing trumpet.

"Push from your diaphragm!" the band director would shout in order to get more volume from our instruments.

I thought of being in the army and volunteering for burial details. There was nothing more rewarding than playing Taps at a military funeral.

Before cancer I had talked to Nila about playing softball again in the men's fifty and up league. I wanted to join the wellness center and get in on some basketball pick-up games. I even thought of going to the Veterans Administration and seeing if I could volunteer again for the local military funerals. I would have to practice and knock the rust off. But that would be easy. I would need to be able to push with my diaphragm in order to project a strong sound.

All of those dreams died at the UMC the day I met Dr. Nesbitt.

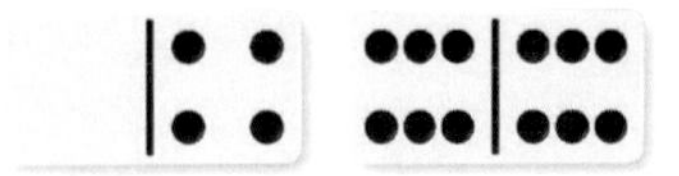

Chapter 16

TAKING MY BREATH AWAY PART II

On November 11, 2018, Nila and I set out again for UMC. It was the day before my surgery, and we wanted to spend some quality time together before the upcoming "very tough" surgery. We rented a Chrysler 300 in anticipation of my return trip home. Nothing was going to be comfortable, but this was the closest we could get. The trip this time was less eventful, and Mother Nature provided brisk but beautiful weather. Traffic was mild, and we were able to enjoy the Sunday drive.

We checked in to the same Holiday Inn and set out to find the destination for my surgery. UMC was spread out around the east side of the city, and tomorrow would be our first visit to the main hospital.

We found a great place to hang out and eventually have dinner. A little bit of Crown helped to take the edge off. We had a great conversation and headed back to the room. We had to be at the hospital to check in at 6:00 a.m.

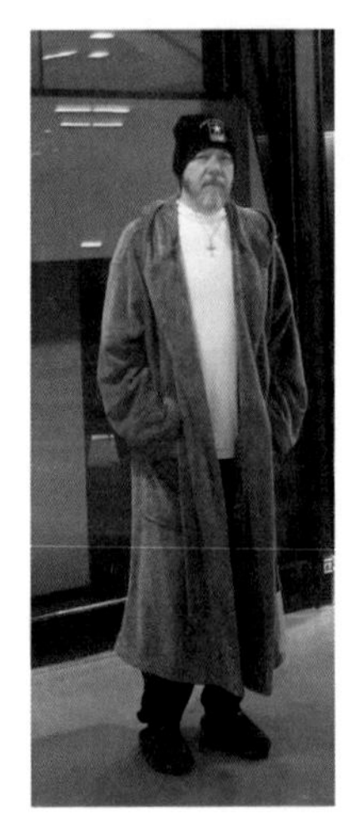

It was a challenging night for me to sleep. The bed wasn't friendly to my aching body. The night sweats from my lowered testosterone, compliments of the $4,500 Lupron shots, woke me four or five times. It was impossible to set the room temperature for that. Once awake, it was thoughts of the upcoming surgery. My labored breathing remained at the forefront of my mind's thinking.

4:45 a.m. came, and I got up, ready to go (I hadn't been asleep anyway when the alarm buzzed). My thought was that at least I would get some sleep soon enough. It would be pain free at first, followed by painful, medicated sleep. Either way, I was ready.

Monday, November 12, 2018, at 5:45 a.m., going into surgery

Check-in was simple—I had done this so many times before. However, the hospital stood out as expansive with beautiful, eye-catching decor. After I donned my stylish, rear-opened gown, I lay in bed awaiting all of my visits from the various medical team members who would prep me. It would be a busy morning.

The nurse came to place my IV. She judged the best place to be the top side of my left hand. However, this is a tender spot that sent pain signals to my brain as soon as the small needle penetrated the skin.

Next came a visit from the anesthesiologist. We talked. Then it was time for my visit from Nurse Nila. It saddened me to see the worry on her face. She tried masking it with a kiss and some upbeat words.

"You're going to do great, hunny bunny. I will see you in just a little bit," she said.

I hated thinking of her sleeping in the waiting room, awaiting the call to see me again. This time, she would have the longest wait to date.

Next came the calming dose administered into my IV. The ride to the operating room (OR) seemed longer this time. My eyelids grew heavy from the comforting drug and my lack of sleep.

Once in the OR, I was placed on the operating table in the supine position, and I gave permission for the hose that delivered heated air to be placed beneath my blanket. I could hear classical music playing faintly from overhead. I caught a glimpse of the ominous robotic machine that would soon be responsible for my toughest surgery, and I looked for Dr. Nesbitt. I never saw him before succumbing to the sandman.

Even though I was not conscious for my surgery, I had done the research to know exactly what would happen.

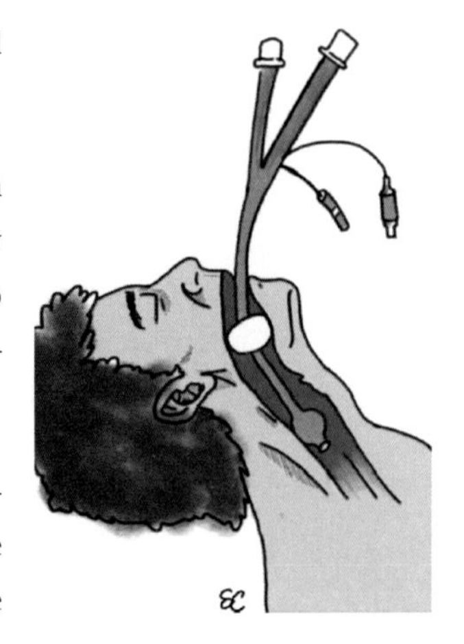

The first order of business was to place a double lumen in through my mouth, down the esophagus, and into my left bronchus. This ventilation system would be used to control my left lung when my right was later intentionally deflated.

Next, I was rolled onto my left side, or the lateral decubitus position, and my right chest area was prepped. Three lateral and posterior incisions were made between the

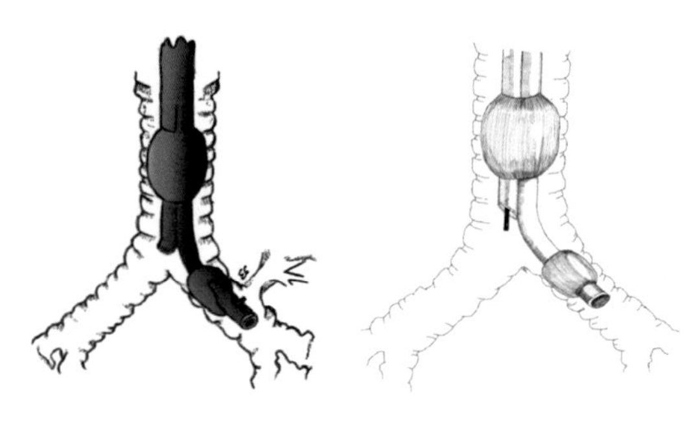

ribs on the right side of my chest, or the intercostal space. The intercostal space is the anatomic space between two ribs. An additional incision was made in my back, right of the spine six to eight inches and between the ribs. All of these incisions still remind me they exist from time to time. But the one in my back reminds me most frequently.

Bupivacaine was injected around the incisions, both subcutaneous (just beneath the skin) and subfascially (beneath the tissue that lies below the skin). Bupivacaine is a newer medication that releases a continuous analgesic to relieve pain for up to seventy-two hours after your procedure.

Now it was time to place the robotic instruments.

Drawing of robotic insertions by Ezekial Cooper

According to Dr. Nesbitt's description in the operative report: "The diaphragm was very patulous and somewhat thinned. It was easily pliable and provided much redundancy for well placement of sutures. In a systematic fashion, parallel U-sutures of pledgeted-ticron were sequentially used to gather and pleat the diaphragm from anterior to posterior. As each suture was placed, it was secured using Core Knot suture tying mechanism. Gradually, the diaphragm became flat and taut. In several areas, additional pleats were created over the initial to enhance the plication. Overall, ten sutures were placed. An excellent and complete plication was accomplished."

Pledgeted-ticron sutures are prepared from fibers of high molecular weight, long-chain, linear polyesters having recurrent aromatic rings as an integral component.

Once the plication was complete, a large Blake drain was inserted posteriorly through one of the incisions. Blake drains are a special type of silicone radiopaque drain used post-open-heart surgery to help patients recover by removing excess fluid around the lungs.

Finally, all areas were inspected, and my right lung was fully re-expanded. The incisions were closed, all but the one used for the Blake drain. This tube would remain inserted for the next three days and created constant wretchedness for me. The double lumen ventilation tube was extubated, and I was awakened after just over three hours of surgery.

A nurse was standing there waiting for me to wake up.

"How do you feel?" she asked me.

My immediate response was, "I can breathe better." I wondered if it was because of the hose feeding oxygen into my nostrils or if the labored breathing was really behind me. "Will you get my wife Nila for me?" I asked her.

After a little while, the staff, confident I wasn't going to succumb to nausea, took me to a private room. The process of transferring me to the bed was incredibly painful, even though I was still under the influence of substantial medications delivered during surgery.

"How in the world will I get up to walk this time? I will go into shock from the pain trying to get up, much less trying to break any records for walking laps," I remember thinking.

The holes in the right side of my chest and the one in my back severely limited the positions available to find comfort. Nila wasn't able to see them, and I had no idea they were there...yet. The Blake drain tube ran down into a graduated container on the floor. Routinely it would be inspected, and the level of fluid documented.

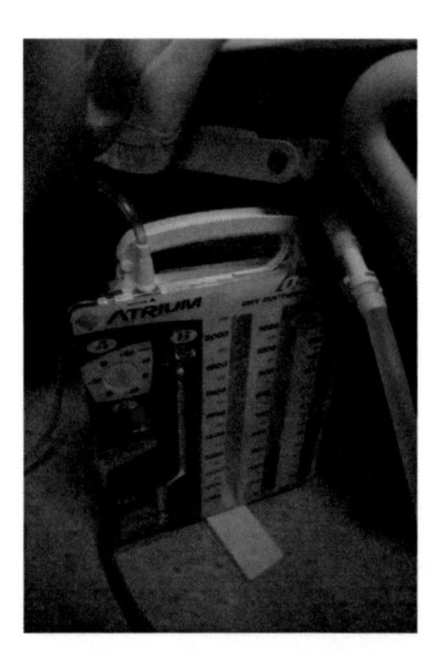

Blake drain

On one such trip to check the fluids, I asked the nurse, "Am I going to have to get out of bed and walk around the halls to be discharged?"

"No, that is not one of the requirements for your surgery," she said. "You only have to get from the bed to the recliner."

"No walking? Heck, yeah! This is going to be easier than I thought," said the optimist on my left shoulder.

At the time, I had forgotten about the Bupivacaine that was releasing pain relief for the first seventy-two hours. The pain reliever used on my diaphragm would take twenty-four hours to wear off. Then, I would feel the full expanse of the ten sutures and the holes that were punctured through my diaphragm when installing them. I should have been less arrogant, knowing that Dr. Nesbitt said it would be “a very tough surgery.” He didn’t mean it would only be tough on him, as he had labored for three hours. He meant it would be tough on me. Minute by minute, the time was approaching when his words would come to fruition.

The first morning following surgery seemed to come sooner than previous surgeries. Constantly being woken up throughout the night always makes it worse. When I was finally able to sleep, it felt like only moments between the nurse’s appearances to check everything out. Then, like a shadow at night, they were gone again, but I was left to fight to get comfortable and try to return to sleep.

It was 7:00 a.m. on November 13, 2018. Shift change at the hospital, and my room filled with bustling activity. Right then, I started to feel the severity of my surgery. I attempted to move around on the bed, yet I was unable. I found myself caught somewhere between weakness and pain that didn’t allow me to move. For the first time, I noticed the catheter and partially filled urine bag. This brought back the appalling memory of my last catheter and the embarrassment of leaving Dr. Hinder’s office with my blue jeans drenched in urine to my knees. I would make sure not to repeat that scenario.

As I tried harder to move in search of comfort, a sharp, piercing pain shot through my chest, and I yelled, waking Nila. If I hadn’t known better, I would have sworn someone stabbed me with a six-inch knife. I was writhing in pain now.

“What the hell have I done, ripped the sutures?” I was thinking. “Perhaps my heart is succumbing to the trauma.”

Then, as quickly as it came, it was gone. Not all of the pain, just the stabbing pain that registered a ten according to the scale of smiley faces on the poster stuck on the wall beside my bed.

Not knowing from where this level ten pain was derived, I chose to remain still. I couldn’t explain it to Nila. I didn’t even understand myself. I was sweating profusely, and not because of a hot flash. Time for my pain medication, and the timing couldn’t have been better.

0
No Hurt
I can feel it
1
2
Hurts a little
Oww..
3
4
Hurts a little more
moderate
5
6
Hurts even more
It's getting there
7
8
Hurts a whole lot
Hurts worst
9
10
worst pain imaginable
EC

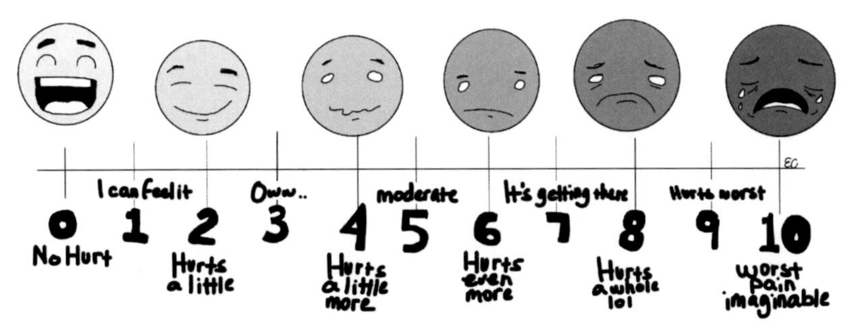

Drawing of pain emoji by Ezekial Cooper

I was able to fall asleep once the oxycontin kicked in. Oxycontin is a narcotic pain reliever that comes in immediate release and time release. The effects can be felt in fifteen minutes and last for six hours. I had the time-released form, and it was given every four hours due to the nature of my surgery and to maintain control of the pain level. The painful experience was exhausting and aided the medication in allowing me to sleep.

An hour or so later, someone woke me. Breakfast had arrived.

"Why did you wake me for this?" I asked. "I'm not touching that." If I could have turned away from the food tray, I would have.

Nila tried to prepare my table for me to eat, but I was an unwilling participant.

Inside of my mouth, on the bottom and behind my teeth is a large bone growth called mandibular tori. Many people have mandibular tori (about 10 percent of the North American population). These are common bone growths located on the inside of the jaw, between the gums and under the tongue. Mine are abnormally large and almost form a solid, continuous platform across the area beneath my tongue.

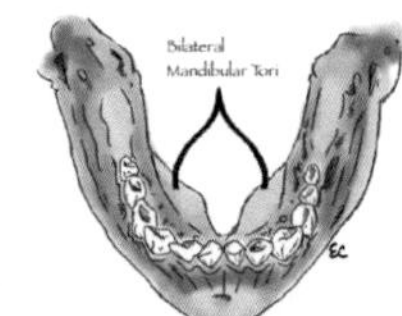

Drawing of normal mandibular tori by Ezekial Cooper

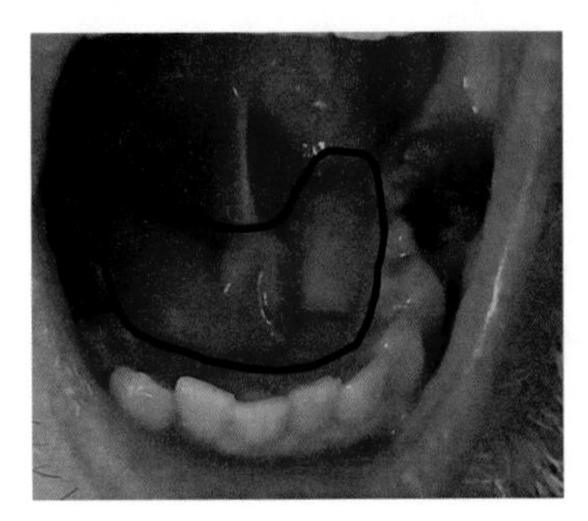

Evidently, when the double lumen was inserted and (somewhat) secured in place, my oversized mandibular tori wasn't cooperative in sharing the space in my mouth. I now had multiple cuts in the surface of the tori. According to my tongue, it felt like what a shark's gill looks like.

My mandibular tori

I tried drinking some of the orange juice that came with breakfast. My first drink burned and stung instantly. This told me the degree of the cuts in my tori left by the ventilator. I quickly chased the acidic juice with water to calm the burn. Instead of breakfast, I asked Nila to get my phone and start going through my emails.

My mindset was, "Foam Products didn't close in observance of Perry's surgery." I had work to do. I had a problematic manager and needed him to know I was still tuned in.

We finished running through the emails, and my medication was delivered again. I was doing things.

"I want to get up and into that recliner," I told Nila. Her eyebrows rose, and her mouth fell—I had surprised her, but my tone told her I was determined.

"How can I help?" she said.

"I have no idea," I said. "Remember earlier when I moved and yelled..."

"Yes," she said, and the vigorous nodding of her head told me she didn't need a reminder.

"Well, I'm timing this attempt so that the oxycontin is in the overlap phase: two hours left from the last time I took it and just after I got another dose. I should be good on pain medicine." I kept silently reminding myself that I had plenty of pain medicine, because it was a painful struggle. The recliner was so close to the bed I could have almost fallen into it. I held my breath and bade my Sagittarius spirit to persuade me to tolerate the movements. In my right hand was the graduated container, and Nila had everything else. Finally, I sat down in the recliner, drained of all energy. Exhausted again, but proud.

I sat quietly and thought, "I made it to the recliner. Now I just need to have a bowel movement, get this tube out of my chest, get the catheter out, and I can go home."

Later that day, my daughter Alanna came to visit with her husband Cory. It was so uplifting to see them. It was good medicine for Nila, as well.

Since my cancer diagnosis, this made my fifth and starkest surgery. As I have said, all of the rest of our children live a long way from us. Alanna and Cory were the only people, friends or family, that came to visit for any of them. I still don't understand it all. People in the town where we lived, people who called us "dear friends" or "family," never called or visited. I understand UMC being a long drive, and during the workweek. However, the other surgeries were local. No visits at our home. Rarely did we get phone calls from anyone except immediate family. It will always be perplexing, and I have given up trying to figure the puzzle out. However, I can never forget.

"I imagine my funeral with a mostly empty room. Perhaps I need to be a better person."

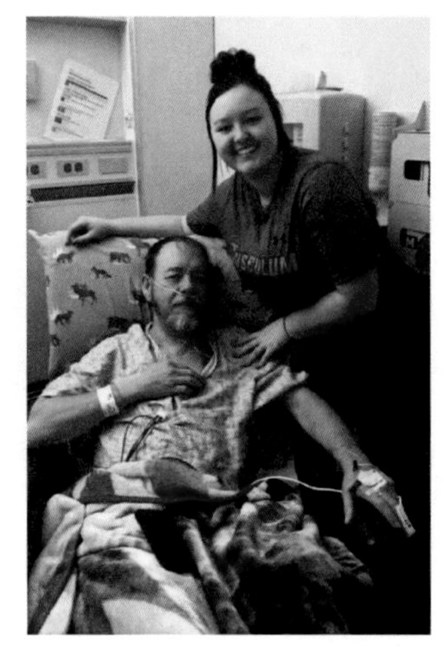

Tuesday, November 13, 2018, with Alanna.
Day 1 after surgery.

At the hospital, the nights grew longer, and the pain became less tolerable. The left side of my body was already getting sore from overuse as I could not lie on my right side or put any pressure on the right portion of my back. Getting up and into the recliner was my only reprieve. It was often short lived.

On day two after surgery, I was sitting in the recliner. The nurse came in and performed her normal routine. This time she had a surprise. It was time to remove the catheter. Since I was in the recliner, it was necessary that she pick up the container in which my Blake drain fed. After removing the catheter and documenting the level in the catch container, she left. I moved slightly to position myself more on my left side and pulled my pillow into a comforting position. Then it happened again. The number ten smiley face.

The pain instantly made me yell and begin to squirm, searching for relief. This time it felt closer to an eleven because the additional surgery medications had long worn off. Nila jumped up to call for help, but they already heard me yelling.

The staff kicked into action, checking my vitals and asking questions. I felt as though I were having a heart attack. Out of all the pain I had experienced throughout my life, this was the new number one.

Unable to determine the cause, the staff called in the emergency trauma response team. The pain was relentless. It wasn't radiating from the incisions or the diaphragm area. It was all in my upper chest. The pain felt akin to how I conceived a knife stuck in my chest would feel, the blade being turned clockwise, then counterclockwise, and repeated.

The team jumped into action, hooking up a mobile EKG and testing vitals, but could not determine the root cause of such prodigious pain. One of them grabbed the drain container, and, for a split second, the pain subsided. Then it returned. Then subsided. I reached to my right side, where the drain tube exited my chest and held the tube in place. It wasn't the right place, and the pain was once again consuming me. I managed to move the tube slightly forward and aft until I found the sweet spot where the pain was relieved.

I had found the problem. Not a doctor. Not the nurses. Not the emergency trauma response team.

The drain tube was located in the pleural cavity. The pleural cavity, also known as the pleural space, is the thin, fluid-filled space between the two pulmonary pleura of each lung. A pleura is a membrane that folds back onto itself to form a two-layered membranous pleural sac. The outer pleura is attached to the chest wall but is separated from it by the endothoracic fascia. The inner pleura covers the lungs and adjoining structures, including blood vessels, bronchi, and *nerves*.

What I discovered was that when the drain tube was moved, it might or might not find its way onto one of many raw nerves in the pleural cavity.

I immediately requested the tube be heavily taped in place.

The trauma team said, "Your EKG and vitals look good. Your heart rate and blood pressure are elevated, but that is likely due to the pain reaction. Do you need anything else before we go?"

"Elevated because of my pain response? You mean the part where I felt like I was dying from a full-blown heart attack?" ran through my mind. "Thanks for the tape. I'm good now."

How could it be that nobody anticipated this? Was I the only person in history to experience this? I suspect that is not possible. No way. To me, this was avoidable agony.

I was given some additional pain medication and fell immediately asleep in the recliner. I wish they could have given Nila some medications. I'm sure that at some point she thought she was watching me die. She was extremely panicked and scared.

Later that day, Nila and I ran through the email threads and caught them up. I even made a call to each plant to talk to the key people about how things were going. I also called and checked in with my boss, Erik. There was no reason to share the details of my experience thus far.

I only said, "Things went well, and I hope to be back at work next week." As usual, he advised me to "take it easy and get some rest."

I had an app on my phone that allowed me access to cameras at the plants, and I enjoyed seeing the operations running. They also reminded me of work that needed to be done in Calhoun as I watched some of their struggles. Work matters allowed me to focus on things other than the pain of recovering from my surgery.

The soreness of the surgery had begun to join the myriad other pains by this point. The Bupivacaine had long worn off. Breathing was labored again. But this time it was due to the sore, swollen diaphragm that stirred each time I took a breath. Sleeping was almost impossible, and the hours and days ran together. I longed for my downstairs recliner, my animals, and Nurse Nila to be at Olgia Lane.

Day three finally came. I had stayed well hydrated, and the Gas-x pills were a saving grace for the bloating and pressure it applied to the surgically sewn diaphragm. The weather report was calling for snow, and the trip home included some higher elevation areas that could be treacherous. I wanted to be unhooked, tubes removed, and checked out.

The nurse checked everything out and asked about a bowel movement. I lied once again without hesitation. A doctor visited and reviewed my chart. Everything was a go, and the doctor left the room. The nurse stayed and removed my IV. It was another painful experience due to the location. The top of my hand had already bruised.

An hour or so later, another nurse entered the room. "Are you ready to go home?" she asked gleefully. "And give up this luxurious recliner?"

I replied sincerely, "Yes, I am beyond ready."

"Well, first we need to get that drain tube out," she said. "I'm going to warn you. It is really going to hurt."

Anxiety kicked in as I thought of the drain tube being removed after my prostate surgery. My mind bounced from that to the number ten smiley face when the tube had only marginally moved previously.

The tape was removed, and the nurse verbally prepared me for the procedure. I didn't realize I had grabbed the tube to hold it in place. It was just an unconscious reaction.

"Let go of the tube, please," she said. I thought her voice sounded sickly sweet. I slowly pulled my hand away as her hand replaced mine.

I grabbed her wrist and said, "Just a minute, please."

"Come on, Sagittarius, suck it up and let's do this. Don't be a wimp in front of Nila. You've already lost your manhood. Show some fortitude and don't scare the s**t out of her again," I said to myself by way of mental preparation.

I released my grip, and the nurse immediately pulled. The tube dragged along the inside of the cavity and randomly moved across nerve after nerve. The needle on my pain meter was bouncing from five to ten throughout the process. One pull, two pulls, three pulls, and it was out. Again, exhaustion overcame me.

Nila was given instructions. For me, it was as though they were standing in another room. I was trying to recover from the event, knowing I had a seven-hour car ride home. The nurse then left.

Nila helped dress me, and I sat back down in the recliner. She left to retrieve the car. A male nurse entered with a wheelchair and helped me transition over. As he pushed me along the hallway, there was an effort on his part to make upbeat small talk. I wasn't in any frame of mind and only responded with short replies.

We arrived at the exit, and Nurse Nila was waiting. The temperature was freezing, and it had begun to snow. The cold breeze felt comforting somehow.

The male nurse helped me into the car. It was a tremendously difficult task. Once in the car, the trick would be to protect my wounds from the seatbelt and to keep my body from fluctuating around during the ride.

Once secured, with my pillow as a cushion, we headed home. We didn't make it five miles until I asked that we pull over. The weather and traffic made me extremely tense. I know Nila thought I was overreacting, but I couldn't control the emotions of it all.

"You think that tube hurts? Just wait until we slide off the road or get T-boned by another car. That will be a fourteen smiley face," was the psychological mind game going on in my head.

I had aggravated Nila, in addition to the stress of her driving in heavy traffic and snow. We pulled into the parking lot of the familiar Holiday Inn, and Nila secured a room for the night.

"At this rate, I won't be home for two weeks. I have to do better tomorrow," I remember thinking as she was inside getting the room.

I was unable to find a comfortable position in the bed. Why should I? It hadn't been comfortable a few days earlier before the surgery.

I spent the majority of the night in a chair and using pillows to help protect my right side and back. Morning came, and I watched as the room lightened from the sunrise. I had mentally prepared myself for the upcoming journey.

Nila was tired, of course. I can't say enough about how hard this must have been on her or about how eternally grateful I am for having her with me.

We waited until the heavy traffic time of morning passed and then we headed home again. The ride was incredibly long. The higher elevations were testy at times due to the weather. Nila was still unhappy with my prior day's reactions to other cars on the road. I did better on this day, but not great. We hardly spoke. When we did, it wasn't cordial.

Under normal circumstances, I have difficulty being a passenger. It is a lasting impact from my prior car accidents. Try as I may, the anxiety always wins. It is all about not having any control. No brake. No steering. No control. It isn't fair to Nila, but after twenty-nine years together, I still can't control my reactions to what I see happening. It is an unfortunate condition and the reason Nila always lets me drive.

Finally, we were home, and Nila helped me from the car. She had put Thor in the garage and unlocked the basement. We slowly walked around the house again, avoiding the inside stairs. I walked in and saw my recovery spot. Before I made it to the recliner, Sparky and Mr. Mitten showed up to greet me. I parked myself in the recliner, and Nurse Nila covered me in my favorite flag blanket before administering some much-needed medication. Work emails or calls would have to wait.

Sparky sniffed around and determined quickly that I wasn't well. He gave me a gentle lick on the ear and curled up beside me. Mr. Mitten gave me a few loving licks with his sandpaper-textured tongue and lay down on the other side.

My shoulder still lacked its ROM. Although I really needed to place it under my pillow, I had to lay it across my chest and hold it with my right hand.

Monday, November 19, 2018, just one week from my "very tough" surgery, I returned to work. Nurse Nila chauffeured, just as she had in times past. It was going to be a four-week recovery.

My follow-up visit at UMC was December 11, 2018. The report stated, "Incisions are healing. Pain comes and goes, but not bad. Breathing is much better; as stated after surgery, could tell a difference when he woke up."

On Friday the 13th of October 2017, Dr. Hinder inserted a robotic instrument into my abdomen in several locations. One of those locations, on the upper right side, was in a place that many physicians have told me was way too high. I firmly believe this was the day my breath was taken away and the resulting end to some of my favorite things in life.

Just over a year later is when the domino effect occurred. It was a "very tough" surgery that created four new and very large scars. It also gave me ten internal sutures that would bind my right diaphragm for life. This was when Dr. Nesbitt gave me some of my breath back.

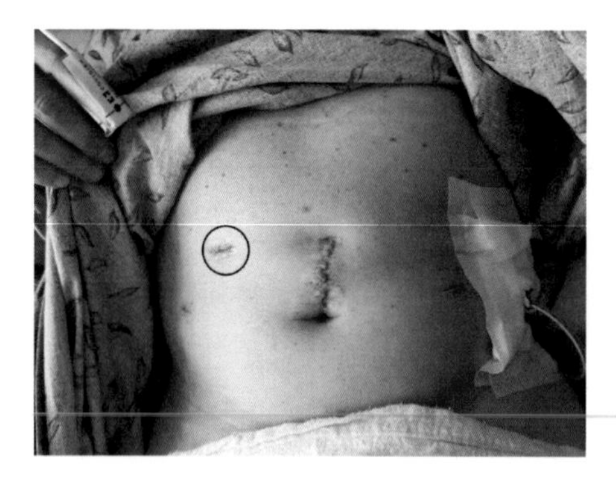

Robotic entry from prostatectomy

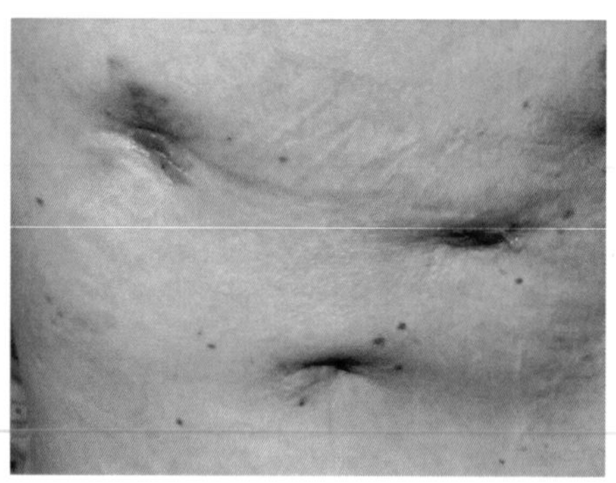

Scars on right side from robotic entry during diaphragmatic plication

I have known this song since I was young. But at the period in my life after my diaphragm surgery, prostate surgery, and ongoing cancer battle, I have come to feel more like the person who wrote it, rather than the listener.

LATE LAMENT

The Moody Blues 1968

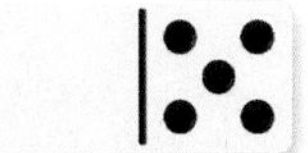
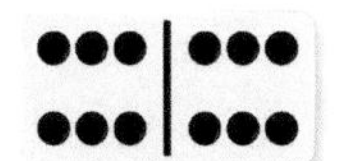

Chapter 17

WHAT'S SED BEARS REPEATING

If you lined twelve people at the top of a cliff, one of each sun sign, Sagittarians would probably be the first to jump, content that something, somehow, would prevent them from going splat at the bottom. And something, somehow, probably would.

What is SED? What is CRP? For that matter, what are all the abbreviations on a lab report from a blood draw? It turns out they matter. Well, duh!

So, after the long episodes of surgeries, recovery, therapy, and don't forget radiation or the Lupron shots that reduced my testosterone to nearly zero (three hundred is the normal minimum), I had worked my way through the months of perpetual recovery. I felt bad. I was super fatigued, but that was par for the course these days.

It was January 2019, a new year with a new outlook. But the outlook was grim beneath the facade that was my outward expressions. My visits to SCC in June, September, and December 2018 all produced PSA numbers of .9. This meant my PSA had not been reduced to an undetectable number. I still had cancer.

"The imperfect surgery, radiation, and quarterly Lupron shots haven't worked. I need to find another way not to die."

This led me to see two of my favorite doctors of all time, which is saying a lot when you have seen the number of doctors I have. I will not name them, but they will know who they are when I share the story of what they did for me.

I will refer to them just as Dr. R. They were instrumental in my health and maintenance from the time I moved to Johnson City, TN. I was given their cell phone numbers and told to "call any time" I needed them, even if the office was closed. Today I consider Dr. R as friends. If they were to call me for anything, I would be there.

Dr. R received copies of all my medical work, X-rays, etc. and evaluated them. I welcomed their perspective and teaching. So, I went to them to help me find an alternative path for my cancer battle. Not surprisingly, they had an option.

In the US, stem cell injections into a joint, such as the knee, are legal. Stem cells are undifferentiated or partially differentiated cells that can differentiate into various other types of cells and proliferate indefinitely to produce more of the same stem cell. They are found in both embryonic and adult organisms, but they have slightly different properties in each.

In mammals, roughly fifty to a hundred and fifty cells make up the inner cell mass during the blastocyst stage of embryonic development, around days five to fourteen. These have stem-cell capability. When they are isolated and cultured *in vitro* (such as a test tube), they can be kept in the stem-cell stage and are known as embryonic stem cells (ESCs).

Blood taken from the placenta and umbilical cord of newborns is a type of allogeneic transplant. This small volume of cord blood has a high number of stem cells that tend to multiply quickly. Cord blood transplants are done for both adults and children. As of 2017, an estimated seven hundred thousand units (batches) of cord blood have been donated for public use. And even more has been collected for private use.

In some studies, the risk of cancer not coming back after a cord blood transplant was less than without the transplant.

All the data surrounds the use of stem cells to fight cancer-related diseases, primarily bone marrow transplants. In this scenario, the best outcome occurs when the donor is a relative or a closely matched donor. The stem cells are given intravenously after recovery from the first chemo treatment. A second chemo treatment is usually administered within six months of the first. But Mr. Skeleton had avoided cancer thus far, and none of this applied to me. I wasn't having chemo. I didn't have a matched donor. But that didn't stop us. My body aches and pains appeared to be the new norm for me. My PSA was stuck at .9. I felt miserable, and life wasn't very much fun any longer.

So, Dr. R ordered allogeneic stem cells. They also paid to bring in a specialist to administer them intravenously. I would have needed to travel outside of the country for this treatment had they not been willing to do this for me. It is something I do not take lightly.

Regardless of the outcome, I am forever indebted.

After the procurement of stem cells, the storage process begins by lowering the temperature to -40° Celsius. Then the stem cells are stored at -196°C (minus 320° Fahrenheit) in cryogenic freezers.

On the day my batch of stem cells arrived, I was excited and anxious. We went into a small room where privacy could be ensured. The nurse put the IV into my right arm, and a rapid drip of saline began to flow. Then, the vial was removed from the special packaging that kept the stem cells at the proper temperature.

The vial was removed, using gloves to prevent frostbite, and the nurse began warming it. The vial was rolled back and forth between the palms until the perfect temperature was achieved. The stem cells were injected into the IV tubing, and two minutes later, I was done.

Within a couple of hours of receiving the IV, I was exhausted. I had been told fatigue could be a side effect. By 4:00 p.m. I was asleep and didn't wake until the alarm clock sounded at 7:00 a.m. the next day!

Within only three days, I was feeling more energetic, and some of the joint pain had subsided. But what I really wanted to know was the impact, if any, on my PSA. My next appointment at SCC was in two months, March 2019.

After waiting four months, it was finally time for my appointment with a rheumatology doctor. It turns out there were only three rheumatologists in the whole Tri-Cities area.

On January 13, 2019, I went to see Dr. Chaffy. I accepted this appointment date because it was the first available appointment when I called in September 2018. It surely wasn't my choice for it to be on the thirteenth.

When Dr. Chaffy entered the room, she was accompanied by four interns. She apologized and asked my permission for them to observe. I agreed.

I talked through my explanation for being there and how the pain had increased over time. I was very detailed and explained how I had thought it was originally just the surgeries and recoveries. I also shared my SED rate, CRP, and RF numbers. It was obvious she was pushed for time as she immediately began her routine check while I explained my reason for being there. She looked at my hands, inspected my knuckles and finger joints, and quickly moved to my hips and ankles.

After about ninety seconds of inspection, she announced that I did not have any signs of rheumatoid arthritis. She scheduled me to have some blood work and swiftly exited. The whole experience was the equivalent of anxiously awaiting a new movie release for four months, only to leave the theater disappointed.

One day later I went to a local medical center for my lab draw. I entered the building at the same location as I had done thirty-eight times previously for radiation. I had hoped to never come through those doors again. I passed the receptionist and proceeded down the hall and past LN231. I wondered if I might see Dr. Channeler by chance.

"I remember you," I imagined he would say. "You're the guy in the 65 percent chance of rain region."

But I did not see Dr. Channeler. I continued to follow the signs until I arrived at the lab.

Dr. Chaffy's office called the following day and asked me to be back in the office on the seventeenth. This was concerning to me because of the expediency in scheduling my follow-up, considering the long wait for my initial appointment.

Once again, we were unprepared for what was coming. The annotations on my lab accession read: "The screening HCV, or hepatitis C antibody test came back positive. The viral load needs to be checked for active infection. I will put in an order for the hepatitis C viral load."

This teleported us back to the first time I had a positive HCV test. This time, there was no crying upon delivering the news. We knew there was a chance it was a false positive again. But what about the process where we must keep apart and not share eating or drinking utensils?

It turned out that a lot had happened with hepatitis C since our first false positive. Nowadays it is curable with medication, and it is not the danger once thought. It is not uncommon for a person to have hep C and never know it. The body sometimes overcomes it naturally.

This was a relief, but there is always the conversation about how it could have happened. Those conversations were uncomfortable, and my mind was racing, trying to figure out how I could prove I hadn't done anything to contract hepatitis or be positive.

On January 22, a week later, I returned to Dr. Chaffy's office for the results. The annotations from my test read, "No hepatitis C virus was detected, so the HCV positive shows he was probably exposed in the past and has cleared it, but there is no active infection at this time based on this test."

My inflammation markers were all still elevated. I was scheduled for a retest on February 25, 2019.

The results of the lab draw confirmed what I already knew. The numbers repeated a previous test. The annotations read, "The rheumatoid factor remains stable at 201 (flag reference range 0-15). Confirmation of repeated values of 61.8 CRP (flag reference range 0-5) and 79 SED Rate (flag reference range 0-15). See primary care physician for further evaluation as there is no rheumatologic explanation at this time."

So, now that I had clarified this little detour, and my rheumatologist decided I did not have RA (rheumatoid arthritis) because of her ninety-second inspection, I was ready to proceed with plan B.

I researched rheumatologists outside of the Tri-Cities area and found a university rheumatology department. This university was not dissimilar to many schools in the fact that it had a thriving medical segment of the curriculum. My research found this university rheumatology department to be a good target to execute plan B.

It was an inconvenient ninety-minute drive. I wasn't completely sure why I didn't believe Dr. Chaffy when she wrote, "There is no rheumatologic explanation." Perhaps it was the brief evaluation and the way she seemed pressed for time. I was prepared for my new rheumatologist, Dr. Raj, to give me the same news. But if that were the case, I felt what I was told bore repeating.

Unbelievably, the earliest appointment for a new patient would be September, more than six months away. Rheumatologists are in short supply and high demand.

For now, it was time to see Dr. Famoyin again. I had gone for a few months without any iron infusions. I hoped that was a positive sign that my body was able to maintain on its own. But that wasn't 100 percent true.

Dr. Famoyin entered with his usual upbeat demeanor.

"How are you feeling, Perry?" he asked with a big grin on his face, extending his hand to me. "And how was your last visit to SCC?"

After shaking my hand, he sat in the other chair in the exam room and listened intently as I answered his questions in my normal, detailed manner. I talked for a while, finally winding down to talk about what had brought me here, my fatigue.

"I'm feeling tired again, Doc. I was encouraged when I felt well for as long as I have. I was hoping it meant I was doing this on my own," I began.

"It takes time. The fact that you have been able to extend the time between treatments is absolutely a positive sign," Dr. Famoyin responded. Then he continued with a chuckle, "I know you are impatient and want these things fixed immediately. But the body heals in God's time, not ours. We will get a lab draw today and see how things look."

I moved on to my more pressing concern: my PSA.

"According to my last three consecutive visits to SCC, my PSA is stagnant at .9," I explained. "It is very concerning to me because I know it should be undetectable after surgery, radiation, and this amount of time."

I continued, "It tells me I still have cancer, and my time is shorter than I had hoped. I can't stop thinking about what Dr. Channeler predicted. He made me angry, and I wanted so bad for him to be wrong. Perhaps my anger was unwarranted."

Dr. Famoyin's response was philosophical and very deep. I listened absorbedly as he spoke from a nonmedical perspective. I would say it was from the heart.

He said, "Mr. Perry, what if someone were to tell you that, in ten years, there would be a flood? Not just any flood, but a historic flood. And, because of this, you start to build a boat. Every day you work on building your boat. Then, after ten years of working on your boat, every single day, the flood doesn't come. Will you not have wasted your ten years building the boat?"

"I get it," I responded. "Somehow, I need to figure out how to stop working on building a boat. Worry only makes things worse, but I keep trying to cover all the bases and explore all the options."

Dr. Famoyin closed by saying, "It is easier said than done. I understand. But you must work on enjoying today as hard as you work at preserving tomorrow. Besides, tomorrow isn't promised to any of us."

I proceeded to the lab. A few minutes later, my results were complete. Dr. Famoyin confirmed that my iron had, once again, found its way to the lower end of the range.

I wrapped my arms around Nila and kissed her.

"Go home," I told her. "There's no reason for you to have to stay here for two or more hours while I get my infusion. I'll be fine, and I'll call when I am close to being done."

As I sat in the recliner with the slow drip of iron solution pushing into my right arm, I focused on work and emails. I felt guilty over my personal concern when I looked around the room and saw many who appeared worse off than me.

I was very concerned about our Georgia division and the lack of time I had spent there. I had experienced problems in the past and was troubled that history might be repeating itself.

Once in the past, an employee was not being productive or successful. I had hired him many years prior and mentored him. He was a veteran, and I had a lot of respect for him and confidence in his abilities.

But something was amiss with him. His performance was down. During conversations we had, he had become defensive and unproductive. The rumor mill had concerning stories floating around.

On July 12 that year, long before my cancer diagnosis, I had a scheduled meeting with the employee to discuss the issues. I was detained at the other plant in Tennessee and got off to a late start.

While en route, I received a call. The employee was sitting in his office, asleep, with a gym bag in his lap. I was sent a picture.

He was in the middle of the floor, not behind his desk. The chair's back came up just above the midpoint of his back. His head was laid back and facing the ceiling. I asked that the other employee try to wake him and see what his condition might be. After several attempts, the sleeping employee was startled and woke up. In doing so, he dropped a loaded magazine for a pistol onto the floor.

"What is that for?" the other employee asked.

The employee replied, "It fell out of my pistol."

He then proceeded to show his pistol to the employee who had found and woke him. Eventually, the pistol was taken out of his hands and secured.

The other employee asked him, "What in the world are you thinking, bringing a loaded gun to work?"

"Perry has got to go," he responded.

He had intended to kill me that day. But it wasn't my day to die.

March and June 2019 were my scheduled dates at SCC. "Is my PSA still holding at .9?" I wondered. "Or did the stem cell experiment pay off?"

After three consecutive PSA results being .9, the results in March 2019 revealed my PSA had dropped t0 .6. This was a 33 percent drop, but it was not undetectable. I received my quarterly Lupron injection and Prolia for Mr. Skeleton.

Three months later, I returned to SCC again. I did not have high hopes and had conceded to the fact that I would never be cancer free or have my PSA undetectable.

Once I got my new bracelet, I headed across the hall for my blood draw. As I sat waiting, I glanced down at the bracelet and was surprised what I saw. It read, "Lowell Muse," not "Perry Muse." I immediately stood up and made my way back to check-in. I did not want Lowell Muse's treatment plan. He might not be fighting the good fight. He might not be on a plan to make the tree of life.

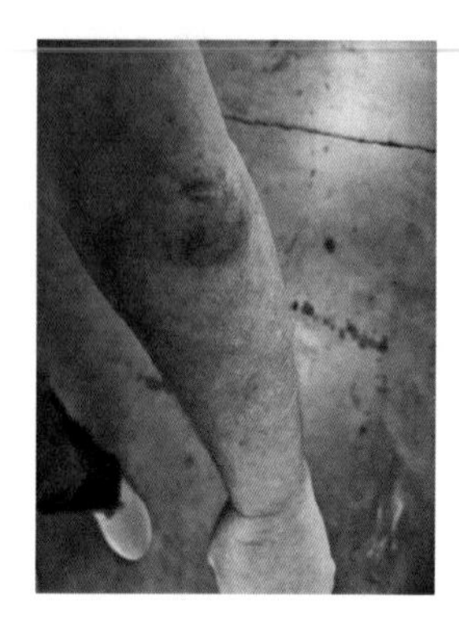

Once I had the correct bracelet on, I returned for my blood draw. The nurse struggled to draw blood this time and had to resort to using the top of my left forearm. It was extremely painful and bruised immediately.

"If this is any indication of how things will go today, I can plan to work on building my boat on the ride home," I thought.

Bruised forearm after IV

But I was wrong. This time, less than six months after my IV in the back room of Dr. R's office, Dr. Taha announced that my PSA was <.014 (undetectable) and pronounced me "cancer free!" My Lupron shots ended. Dr. Taha asked me to pose for a picture to go on his wall of cancer survivors. This time, I did not crop myself out.

There are many days that I pick up my phone, open the daily horoscope app, and tap Sagittarius. Although I put my faith in God, I find it interesting to read my daily horoscope. This particular app really hits the nail on the head a lot of days. It has been pretty amazing.

September arrived, and we made the trip to the university rheumatology to see Dr. Raj. He entered the room and sat down. Dr. Raj was soft-spoken, and he listened as I caught him up on all things medical for Perry Muse.

I concentrated on the pain in my hip, shoulders, back, and neck. I explained the limited ROM.

Daily / Weekly / Monthly
Sagitarrius
11/22 to 12/21
Alias: The Archer
June 6, 2019

Is there light at the end of that tunnel you may feel you've been traveling through, Sagittarius? Could it be filtering in through an opening you can see ahead in the distance? Yes, things are definitely getting brighter for you now, so stop worrying and wondering what could go wrong. Let it sink in that things are changing for the better for you. Remind yourself of this whenever a fearful or negative thought enters your mind - even if you don't fully believe that things really are getting better. The more you hope for and believe that the best will be, the faster it will happen.

"As you can see, I cannot turn my head very far in either direction," I explained as I demonstrated. "If I am in a car, I have to turn my whole body in order to see in each direction. If I sit for too long, Nila has to help me get up." I recited the numbers associated with my inflammation markers. "My SED rate numbers and other markers have repeated consistently over the past year," I explained. "At night I cannot sleep due to the pain in my shoulders and hips. The pain of trying to roll over in bed makes me moan and cry out. I am taking ibuprofen and naproxen around the clock just to be able to function," I stated as I concluded my medical history report.

As bad as it sounds, anyone other than Nila probably didn't know about all of my pain. At least that was the Sagittarian plan.

Dr. Raj asked permission to check me. The method and procedure mimicked what I'd experienced with Dr. Chaffy, but Dr. Raj was more methodical.

"I don't see any signs of rheumatoid arthritis," he began. "You do not have swollen joints in your hands or signs of fluid accumulation in your ankles," he continued. "You have all of the classic symptoms of polymyalgia rheumatica (PMR)," he calmly shared.

Once again, Nila and I were unprepared for the news. Dr. Raj did a great job of maintaining a calm tone and explaining the diagnosis.

"This is not life-threatening," he explained. "PMR typically affects people in your age range. We do not know what causes the onset. However, within one to two years, it usually goes away just as mysteriously as it came. We will treat it with prednisone, and you should feel relief from the symptoms within the first few days," the doctor concluded.

I was given a paper explaining PMR before leaving the office. It convinced me that Dr. Raj had correctly diagnosed my condition, and there was, in fact, a rheumatologic explanation.

Polymyalgia rheumatica affects the larger muscles of the body. A person who has PMR may first start to notice aches and stiffness in the larger muscles of the upper arms and throughout the shoulders. Similar aches and pains may occur in the hips and in the neck as well. This pain may make it difficult to raise your arms over your head, to get out of a chair, and even to turn over in bed. Most of the time the stiffness or soreness will be the worst in the morning and will ease up a bit during the latter part of the day. Some of the other symptoms of the condition include noticeable swelling and inflammation. The tendons may be tender to the touch, and there may be swelling in the wrists, hands, feet, and ankles. Some people complain about a loss of appetite and may feel depressed and tired.

A person who is suffering from PMR may notice the symptoms of the condition long before they are diagnosed with it. One of the things about this condition that should be noted is that it is often not diagnosed until later. The main reason for this is because most people will simply write off the pain and other issues associated with the condition as just a sign that they are getting older, and their parts are not working the same as they once were.

The most useful blood tests that are used to diagnose polymyalgia rheumatica include C-reactive protein and sedimentation rate. Currently, the only treatment that is provided for people who are suffering from polymyalgia rheumatica is to use prednisone. Prednisone is a steroid medication. It will typically begin to work within just a few days. In fact, prednisolone is so effective at treating polymyalgia rheumatica that if a person does not see some improvement in their symptoms after the first week of using the medication, the diagnosis of polymyalgia rheumatica may be questioned. Most of the time a dose between five to eight mg per day will be maintained. Treatment may be able to end after two or three years. However, there are some people who must use the treatment for a lot longer and at times for life.

Other than the swelling and loss of appetite, this perfectly described my condition. It now made better sense why turning over in bed was so very painful. Everything made sense.

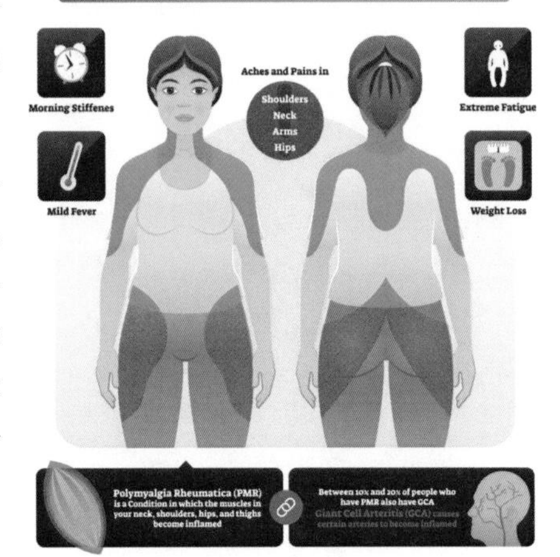

Dr. Raj wrote a prescription for 10 mg/day of prednisone. Over time he wanted me to reduce the amount, 1 mg at a time, over two-week intervals, and find the minimum dosage that provided the needed relief. I didn't realize it at the time, but this would be an experiment with consequences.

Lastly, I was scheduled for a bone scan.

"It didn't take long for Dr. Raj to be concerned about Mr. Skeleton. The result will determine if I will be building my boat," I thought.

The holidays came and went. This year, though, I found myself to be profoundly more grateful and spiritual. It didn't happen all at once. It was a slow evolution. I hadn't grown in faith because I thought I was going to die from cancer. My perception of the world and what was really important found its way to the forefront, skipping past improvident things of the world. It was slowly becoming the face of who I was now.

My eldest Saint Bernard, Sebastian, and I were a therapy team, and we worked every chance we got. Nila and I were both in very festive moods and spent time with friends and family when possible. The curvy road of life had begun to straighten.

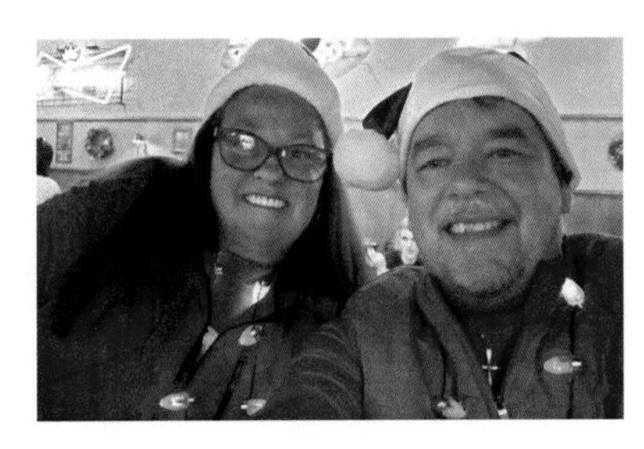

December 2019

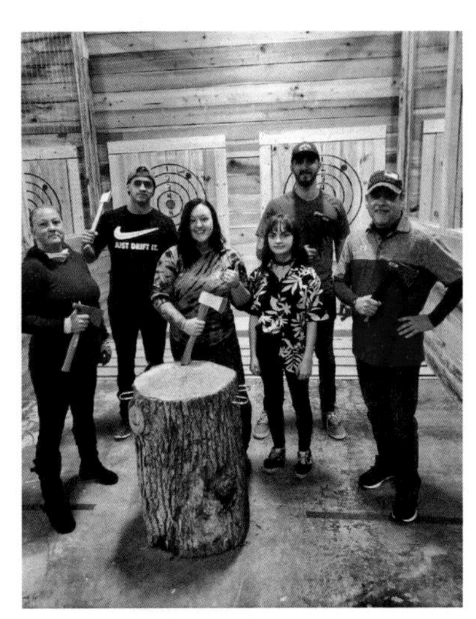

November 2019

On New Year's Eve 2019, Nila and I made our way back for my bone scan. This was a different location on the university medical campus from where we saw Dr. Raj.

As we pulled into the parking lot, my stomach sank. The sign read "University Cancer Institute."

The first thing I saw when we walked into the waiting area was the "Wall of Hope." It was in the same genre as the Tree of Life at SCC, or the wall of cancer fighters. According to Dr. Taha, I had been cancer free for six months. The morbid thoughts hadn't evacuated my mind completely, but I had spent less time building my boat. The facility and Wall of Hope took me back to a recent time in my cancer battle. I would have fared better without the experience.

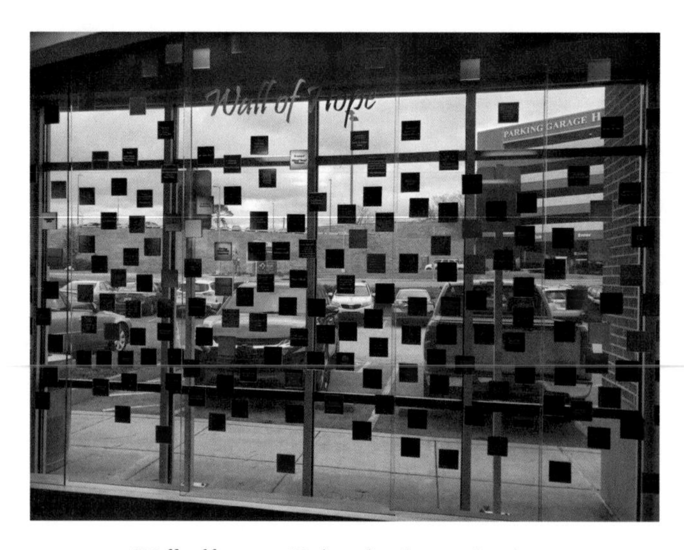

Wall of hope at University Cancer Institute

All the time leading up to my bone scan, I had been concerned about whether we would find out that some of those really mean cancer cells had slipped into Mr. Skeleton. But that wasn't what I was there for at all.

I was scheduled for a dual-energy X-ray, not a nuclear bone scan.

Dual-energy X-ray absorptiometry (DXA) is a means of measuring bone mineral density (BMD) using spectral imaging. Two X-ray beams, with different energy levels, are aimed at the patient's bones. When soft tissue absorption is subtracted out, the BMD can be determined from the absorption of each beam by bone. DXA is the most widely used and most thoroughly studied bone density measurement technology.

The DXA scan is typically used to diagnose and follow osteoporosis, unlike a nuclear bone scan, which is sensitive to certain metabolic diseases of bones in which bones are attempting to heal from infections, fractures, or tumors.

Dr. Raj had prescribed me prednisone for my PMR. High doses of prednisone over time will thin out the bone density. This can lead to easy fracturing.

The results are notated as a T-score. My left femur had a T-score of negative 1.3, osteopenia. My left femoral neck had a T-score of negative 1.8, osteoporotic. Major fracture risk was determined to be 7–12 percent over ten years. Hip fracture was 1–2 percent. The report impression stated, "Osteopenia of the femoral neck. Fracture risk is moderate."

Osteopenia is reduced bone mass of lesser severity than osteoporosis. Overall, the report was good. The five thousand units of D3 per day, and the twelve hundred units of calcium, coupled with the Prolia, seemed to have my bones in good shape to handle the prednisone.

The first day taking the prednisone was like a super caffeine ride. I felt great, with high energy, but couldn't sleep a minute. I would have to be sure to take it early each day if I was going to be able to get needed sleep.

Within a couple of days, I felt as though the inflammation was all but gone. The Sagittarius in me immediately started planning an exit strategy.

"If those really mean cancer cells are still hiding in me, I will need to get off the prednisone. Mr. Skeleton needs to be in tip-top shape should the day come that they find him."

But, for now, I was "cancer free." Nila and I were enjoying every day together. Although I still spent some of my time building a boat, it no longer consumed me.

Daily / Weekly / Monthly

Sagitarrius

11/22 to 12/21

Alias: The Archer

December 31, 2019

There are some people who own a boat, but they rarely go out on the ocean or a cruise on the river. They leave the boat docked, and they barbecue, or sunbathe, or enjoy cocktails while watching the sunset.While all of that may be nice, Sagittarius, it may seem a shame not to fully use and enjoy all the boat has to offer. You are adventerous, but in some way in your life now, you have been stuck at the dock. But you can untie that knot if you wish and sail away. Keep that in mind.

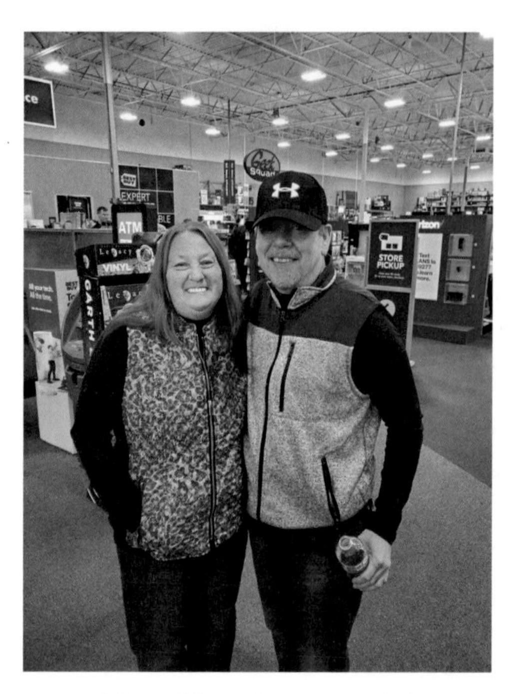

Nila and Perry, January 1, 2020

I was told, "You are cancer free." Life was better, but as I pondered the events to date, I come to realize the lyrics to this song were honest.

BRUTAL PLANET

Alice Cooper, 2000

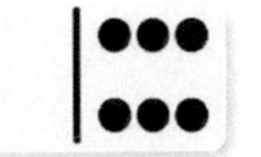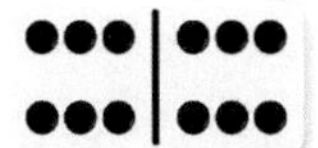

Chapter 18

FREE ISN'T REALLY FREE

Sagittarians are very kind and generous. They never expect favors in return.

In late January 2019, a few members of my company flew to Las Vegas for the annual trip. I worked a booth with my boss, among other coworkers, at the floor covering show. I had missed the previous year, so I felt this was an important trip for me—I needed the team to know I was back!

It was a real test of my physical endurance. The time change, which I had always found challenging, taxed me even more this year due to my new fatigue. The walk from my hotel, The Luxor, to the Mandalay Bay Convention Center, seemed like an expedition that stretched longer each day. I walked it for four consecutive days, including the setup day. During the show, we spent a great deal of our time standing in the small booth. I quietly ate extra OTC pain medication in order to sustain it for three days. There were also the evening business dinners or early morning breakfast meetings that only made the day longer.

Mental staying power was also tested. I needed to be sharp while talking to visitors and customers who stopped by. During the infrequent moments of downtime, we would have impromptu executive meetings with Jim (VP of Sales), Rick (director of R&D), Kevin (National Sales), and my boss, Erik. In order to hone my mental acuity, I drank extra coffee in the morning and had plenty of 5-Hour Energy drinks the rest of the day.

Nila loves the trips to Las Vegas. The trip is free for her. She freely wanders and explores all day while I am working at the show. On the last night after the show, Nila and I went with Rick and longtime friend Sparky Roberts down to Fremont Street. Freemont is old Vegas revived. Live bands play. You can hear the music coming out into the street from the various restaurants and clubs. You can find all kinds of street performers: dancers, jugglers, singers, musicians, posers. There are even zip lines.

"We should take the highest one!" Rick said.

I felt the same way. I wanted to chase the adrenaline dragon.

The highest, longest zip line zipped just beneath the huge video screen canopy and would be the best view.

Thankfully there was an elevator to the top of the zipline platform. Before I knew it, we were strapped into the harness.

However, when the time came to self-launch, I wasn't sure I had the physical strength to pull myself over the edge. The week of work had worn me down. But Sagittarius wasn't about to let a little pain and stiffness stop the race to the other end of Fremont. I didn't beat Rick to launch, but it was still a victory for me. Once launched, there I was, flying again. The breeze rushed into my face and blew through my hair.

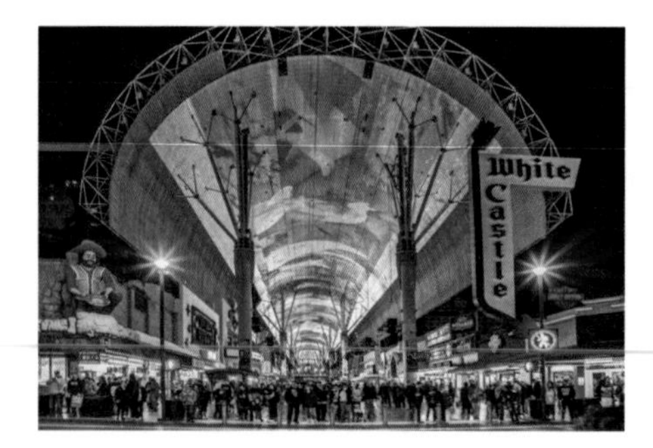

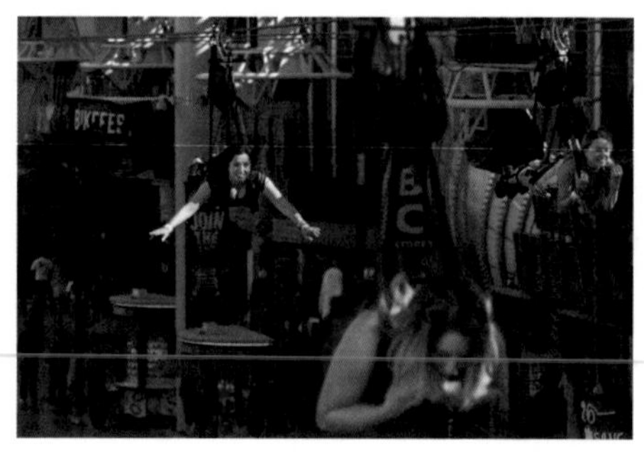

During the same trip, Nila and I went to see the Criss Angel show in Vegas on January 30, 2019, at Planet Hollywood. I was completely enthralled by the show. My mind was blank except for the wonders of magic on stage. But then, he announced that his son has leukemia, and he has a foundation to support children with cancer. During the show, he took time to advertise this program and request donations from the crowd when everyone departed from the show.

I cried openly, watching the advertisement, and decided I wasn't doing the best thing with my therapy dog program by primarily focusing on veterans. I needed to focus on children with cancer. My mind was only distracted for a short time before cancer took center stage again.

On the way out, I made a donation. I couldn't possibly imagine what it would be like as a father to find out one of my children had cancer. I doubt I could handle it.

This was not the only trip we had been on since my diagnosis. We managed to work in another vacation trip. April-18, we took our daughter and son-in-law to Cat Island, Bahamas. This was just after the completion of my radiation and the haunting consultation with Dr. Channeler.

I couldn't swim, snorkel, sleep, or get comfortable. But being with family and away from home was good medicine. We did take a private boat ride to a protected area of the ocean in a secluded inlet. This was referred to as daycare for many species that needed protection early in life. There, turtles were caught and tagged.

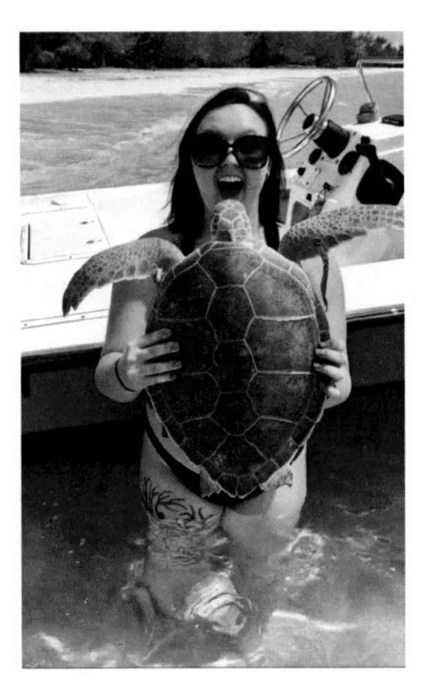

Daughter Alanna with a sea turtle, Cat Island, April 2018

A year later we went to Jamaica with some friends. We used reward miles from flying and rewards points from hotel stays so that the flight to Atlanta and the overnight hotel stay were free.

The trip to Jamaica was long but medicinal. Our son Shane and his wife Monica were able to join us. I felt free of cancer and all of the health issues that were the domino effect. But I wasn't free. I ran away, and it all followed along, slipping morbid thoughts into my mind after an evening of sipping Crown Royal when no one was around.

We hear the term "free" a lot. We are accustomed to hearing about "free" deals all of the time. "Buy one, get one free," or "visit nine times and your tenth visit is free." Another one is "Buy an entrée and get a free dessert." And "Use your rewards points for a free flight."

But let's think about it. Could it be true that if you buy one, you get one free? That means if one million were sold, then one million would be given away. How could a company stay in business if it gave away 50 percent of a product?

The answer is simple. They don't. The slogan "buy one, get one free" is a marketing tool. The price of the "free" item is baked into the price of the one we are paying for. So why do they tell us one is free? The simple answer is that it makes us feel good, like we got a great deal, and we are happy with the purchase.

A freelancer is an independent worker who sells his/her services to various clients, without being officially employed by any of them. In this case, the definition of freelancer says the person "sells services." That isn't free, but I understand the term.

When I began taking the prednisone, I had been in miserable shape for more than a year. I couldn't stand without pain. I couldn't get up from sitting without help...and pain. I couldn't sleep because of the pain. But as soon as I began my prednisone regiment, I became pain free. It was like a miracle drug! I never thought a tiny white pill could free me.

An unexpected side effect was energy. It was false energy, but I cared not. I went for days without touching a 5-Hour Energy shot. I was able to zoom through the day like a younger man, being productive and checking off boxes at work. I was able to make the trips to Georgia and work without freezing up on the ride down. I was again able to put in fourteen-hour days to stay on top of the business of Foam Products.

But being pain-free and fatigue-free came at a cost. It wasn't free at all. Since my cancer diagnosis in mid-2017, the doctors had worked on strengthening my bones. It took some time to realize that almost every doctor was concerned about Mr. Skeleton. I had three Prolia shots before I even knew I had one. The purpose of the five thousand units of vitamin D3 per day and the twelve hundred units of calcium that accompanied it didn't register at first. I just thought they were good for me.

Generally, the higher the dose of prednisone you take and the longer you take it, the greater the risk of osteoporosis. However, even low doses interfere with healthy bone growth. Corticosteroids also can dramatically weaken bones and lead to osteoporosis. And therein lies the cost.

"I'm pain free, but not without Mr. Skeleton paying a price," I thought. "I've got to give up the prednisone so my bones can be strong enough to fight another day."

Prednisone is used to treat conditions such as arthritis, blood disorders, breathing problems, severe allergies, skin diseases, cancer, eye problems, and immune system disorders. Prednisone belongs to a class of drugs known as corticosteroids. They decrease your immune system's response to various diseases to reduce symptoms such as swelling.

To stop taking prednisone requires some strategic planning and execution. The printed warning that accompanied the prescription read, "Some conditions may become worse when this drug is suddenly stopped. Also, you may experience symptoms such as weakness, weight loss, nausea, muscle pain, headache, tiredness, dizziness."

Then there are the side effects. Some stood out more than others. The warning continued: "Tell your doctor right away if any of these unlikely but serious side effects occur: **muscle pain/cramps**, irregular heartbeat, **weakness**, swelling hands/ankles/feet, unusual weight gain, signs of infection (such as fever, persistent sore throat), vision problems (such as blurred vision), symptoms of stomach/intestinal bleeding (such as stomach/abdominal pain, black/tarry stools, vomit that looks like coffee grounds), **mental/mood changes (such as depression, mood swings, agitation)**, slow wound healing, thinning skin, **bone pain**, menstrual period changes, puffy face, seizures, easy bruising/bleeding."

I was counting on the polymyalgia rheumatica being a short-lived condition.

Dr. Raj said, "It usually lasts one to two years."

I mentally counted in my head—I was sure I was close to two years.

"Prostate cancer is slow-spreading. I will stay on the prednisone a little longer, until the PMR is over, and then wean myself off and focus on strengthening Mr. Skeleton," I schemed.

As I said, to stop taking prednisone requires some strategic planning and execution. Not impatience and strong will. I would learn that lesson soon enough.

For now, there was work to do, and I felt great. I made business trips to Massachusetts, Ohio, and North Carolina in the fall of 2019. I even joined the Georgia Division of Foam Products in a 5k run!

It was the United Way Unity run. We had quite the group to volunteer. Due to my paralyzed diaphragm, I knew I couldn't run the entire 5K, but I wanted the challenge. For years after getting out of the army, I ran five miles per day. That was in a past life now. My muscles were weak, and my right diaphragm was sewn to the inside of my rib cage. But I was "cancer free."

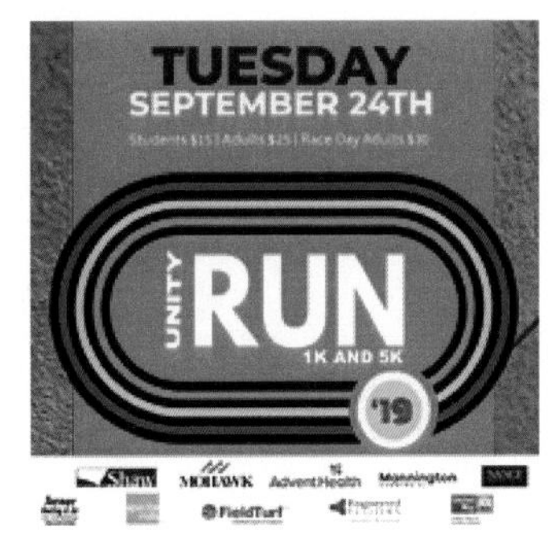

Unity Run flier

We lined up and started the run. I lost myself in the huge crowd in order to avoid embarrassment in front of my coworkers. I was only doing the airborne shuffle, not much of a run, but not walking. By the end of the first straightaway, I was longing for the end and gasping for air.

Breathing was especially hard in the humid Georgia heat. I constantly set goals of getting from one shadow to another. Slowly and methodically, I shuffled my feet one after the other. Sagittarians do not quit. It was never an option.

"I survived all of the surgeries and radiation but volunteered to die on the side of the road in the name of unity and a 5K run," I quietly fussed.

At one point I wondered how many more people could possibly be behind me. I was constantly being passed. Then here came Mark Williamson, the husband of our VP of Finance, Stephanie. Stephanie was the first person I ever met at Foam Products.

Mark was fast walking and outrunning me! He slowed down a bit and shared some conversation. It took my mind off the pain and struggle. Perhaps he saw how close to the edge I was. I imagine I looked like each step could be the last.

Mark ended the conversation with some encouraging words, and off he went. I always appreciated that moment. I hope he didn't think I was inauspicious. I couldn't run, breathe, and talk. The timing was perfect, though, and I needed that conversation, that distraction from the pain and difficulty breathing.

When I reached the halfway point, I was incredibly disappointed. How could I only be halfway? How in the world would I ever make it to the end? And then I would see another employee, or a stranger with a sign on the sidewalk, encouraging me to motor on.

By this time in the 5K, I was walking about 50 percent and running about 50 percent. I used the methodology I learned in air assault school in the army. Run when it is level or downhill. Walk if there is an incline.

I passed some onlookers who had water on a table. I grabbed a cup, but didn't have enough air to say "thank you" and ran by. I turned up the cup of water and welcomed the coolness of whatever didn't make it into my mouth.

As we neared the end, there was a crowd that lined each side of the street. I didn't make eye contact but used the cheers like adrenaline. But I needed real adrenaline to make it up the slight incline to the finish. Where was the prednisone when I needed it!

With the finish line in sight, I scanned the crowd and saw exactly what I needed to get me to the end. There was Nila Muse, rooting and cheering for me like she always had before.

Through all of our years together, when I played sports, Nila was my biggest fan. She made me find the absolute best somewhere deep down inside. She made me run faster, jump higher, shoot straighter, hit farther, and score more often.

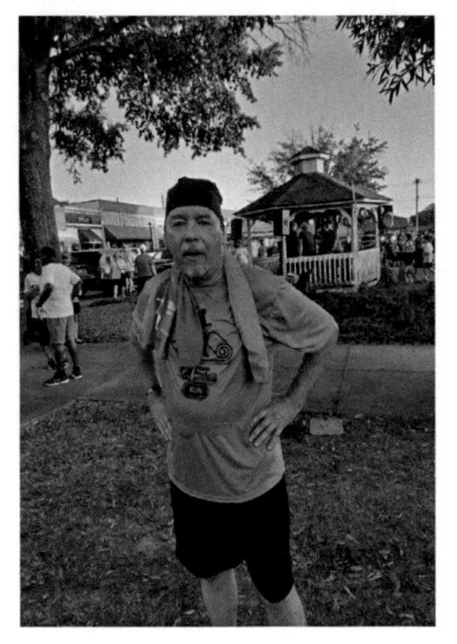

So, seeing Nila in the crowd, yelling, "C'mon, baby, you got this!" made me finish strong. Not just strong. I had finished the 5K alive!

In January 2020, I continued my march forward. I joined my boss and traveled to Hannover, Germany, to a huge floor covering show. This time, we were not working at a booth but were visitors. We had some meetings set up and an after-hours party to attend, compliments of one of the companies we were there to visit.

Perry after the 5k Unity Run on September 24, 2019

After being told I was "cancer free," I wasn't as excited as everyone around me. I kept recalling a visit to Dr. Famoyin when I was alone with him for one of my routine appointments. I vividly remembered Dr. Famoyin saying, "You will never really be cancer free. You will always have the cancer tag."

What he meant and what the little guy was whispering in my ear were two different things. He *meant* that every time I sneezed and went to the doctor's office, the first thing they would see was that I had cancer.

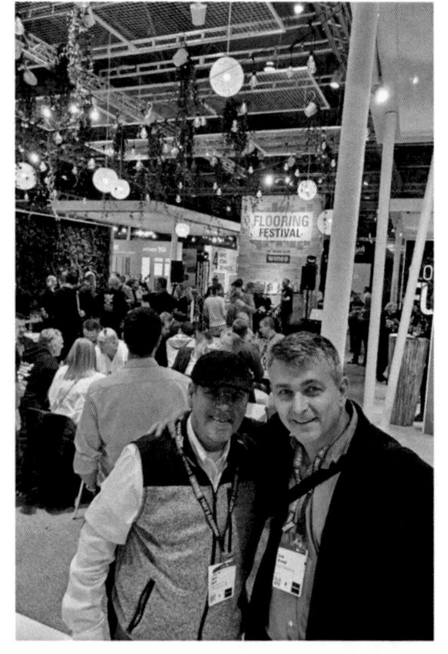

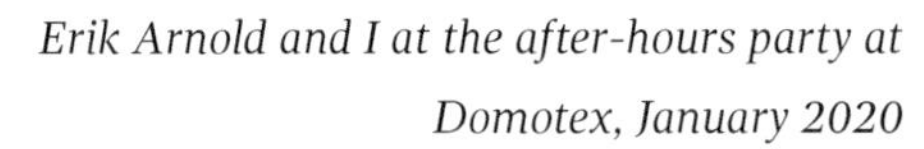

Erik Arnold and I at the after-hours party at Domotex, January 2020

But what I heard was: "*You will always have cancer. It is just undetectable right now.*"

I always appreciated Dr. Famoyin's honesty. He was sincere and truthful. Sometimes the truth is painful, especially when it is not what you want to hear. I don't believe a person can fight ferociously without truly understanding the opponent. I also needed it to live more freely.

Some people are blessed to be truly cancer free. But for me, "cancer free" is one of those psychological things one says so the patient can celebrate and stop stressing. Just like the name of the road that leads to the Specialty Cancer Center: Celebration of Life Drive.

In my heart, I knew free wasn't always free.

My cancer battle had become a roller coaster ride of emotions. In 2021 a new song played on my Sirius XM app from a band I had seen live many years earlier. As I listened to the lyrics, I started to cry.

FLOWERS ON A GRAVE

Bush, 2021

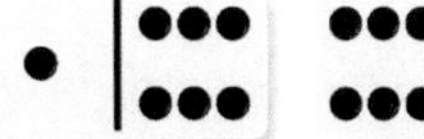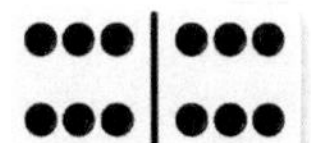

Chapter 19

THE DAY THE EARTH STOOD STILL / EVERY FIVE SECONDS

Sagittarians love to socialize just as much as they hate to procrastinate. You will always feel their presence at gatherings and different events.

After stopping my Lupron shots in June 2019 and being pronounced "cancer free," I was feeling as though I could start a new chapter in my life. All of the surgeries and the healing were behind me (at least as far as I knew). Sleeping was still an issue, and although OTC medications helped, I wanted to get back to zero meds. It was time to get back in shape.

The local wellness center had a huge basketball court and a hot tub. Those were both inviting to me. So, Nila and I got a gym membership and formulated a plan.

We scheduled our visits when we expected there weren't going to be many people there. And it worked. Most times when we visited, the basketball court was vacant. That was perfect. We changed clothes and grabbed a basketball.

Nila and I started out by standing ten to fifteen feet apart. We just passed the ball to one another, allowing it to bounce once each time. It was an exercise in stretching and trying to break all of the rust loose.

We would hold the ball over our heads and bounce pass it. Then we would shift to using the left arm and the right arm, varying the position between throws. Meanwhile, as the rust broke loose, we ventured farther apart.

This routine went on for about thirty minutes until the pain eased and the ROM increased. It was wonderful to exercise again, albeit in baby steps. The pain was welcomed as I knew it was all part of the journey back to normalcy, and not a product of being broken.

Then, I got the bright idea of trying and shooting some baskets. It was always fun to shoot and play around with Nila. The Sagittarius in me never missed an opportunity to show off a little in front of the love of my life.

There would not be any running around now though. I didn't have two fully functioning lungs any longer. For now, I would settle for standing stationary.

"Patience, Sagittarius," I told myself. "One step at a time."

But there wouldn't be any showing off today. I started off by standing just beneath the goal and off to one side. As I shot, no, threw the ball at the backboard, I began to realize how far from normal I was. The goal looked higher, and the ball felt heavier.

As time passed, I ventured a few feet away and a few more. Then, I had the bright idea I would go to the free-throw line before I was too tired.

As I positioned myself at the line and dribbled the ball, I remembered my routine from days gone by. I had always played point guard, and shots around the foul line were in my wheelhouse. I focused on my stance and the positioning of the ball in my hands. Once set, I stared at my target, which was the front of the rim. I raised the ball and launched it.

To my dismay, the ball fell short by quite a few feet. I tried several times, all with the same result. Nila offered words of encouragement, as I am sure she could see the embarrassment and disappointment on my face.

"Cancer and its domino effect made me an old man. Maybe they need to lower the goal like they do for little girls," I thought in disappointment.

In the end, I positioned myself just inside the dashed circle and in front of the goal. I lowered the ball to my waistline, the way I had to when I was just starting to play as a kid. I bent my knees for extra leverage, used my right arm, and launched the ball.

This time the ball bounced off the front of the rim. Nila rebounded, and I repeated the exercise. After several attempts, and using all of my strength, the ball went in.

I decided to stop on a positive note.

We continued to go to the wellness center regularly. We usually went through the same routine, passing the ball and loosening up before going over to shoot. As time passed, I was getting stronger and better. I added resistance bands and eventually started lifting weights during my routine. Nila used the stationary bikes, gazelle, and elliptical machines. I was so thankful for the hot tub. The aches and pains of working out were truly magnified by my condition.

After several weeks of the same steps, we returned to the basketball court one day. Every week I worked my way back toward the free-throw line, one small step at a time. On this day, I found myself standing behind the line and going through my routine again from days gone by. This time I positioned my hands on the ball and stared down the front of the rim. Everything around me seemed to go silent. I shot, and the ball hit the front of the rim. A couple of tries later, it was nothing but net!

Nila and I celebrated with high fives and a hug. Anyone watching would surely wonder what the celebration was all about. We didn't care. We both knew it symbolized much more than just making a free throw.

2020 was off to a good start. The trip to Germany with Erik went well, except for one issue leaving.

Evidently, my plane ticket was marked as a "flight risk." It didn't say so in printed words but in code on the ticket. I was pulled aside and searched, going through the initial gate in Hannover, Germany. From there, we took a short flight to Denmark. There I was searched a second time.

Finally, we were at the gate and boarding for the United States. This time I was pulled from the line and taken aside. Keep in mind, everyone else was boarding the plane directly behind me.

A Delta manager came over and explained, "According to your ticket, you are on a watch list. This is now out of my hands."

A lady wearing a red outfit introduced herself as a Delta liaison for the United States. She sat down beside me and asked me to confirm that I owned the bag in front of us, my carry-on bag. I confirmed, and she began explaining the process.

"I am going to ask you some questions. I will use your answers when I contact the United States. We will need the United States to confirm that you can reenter," she began.

Then she continued, "Someone will be coming to inspect your bag."

About that time, an officer showed up with his K9. He asked, "May I have permission to search your bag?"

"Sure," I said, "anything you need to do. I just don't want to miss this flight. My coworkers are already on board."

Then the lady in red proceeded to ask why I was there, where I stayed, how I traveled, and if I'd left the country for any reason during my visit.

I answered all of her questions without pause. I also explained that I had a Delta SkyMiles number that would show my flight history. I followed by telling her that I was TSA (Transportation Security Administration) precheck certified.

A TSA precheck is applied for in order to minimize the security check at the airport. There is a background check performed to ensure a person is eligible. If your record is squeaky clean, you qualify with a small fee.

Being TSA precheck allows you to take a special, usually shorter, line through security. In this line, a person is not required to remove their shoes or belt. This is because the background check deems you not to be a risk.

Yet here I was. About to miss my plane due to being tagged a flight risk.

The officer took my bag and disappeared. I had been very relaxed and calm up to this point. I didn't want to give off the wrong vibe. But this immediately made me nervous.

"Why couldn't he inspect my bag in front of me?" I wondered. "I hope this isn't a setup. I don't want to see the local jail."

The lady in red left, and I sat alone. The plane had completed boarding, and it was looking as though my coworkers would be going home without me.

A few minutes later, the officer returned with his K9 and my bag. "Thank you," he said. "Your bag is good."

Shortly afterward, the lady in red returned and notified me the United States would allow me back. She explained the mistake involved a passport number very similar to mine.

"My apologies for the delay. Have a good flight," she said and then turned and left.

I grabbed my bag and boarded the plane. I sat down and chuckled to myself, "Out of all the people on this flight, of course this happened to me."

Not too long after my experience with the German airport, something happened in our world that reminded me of the 1951 American science-fiction film, *The Day the Earth Stood Still.* The story is set in the cold war era, during the early part of the nuclear arms race. In the movie, a spaceship lands in Washington, DC. The US Army quickly surrounds the vessel.

A humanoid and robot emerge and unexpectedly open a small device. A nervous soldier shoots and wounds the humanoid and breaks what was supposed to be a gift. The gift would have allowed the president of the United States to study life on other planets.

Klaatu, the humanoid, says he has a message that must be delivered to all world leaders simultaneously. The basis of the message is that Earth will be destroyed if the nuclear threats aren't rectified. Otherwise, Earth poses a threat to other planets in the universe.

He is told, "Under the current political climate, that will be impossible."

The earth pauses as everyone tunes into what is happening with the flying saucer. Everyone could be impacted by the visit, as Earth is threatened to be obliterated.

Shortly after my return from Germany, the earth experienced an event just like the movie—everyone paused and tuned in to see what was happening in other parts of the world. However, it was not like in the sci-fi movie. The threat didn't come from a spaceship. It came in the form of a virus.

I was sitting in my office in Calhoun, trying to stay abreast of the news. On January 31, 2020, only a short time after returning home from Germany, President Trump blocked travel from China and issued an executive order blocking entry to the US for anyone who had been in China in the previous fourteen days.

I was "cancer free," but my right diaphragm wasn't functional. I only had partial aspiration ability with my right lung, and so I was tuned in. I did not want to get anything respiratory. Not bronchitis, not pneumonia, and not whatever this novel coronavirus happened to be.

My next trip to our Georgia plant was at the beginning of March. I had begun putting the word out that everyone needed to pay attention to the news about the novel coronavirus or COVID-19. I locked the door to my office and started having everyone call me when needed. I also began using phone conferencing services as an alternative to meeting in groups.

Almost everyone thought I was overreacting.

"Do you really think it's that bad?" I was asked many times.

I told one person, "Yes, my prediction is that the school year will end prematurely, and the military will be called in to assist with the medical needs." And I said that in the very beginning.

Li Wenliang, a doctor in Wuhan, China, was one of the first people to alert others about a "strange new virus." Political tensions were high in the US and with China. In the early part of January, the Wuhan police reprimanded Dr. Wenliang for "making false comments."

In December 2019, Dr. Wenliang received a report of a patient diagnosed with severe acute respiratory syndrome (SARS) coronavirus. On the same day, the Wuhan CDC issued an emergency warning to local hospitals about an outbreak of mysterious "pneumonia" cases.

Li shared a screenshot of the report on the social media platform WeChat and noted to his medical classmates that there were seven confirmed cases of SARS from the Huanan Seafood Market. He posted the patients' examination reports and CT scans.

On January 3, 2020, Li was interrogated and issued a formal written warning for "publishing untrue statements" about the report.

"Any further noncompliant behavior will result in prosecution," he was informed.

On January 8, 2020, Li contracted the virus and published his experience and police report on social media. He died at age thirty-three on February 7, 2020.

2020 was an election year, and the political climate in the United States was very adversarial. It was difficult to determine what the facts were. Schools began closing, and governors began issuing stay-at-home orders.

"I beat cancer, but a novel respiratory virus could be my demise."

Before long, business conditions for restaurants, businesses, planes, and trains came to a screeching halt. The CDC was all over the map with its guidance. Some people wore masks; others opted not to. Meanwhile, the military was called into action to utilize its medical expertise and equipment.

At work, I formed a coronavirus task force team. I wrote a letter identifying Foam Products as an essential business. We conferenced daily and put together documents and protocols to be able to safely work. But we could not control the employees or their habits outside of work.

I was obsessed with watching and reading to learn everything I could about this new threat. The truth was, I was terrified of catching this disease.

During the summer of 2020, the businesses that were still operating had begun to catch up. Employees were wearing masks, and plexiglass dividers were installed to further aid in keeping people separated. All of our protocols were in place. We checked the temperature of each employee daily and asked a list of screening questions before allowing them to work. A designated person at each of our facilities was dedicated to cleaning and disinfecting constantly.

People who were able were allowed to start working from home. I was still cautiously making trips to Georgia, but we suspended our membership to the wellness center long before summer.

It was difficult to stay isolated. The lack of exercise was evident quickly. I began to seize up again. My body began to morph back to a time prior to the gym and passing the basketball with Nila.

I missed being able to take Sebastian on therapy visits to the VA and to nursing homes. I could tell that he didn't understand not being able to jump in the truck and don his vest. It concerned me that he was nine years old now, and I didn't know how long we had left together.

On July 10, 2020, I was making my way back to Tennessee. Sebastian had an appointment at the veterinary hospital. It was a routine checkup, but I liked hearing the reports and providing reassurance to Sebastian when we went in. All of the previous reports were the same. "Sebastian is in great health. Other than needing his teeth brushed, anyone who didn't know him would never guess his age," the doctor would say to us.

When I drove into the parking lot, Nila was already there. Sebastian had gotten out of the vehicle and collapsed in the parking lot. The vet techs rushed out with a stretcher, and we all rolled Sebastian onto it. My heart was racing.

"What is happening?" I said aloud. Sebastian started having a seizure before we could get him up. He weighed a hundred and thirty pounds.

Minutes later, the doctor came out to the waiting room.

"We did an ultrasound but could not see anything at all," the doctor said hurriedly. "We inserted a needle, and his stomach was full of blood. We don't have much time; do you want us to operate?"

"Of course, yes," Nila and I responded immediately and in unison. "Whatever you have to do."

Moments later, he returned. "I think it's too late," the doctor informed us with a grim tone. "We got him shaved, and he had another seizure. I don't think he will make it through surgery."

We went back to see Sebastian. It was hard seeing him lying on the table, unresponsive. Nila and I hugged and kissed him repeatedly while whispering loving thoughts. His tongue slipped from his mouth, and he began to shiver as another seizure approached. We immediately gave permission for the doctor to administer a final shot.

As the shot was administered, I saw Sebastian's life leave his body. I remembered the words of my granny, "You know, Perry, it doesn't hurt anymore." I knew the same was true for him.

Nila and I turned to one another, held each other tight, and cried like little girls.

We never recovered from losing Sebastian. It was so unexpected. It was so ugly and shocking.

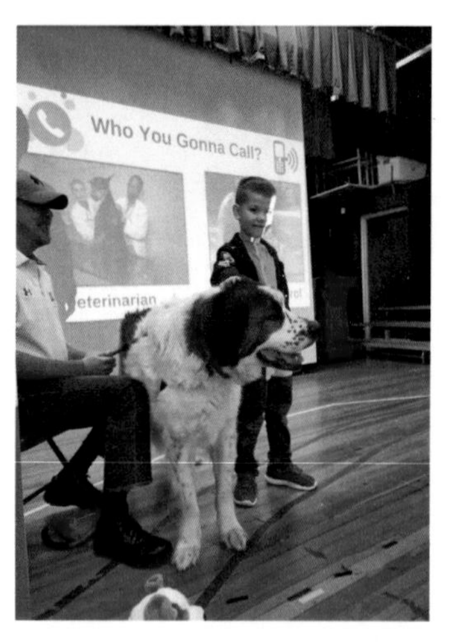

But Sebastian left us with some incredible memories. He did wonderful work on this earth and touched many lives. Boys and girls, veterans, the elderly, friends and family all loved Sebastian. He was one of a kind, and I am sure God has a special place in heaven for him.

We had him cremated, and I think of him every time I pass his urn. We have pictures on our phones, computers, and walls. He will surely be missed by many.

Sebastian working with the Humane Society to teach kids about dogs.

Written by Perry Muse

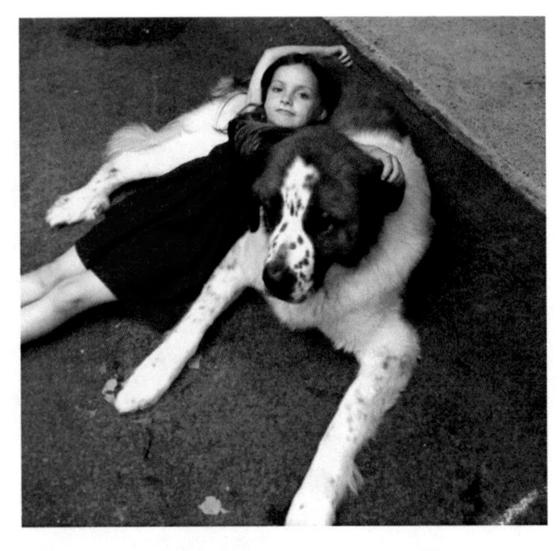

Sebastian with granddaughter Ainzlee.

Losing Sebastian was difficult in an already difficult environment. There was an outpouring of love from fellow therapy dog teams who knew him.

Shortly after the unexpected tragedy, I had a visit with Dr. Famoyin. Although the PMR continued to plague me with inflammation, pain, and weight gain, things were definitely on the uptick with the way I felt. I could tell my testosterone was inching up, and it improved my energy. I spoke to him about my interrupted sleep and dreams.

"The other night I dreamt someone was knocking on the front door," I shared. "It was daytime, and I had no worries opening the door. When I turned the knob, an intruder rushed toward me and placed a grocery bag around my face. There were others in the house, but I couldn't make a sound to alert them."

I continued, "I tried to breathe, but I could only suck the grocery bag into my mouth. I tried once more and woke up. I was panting, and my heart was racing."

"Oh my!" Dr. Famoyin responded. "No wonder you can't sleep if you are having those dreams."

Then he surprised me. "You are not a typical candidate for sleep apnea, but I think we should schedule a sleep study," he suggested.

"I'm on board," I replied without hesitation.

But I had other things going on in my life at the same time. After losing Sebastian, Nila and I thought again of our dream. We had always wanted to open a business of our own. In late July, we had an idea. We scheduled a meeting with our longtime groomer and pitched the idea to her.

On August 12, 2020, we opened Fairy Tails Pet Grooming and Daycare. It took a lot of help from a close personal friend and a lot of work on our part. Nila loves dogs, and she is wonderful with them. It just made sense. And it felt right to dedicate the salon to Sebastian.

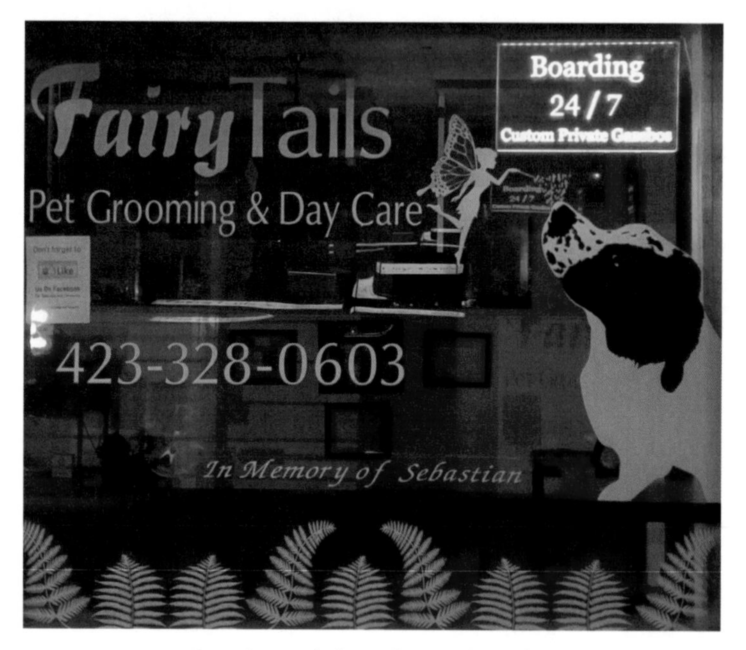

Storefront window of grooming salon

With all of the work getting the pet grooming and daycare facility going, I did not forget about my sleep apnea test, and through Dr. Famoyin's referral, I was prescribed a home apnea test. A home apnea test is basically a breathing monitor that records your breathing, oxygen levels, and breathing effort. The test kit came in the mail, and the test lasted one night.

A few days later, the results were in. I had sleep apnea. According to the study, I stopped breathing on average twelve times per minute.

"No wonder I am always dreaming of drowning or smothering. I literally stop breathing twelve times a minute!" I realized. "If cancer doesn't get me, I'm going to suffocate one night."

I was prescribed a CPAP (continuous positive airway pressure) machine. It took some time to find a mask that was comfortable for me to wear. I understand why people give up on these. They can be uncomfortable and can even feel smothering at times until you get accustomed to wearing the mask.

Data is collected over time, and the machine adjusts based on your needs. This means wearing the mask, and trying to sleep, even when the pressure may not be optimum.

I changed my mask and found one better suited to me. I would go to sleep and see seven on the indicator. Sometimes I would wake up in the middle of the night and see twelve. I could feel the pressure increase. Oftentimes, it was the increase that woke me up. This meant the machine had determined more pressure was required to force me to breathe.

Overall, it was a good call by Dr. Famoyin. Over time I slept better. I was in a deep sleep and dreaming, but not horror movie dreams. I could tell the difference when I woke up.

COVID was still a big threat, and I still had some type of issue with my breathing. Otherwise, why would the machine need to adjust to twelve, or even as high as seventeen, in order to force air into my lungs? It wasn't my lung that was a problem. It wasn't the machine. I couldn't put my finger on it yet. But at least I no longer stopped breathing every five seconds.

I volunteered for a Compassion International event to get children around the world sponsored. I have been a sponsor for 10 years. This was a concert event. When the band played this song, the lyrics ran through me and gave me new strength.

IT'S NOT OVER YET

For King and Country, 2014

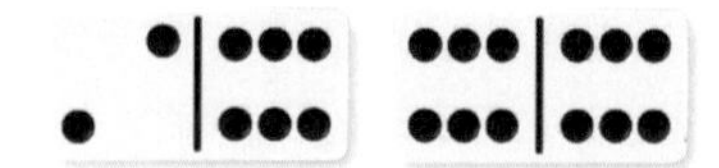

Chapter 20

MR. SKELETON AND THE SACK OF GRAVEL

Sagittarians never want to slow things down. They are restless and impatient. Sagittarians sometimes act in a careless manner, taking risks that can put them and others at risk.

May 3, 2020. I had weaned myself off prednisone for at least the third time because of being so concerned about the effects on my bones. Each of the two times prior, I stopped after dropping my dosage to 3 mg a day for a week. This time I seemed to feel fine and thought perhaps the inflammation was finally over. Within a week, I knew it was not over and was forced to resume the medication. I wanted to be off the medicine because I had reached a point where it was unpleasant to see myself undressed in the mirror.

At the time of my motorcycle crash in 2009, I was working out regularly. I was fit and strong. However, my recovery period and the treatments took my body mass. My muscles withered away. My energy vacated. My body was scarred. My manhood was terminally broken. My urine slipped out when I had too much water or some relaxing wine. The prednisone caused me to gain belly fat, giving me an old man beer belly. I hated the sight of it. Nila was officially married to an old man, without much to look at. I was ashamed of what I had become.

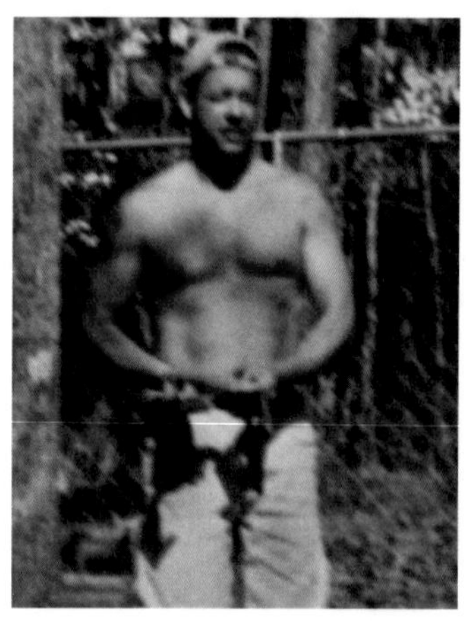

It had only been a couple of months since we suspended our membership at the wellness center, but my body told a different story. COVID forced me to be isolated more often, and I was afraid I was headed in reverse.

Perry 2009

Perry 2020

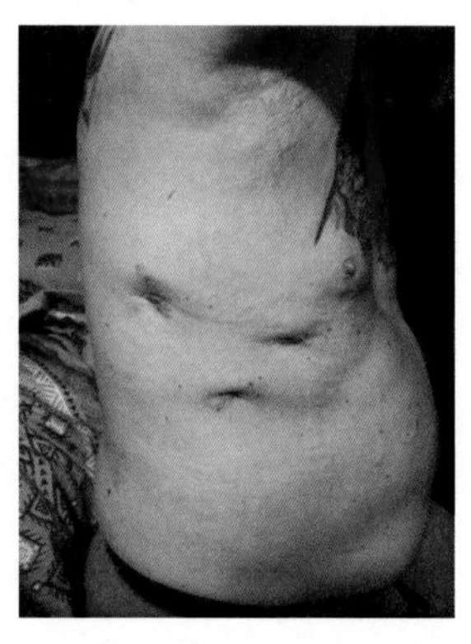

The last time I stopped the prednisone, it took a couple of days for the pain and stiffness to start sneaking up on me. At the same time, I had become more active outside. It was the beginning of spring, and we had a lot of yard work after a winter in the forest. As the aches, pain, and stiffness came, I mentally convinced myself the extra labor following a winter off from strenuous yard work was the obvious culprit. It's like getting back into the gym for that New Year's resolution. You must endure those first days of pain. You have to suck it up if you want that gut to go away and get those muscles back. No pain, no gain!

After a week, I knew it was more than exercise. That familiar pain in my neck, shoulders, hips, and lower back had returned with a vengeance. I found myself once again struggling to stand up straight. I was forced to turn my whole body to look left or right. I was in need of Nila's help to get out of the chair if I sat through a movie with her.

I was extremely self-conscious at work. I made it a point to hold my head up and walk straight. It was the most painful posture, but one I had to adopt to look normal. I did not want to give away that I was in trouble...again. This was just a repeat of what I had been doing for a couple of years now.

I made sure to minimize how long I sat in meetings. Many times, I would stay seated as though I was working to finish up notes until everyone was gone. I did not want them to see the fifty-nine-year-old guy getting up like an eighty-year-old guy. If I was meeting with outside clients or vendors, I would load up on naproxen or Tylenol Arthritis. It would hold me to the end and allow me to minimize the pain of standing up and walking.

Occasionally, someone would ask if I was okay.

"Sure, why?" I would always reply (as if I didn't already know).

"Because you look like you're walking a little funny."

"Oh, I just slept wrong and got a little kink."

As I walked away, I morbidly thought, "Or, cancer is in my bones, just like Dr. Channeler said it would be. I have all the pain, just no fractures yet. But those really mean cancer cells are working on it."

I felt like this particular time was the worst. I had teleported back in time and felt nearly crippled. How could I be approaching one year "cancer free" (remember, free isn't really free) and be in this rough state? I made an appointment and went to see Dr. Raj. After a quick assessment, he prescribed 20 mg prednisone. I had upcoming travel to Florida for an important wedding. I imagined in my current state that riding, flying, and a wedding would be devastating and painful. The 20 mg prednisone worked, and I was back in action almost after day one. I managed not to miss work and not to miss the wedding.

So, I learned my lesson and worked my prednisone dosage back to 5 mg a day quickly. If you consider this had already happened two times, you would think I would have a better plan. Nope, not Sagittarius. I thought back to the warning that accompanied the prednisone. "Some conditions may become worse when this drug is suddenly stopped." So, as I mentioned, I jumped from 3 mg per day to zero on May 3. On the afternoon of May 5, I began to feel a rapid progression of symptoms returning. What had taken a week the last time only took two days this time.

By early evening, I was in so much pain I had to resort to taking a leftover pain pill from my last surgery. I hated pain pills because they obscured my ability to rate my progress, but no amount of ibuprofen, naproxen, or Tylenol Arthritis was going to help.

"It must be the cancer. This is the most painful yet. Yep, those really mean cells have been working overtime, and the medication has been masking it. I think I am in the 65 percent chance of rain area today."

My appetite was good, my weight was good, but I was in serious trouble. I ate supper and waited for the pill to do its job. At this point, I was definitely clock-watching. I was waiting on the thirty-minute mark when I should have had enough relief to be able to tolerate it. Nila walked by and asked if there was anything she could do.

I replied honestly, "Yeah, shoot me."

She quickly responded with, "I can't do that."

My reply surprised her.

"You have to do it. If I do, it's suicide, and I go to hell. I'm sick and tired of being sick and tired."

Did I want to die? Hell, no. But at that moment I was in a dark place. I couldn't see any light at the end of the tunnel. I wasn't sure if the cancer was hiding in my skeleton, not to be found yet.

"There are plenty of places for cancer to hide in Mr. Skeleton."

It had consumed my mind and body for years. I had made it through work that day, but what about tomorrow? How could I even sleep enough tonight to be productive tomorrow? The earth was starting to move again, slowly. I had important work to do so Foam Products could survive its own life-threatening challenge.

"I have won the battles, but tonight I feel I am surely losing the war."

I found an ear, nose, and throat doctor. His name was Dr. Zajonc. He was a very kind and caring doctor. He wasn't ashamed to say God bless you, and that told me a lot.

Dr. Zajonc examined me and described my problem in a unique way. He said, "You have what looks like a sack of gravel in the back of your throat. You will need to have surgery to remove the tonsils, adenoids, and this sack of gravel. It may be tough to schedule during this COVID situation." The surgery was, in fact, delayed twice.

After dinner on this particular night, the one when I asked Nila to shoot me, my throat began to swell, inside and out. Moving my head back and forth to keep the sack of gravel from blocking my airway was not really working well. As time progressed, the pain pill started doing its magic. My attention shifted to the blockage in my throat. The sack of gravel seemed to be getting larger. I resorted to calling a local emergency room. I told them what I was experiencing and about the delayed surgery. The response was unexpected.

"If you were scheduled for surgery with Dr. Zajonc, it was likely at Mountain Forest Hospital. If you come here, we will likely just have to transport you to Mountain Forest."

Actually, my surgery wasn't scheduled at either place. It was going to take place at a specialty surgery center, the place where I had gotten fried four times in the last nineteen months. I was not going to this ER just to get an ambulance ride to Mountain Forest ER, four minutes away. I guessed that would cost around one grand and would allow more time for this sack in my throat to keep filling up with gravel!

"The EMTs would have a story to tell about giving this guy a breathing hole in his throat because he came to the wrong emergency room. 'Everybody knows we don't deal with sacks of gravel at this ER!'"

Nila took me to Mountain Forest ER. I was taken back almost immediately after my COVID-19 screening. It was odd to see a totally vacant ER waiting room. I told the doctor my issue, and they took a look.

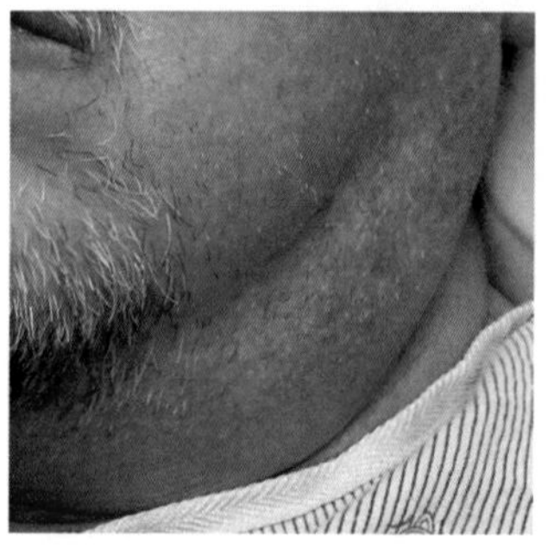

My enlarged throat at the ER

"It is definitely very enlarged. It has a lot of mucus buildup, as well. All of the pollen has probably gotten it aggravated. We will do a lab, a CT scan, and get you some antibiotics," said the masked doctor.

We all had our masks on. I had learned it was very difficult to read people's expressions when they were wearing surgical masks. Their eyes alone did not tell their story. Were they concerned? Was it serious? I could not tell.

Taking blood was uneventful. I pointed out everyone's favorite vein to draw blood from in the fold of my right arm. The port was left in for a future IV, or dose of drugs, if needed. Before going to get the CT scan, I was given a strong steroid injection into the port. I was told it was to reduce the inflammation.

I remember wanting, needing it to hurry. I was fighting the anxiety back and trying to remain calm. For some reason, I was reminded of the recurring dream I had had since I was a kid. One of the thousands of night terrors I had. In the dream, I was underwater, but I could see the surface. I was trying to reach the surface before I inhaled. I *never* reached the surface. I vividly recalled the feeling of knowing it was over, and I was only going to inhale water. When I gave up and inhaled, I awoke with my heart pounding in my chest from holding my breath until the final second.

But this current experience was the opposite. Each time I inhaled and felt the restriction increasing, I wondered, "Is this my last breath, like the last breath I must have taken before I plunged into the water?"

The CT scan was clear. I was relieved of the concern about the possible malignancy Dr. Zajonc mentioned. The super steroid shot had begun to work, and I could feel my airway opening. The obvious swelling on the outside of my neck was receding. Luckily, Dr. Zajonc was on call that night. He instructed me to be at his office when it opened the following day.

Sleeping that night was nearly impossible. A little bit of drama, a little bit of panic, a shot of steroids, and plenty of morbid thoughts. I arrived thirty minutes before time for the office to open. As I sat there and reflected on everything, it hit me. It was a steroid shot that had reduced the inflammation in my throat. For the last month, the sack of gravel seemed to be getting fuller. This was the same time I was weaning off the prednisone, lowering my dosage in small steps.

Prednisone is a steroid that reduces inflammation. That is why it is the go-to drug for polymyalgia rheumatica. This means when I stopped the prednisone, the tonsils revealed how bad they really were. I was anxious to speak with the doctor and tell him my diagnosis. When I did, he chuckled and said, "I believe you nailed it!"

He instructed me to get back on prednisone until I was able to have my surgery in a couple of weeks. No need to worry—I was definitely getting back on the prednisone, regardless of the tonsils. I had to call my boss, like I had every time. I was transparent and shared what had happened over the past eighteen hours. My boss was always very understanding and caring. I just hated to keep sending up red flags that might make him wonder if I was capable and dependable. I had shared several of my Sagittarius traits with him over the years. Hopefully, he knew how true they rang for me.

That afternoon I had an appointment with my blood doctor, Dr. Famoyin. It was a great visit, as usual. It was unfortunate to see how the COVID-19 pandemic had hurt his business. He saw me and took me back before the nurse even checked me in! I had graduated to quarterly visits, so we didn't see one another as often as the old days. Though it was unfortunate that business was slow, it was great to spend thirty minutes chatting. I would have loved to sit with him at a bar for six hours, drinking beer and talking about everything in the world.

That day we covered topics from business to God, with my health mixed in the middle. So, Dr. Famoyin diagnosed my sleep apnea. He was perplexed at the same time because I didn't fit the profile for sleep apnea. When I told him the story of my hospital visit and the realization of what the unintended benefit of prednisone had been, he was beyond amused. It was like Vanna White turning the hidden blocks around to solve the puzzle on Wheel of Fortune. He lit up and began to talk about how everything was tied together.

I responded with, "Like a domino effect?"

He said, "Exactly. It is all a domino effect."

Dr. Famoyin spoke about how God created such a brilliant human body and how everything influences it. Even space. I understood his comment about space. I remembered a documentary about twin brothers. One of them went into space, and the other stayed on earth. It was a study on the impact gravity has on the human body, or the lack of gravity's impact. A Year in Space is a two-part series adapted from TIME's original digital video series about astronaut Scott Kelly, whose 12-month stay on the International Space Station (ISS) tested human limits for space travel and set the groundwork for a manned mission to Mars.

Scott and Mark Kelly were gathered and recruited by NASA to see what the effects of space were and what the potential for changes were if one of them spent a long time in space. Both twin brothers accepted and decided that Scott should be the one to make the space journey. He was sent to the International Space Station for a year while Mark stayed on the ground.

NASA wanted to determine how DNA is affected after spending an extended period of time living in space. There's actual knowledge about physical changes that humans can suffer while being up there, but nothing related to the changes genes go through after spending several months under the effects of a zero-gravity environment.

"Some of the most exciting things that we've seen from looking at gene expression in space are that we really see an explosion, like fireworks taking off, as soon as the human body gets into space," said investigator Chris Mason. "With this study, we've seen thousands and thousands of genes change how they are turned on and turned off. This happens as soon as an astronaut gets into space."

People going to space for a short period usually come back with their spine stretched, muscles shrunk, and their sleep cycle changed. But the effects of long-term exposure had not been wholly assessed before.

While in space, Scott's methylation was much higher than his brother Mark's.

Methylation is a metabolic process that occurs with every cell and organ in the body. It is vital.

This might be because Scott was in an environment where there was barely gravity, so his body had to adjust to it radically. Scott also sent information about his telomeres, which are the caps at the end of chromosomes. According to the scientists, these were longer while he was in space, but then they returned to normal after Scott returned to Earth.

Once we finished our conversation about space, I asked the doctor about my polymyalgia rheumatica. I had read additional material and found the published symptoms perfectly aligned with mine.

I asked him point blank, "Do I have this because of my cancer?"

Without hesitation, he said, "Yes."

From there he explained things in understandable detail for me. This is what I learned. Our immune system is what keeps us alive. Without it, we would surely die soon after we are born. When I developed cancer, my immune system kicked into high gear and created an army to fight the cancer. It is not until the cancer overwhelms the immune system army that it becomes detectable.

"My immune system army fought my cancer for five years before it was discovered. That's all because I was too busy working to have blood drawn once a year. Had it not been prostate cancer, my army would surely have been defeated, and so would I."

My immune system had been on the front lines, fighting this cancer for years. Then, one day, the prostate was removed, along with most (my opinion) of the cancer. This was followed by thirty-eight days of radiation to kill most of the rest (except those really mean cells). In a short period of time, the war was over for my immune system special forces. However, I had amassed quite the army, and they were not going to just quit. So, they turned on me.

The army attacked Mr. Skeleton relentlessly, as though he had fallen drunkenly into a bed of angry red ants. Just as quickly as an accidental crash into the ant hill, I awoke one morning with the army attacking my joints and no prior warning. In a brief moment of time, I went from regular ole me to Mr. Skeleton, a pile of bones under an inexorable assault. *The foot bone's connected to the leg bone. The leg bone's connected to the knee bone. The knee bone's connected to the thigh bone. The thigh bone's connected to the backbone. The backbone's connected to the neck bone.* And on went the childhood song that taught us about Mr. Skeleton's anatomy.

The ants cared not. They were only there to bring pain. Mr. Skeleton was once again consumed with the purveyors of suffering.

This was the onset of an autoimmune disorder. This attack had been merciless on my body. "It couldn't kill the cancer, but it felt like it was killing me." This raised my SED rate and my CRP, my inflammation markers. It is still unknown if my rheumatoid factor was a false reading due to my radiation. But that is likely the case.

So, I explained to the good doctor, "I am afraid of staying on the prednisone. I am afraid of what it is doing to my bones." I didn't mention how I wanted my girly figure back too!

I quoted Dr. Channeler again and expressed that I did not want to add insult to injury by being on the prednisone too long. In return, I got a new Famoyinism (that is my new nickname for the wise and comforting sayings he shares).

"How do you feel when you do not take your prednisone?"

I responded honestly, "I am miserable and in pain. It limits my ability to function and sleep."

He continues, "Then why are you worried about tomorrow? If tomorrow will only bring you pain and misery, then live for today and take your medicine." He continued, "I am sure you have done your homework and you are taking calcium and vitamin D3, right?"

"Yes," I answered. "I take twelve hundred units of calcium to facilitate absorption of the D3 and five thousand units of the D3."

"Of course, you do," was the response. That comment made me proud, like a teacher complimenting the work of his student.

He continued, "Take 5 mg a day and work your way down to where you are taking the lowest dose without symptoms. If you get to 1 mg a day without symptoms, then you may be ready to stop. Until then, take what you need. As long as you are taking calcium and D3, you have no worries about the prednisone at 5 mg per day or less. Live for today. We aren't promised tomorrow anyway."

I felt like a ten-ton brick had been lifted from me. It all made sense now. I would take 5 mg a day of prednisone until after my surgery. Then, I would find the lowest dosage without symptoms and work from there. One day, my immune system army would retreat.

"Unless those mean cancer cells are still hiding and waiting for the testosterone to come back and feed them. Then the army will be called to return and fight another day, but hopefully not in Mr. Skeleton."

The lyrics and music to this song were perfect for this period in my life. They spoke to my feelings and were also a release mechanism for my anger and frustration.

TEN-TON BRICK

Hurt 2007

Written by Perry Muse

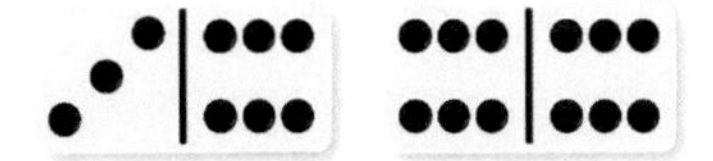

Chapter 21

ANOTHER BRACELET

A Sagittarius seeks truth, beauty, and wisdom, and the only way he can find these ideals is to travel, meet others, and ask some soul-searching questions.

On March 12, 2020, President Trump issued another travel ban, this time from Europe. Two days later, there was another travel ban from the United Kingdom and Ireland.

I was finally called to schedule my fifteenth surgery for Friday, May 22, 2020. I was ready.

I answered a call from the doctor's office three days before my surgery.

Aside from getting all of the normal preoperative information, I got an unexpected directive.

"And you must have a negative COVID-19 test before the surgery," the female nurse said on the other end of my phone. "You must bring the results in writing the morning of the surgery."

"Wait, what?" I asked.

She repeated herself. "Yes, you must have written proof of a negative COVID test on Friday."

I see, I thought. I could figure that out, right? In three days? Sure, I told myself.

It was not as hard as I thought to find a COVID test, and I knew I needed to get the test taken care of as soon as possible. I made an appointment and showed up on time at Mountain Forest Hospital; I followed the signs originally intended for "Ambulances Only." This was just a few weeks after the earth stood still, and everything changed. I donned my mask and presented my credentials upon arrival.

The test consisted of some of the same verbal questions that had become common during the worldwide pandemic. I must test negative in order to be accepted for my surgery on the twenty-second. I felt as though I needed to be negative in order to stay alive. I had been a good boy and worked from home. I rarely got out, and when I did, I wore gloves and a mask to protect myself and others.

The test was quite invasive. To say it was uncomfortable would be an understatement. It was downright painful.

Throughout my life, I've had many accidents that inflicted more than minor injuries.

One time when I was six or seven years old, I was playing behind the neighbor's house with a friend. They had collected a lot of wooden planks that had come from tearing down another house. The long wooden planks had been thrown into a pile. For young boys, this was an invitation to find creative playtime.

The planks were quite long and had bent, rusty nails that protruded. We were oblivious to those. Our game involved standing on one end of a plank while the other person jumped on the opposite end, like a seesaw. This would launch us into the air. The ill-advised plan was to see who could land on their feet on the ground beside the pile. If I had been able to foresee the future and what my ankles would endure later on, I might have thought better about playing this game.

After a couple of times of being catapulted, it got boring. It was my turn to launch. I stood ready and had picked out my landing spot. This time, we decided to increase the challenge. My friend jumped from the nearby porch.

It was a perfect shot and propelled me skyward. This was perhaps my first time flying! However, I was not in control of my body or my destination as I had been in previous turns.

I did not land on the ground as originally planned. The extra propulsion eliminated my body's ability to control its destination. Instead, I landed on one of the planks that had a large L-shaped nail protruding. Oh yeah, we were barefooted.

The nail penetrated the inside of my left foot, right at the ball of the foot, and directly behind my big toe. As I fell from lack of balance, the point of the bent nail worked its way around and sprouted out an inch away from entry. I was hooked.

Chaos set in and my friend ran, yelling and screaming into his house. I was enthralled by what I saw in my foot. His father arrived on the scene quickly.

"Go tell his mother," he ordered his son. Meanwhile, he ran into a small building not far away.

"Stay still and don't move," he told me as he ran off.

He returned with a handsaw. The nail was located close to the corner of the plank.

"Hold on to me and try not to move," he said. I grabbed tight to his leg with both hands. He began to frantically saw back and forth.

It was a minute or it was an hour; time stretched into eternity as the pain in my foot seemed to beat in rhythm with my heart and the steady pull and push of the saw. It echoed in my head as loud as gunfire; I could hear nothing but the saw and the beating of my heart, which was now centered in my foot. Finally, the corner of the plank was cut loose, and it was now attached only to me by a large, bent, rusty nail.

My friend's father picked me up and hurriedly got me to the car. I remember my mom and sister being upset as I was loaded into the back seat of our car.

My sister Gail accompanied me in the back while Mom drove. All of the excitement was like a whirlwind around me. It was almost like a dream.

At the hospital, they put shots in my foot to numb it. At this point, the pain was radiating from my foot into my leg. Once my foot was numb, the doctor used a scalpel and made an incision from the nail's entry point to the exit. Then he slid the corner of the plank, and the nail, out of my foot.

The incision was washed out and stitched up. I also received a tetanus shot. The shot was given to prevent tetanus infection, which is caused by Clostridium tetani bacteria.

During the whole event, I never really felt the pain of the nail physically passing through my foot. I realize now that adrenaline kept me from feeling most of that pain. It was the same when I had my motorcycle accident, and I was lying on the roadside, barking orders to Nila after tumbling a hundred and ninety-two feet along the asphalt.

Adrenaline is great. I wish we could use that for pain relief. But when the nurse administered my COVID test, there was no adrenaline. And when she inserted the cotton-tipped swab deep into my nasal cavity, I felt plenty of pain.

"Errrrrr-ooowwww!" was my response.

I felt as though she had penetrated the nasal cavity and reached brain matter. My eyes poured water, and I squirmed at the discomfort. I had all I could tolerate and reached for her arm. But she withdrew the swab before I could make my move. The test was over.

I tested negative, and the long-awaited surgery was finally going to happen.

The morning of May 22, 2020, finally arrived. It was a Friday morning, and, as with previous surgeries, I liked this day of the week, so I could have a couple of days to recover before the work week resumed.

We arrived at the familiar surgery center, but now there were new protocols.

There were instructions on a sign: "When you arrive, stay in your vehicle and call this number."

A few minutes later, the nurse came out to meet me. Nila was given written instructions, and I was taken away. This time Nila would have to wait for me in the car. I really hated that she would be stuck waiting in the car for so long. She had the option of leaving, and they would call her. But Nila wasn't about to do that.

I was taken back to a room and issued another stylish open-backed gown to put on.

After I was in the bed, dressed in my gown, the nurse started to work on getting me comfortable.

"Would you like some heat?" she asked.

"Absolutely," I replied. She slipped the heater beneath the covers, and I felt the comforting warm air start to blow.

"Can you tell me your name and date of birth?" the nurse asked, business-like. After I answered her question with information that matched the chart she held, she placed an identification bracelet onto my wrist.

IV time was next.

"This is the one everyone usually settles on," I told her after she had gotten out all of the tools for starting an IV. I pointed to my arm. "This is everyone's favorite vein."

"We will see about that," she said, looking at my arm like a cat closing in on a small mouse. She moved her tray closer.

"Make a fist," she said, knotting a piece of rubber around my arm as she felt the skin I had shown her. "Hold your fist tighter," she said, feeling my arm some more, "Yes, this is a good one." And in a few seconds, my IV started with very little trouble on her part or mine.

I had offered her the proffered arm and advice to minimize the chances of multiple tries and what came with the repeated efforts, namely bruises all over me.

"Do you know what you are having done today?" the nurse inquired.

I answered, "Yes, a tonsillectomy and adenoidectomy; plus, he is going to remove a sack of gravel."

The nurse's face was perplexed by the last part of my answer, but she didn't ask me to elaborate.

"Doc has to remove the sack of gravel so I don't suffocate from it blocking my airway every five seconds when I sleep. I had to get my bracelet here. The other nearby medical center doesn't deal with sacks of gravel," I thought to myself with a grin.

I was given something in my IV to relax me. I was a veteran of surgeries and knew we were about to go to the operating room. I didn't allow myself to go to sleep, as was the usual plan. I wanted to experience all that was happening while getting fried before the surgery. I terribly missed getting to see Nila before making the trip down the hall to where the surgery would take place.

We entered the chilly operating room, and a new heating hose was placed beneath my blanket. I felt comfortable and without anxiety. The anesthesiologist finally placed a mask over my face and asked that I take some deep breaths. Meanwhile, the knockout drug was injected into the port of my IV.

I fought as long as I could. My soul seemed to leave my body, but not the room. I recall seeing Dr. Zajonc, but I did not understand his communications with some of the others in the room. Immediately after, I was comfortably numb, and the lights went out in my mind.

Tonsillectomies and adenoidectomies are surgical procedures to remove the tonsils and adenoids. The tonsils and adenoids are masses of immune cells, like the ones found in lymph glands. They are located in the mouth, behind the nasal passages.

If the tonsils or adenoids become infected or enlarged, they can cause a host of problems. Some of the recurrent problems are sore throat, bad breath, or upper airway obstruction that, in turn, causes difficulty breathing.

As with most surgeries, my oxygen saturation was constantly monitored by a pulse oximeter and a continuous heart monitor.

The tonsils and adenoids were removed through my mouth, with no external incisions. The tonsils and adenoids were burned at the base with an electric cauterizing unit. The surgery took just over one hour.

Recovery from the anesthetic took a couple of hours longer than some previous surgeries.

"Between the anesthesia and the electric cauterizing machine, I really did get fried this time," I later thought.

I awoke to not being able to see Nila in recovery. I missed her immediately and felt guilty, thinking of her sleeping for hours in the parking lot.

The nurse went out and gave Nila verbal and written instructions for my home care.

- *When the patient arrives home, he should immediately go to bed.*
- *Rest with the head elevated, using two to three pillows.*
- *Once the patient has recovered fully from the anesthetic, and if tolerable, a light and cool diet is recommended.*
- *The patient may be hungry. It is best to feed slowly to prevent nausea and vomiting.*
- *Weight loss is common.*
- *Avoid hot liquids for several days.*
- *The patient must drink plenty of fluids to prevent bleeding and dehydration. Although it may be very difficult to drink, the patient will have less pain overall.*

Nila was informed that there was more to the surgery than originally anticipated. The tonsils and adenoids had been removed as planned. The sack of gravel had come out as well. But the doctor noted my uvula was also enlarged. Therefore, Dr. Zajonc had removed most of it. It was a good call. Besides, it's not as if he could have woken me up and gotten my opinion.

The uvula is the teardrop-shaped piece of soft tissue that hangs down the back of your throat. It's made from connective tissue, saliva-producing glands, and some muscle tissue. When you eat, your soft palate and uvula prevent foods and liquids from going up your nose.

So, the nurse helped me into a wheelchair, and Nila was waiting outside at the front door. I was grateful for the warmer conditions, compared to the snowy day we'd left UMC after getting some of my breath back.

The routine was the same at home. Nila helped me make my way to the recliner, and we were met by Sparky. I immediately thought of Mr. Mitten and missed him.

Although Mr. Mitten and Sebastian were no longer with us, we had a new Saint Bernard puppy named Hooch. He was eight months old at the time of my surgery and a tad rambunctious. I was grateful to have family staying with us to keep Hooch away. It was also good medicine to have the occasional visit from our granddaughter.

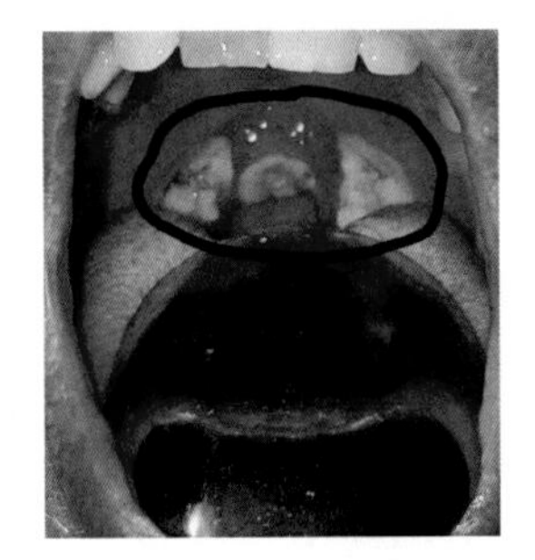

Visible scabs in throat after surgery

At home, I asked Nila to take a picture of the inside of my mouth. It was very difficult. I used a spoon to hold my tongue down. In the back of my throat were now three white patches where the cauterizing unit had burned my throat after Dr. Zajonc removed my tonsils, adenoids, and a portion of my uvula.

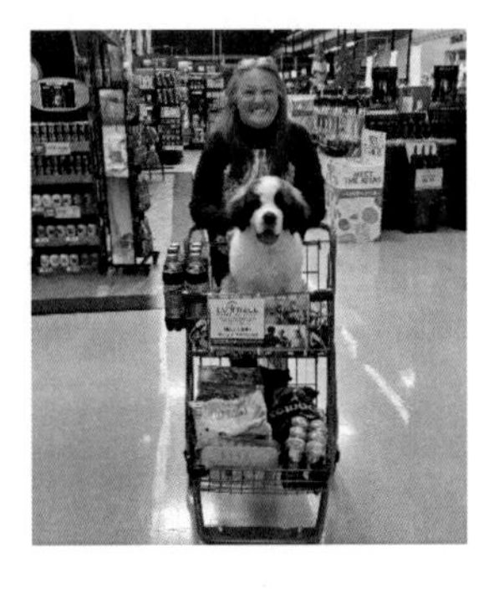

Nila with Hooch at eight weeks old

After taking the picture, I asked Nila for my phone. I needed to catch up on Friday's emails before going back to sleep.

The first night after surgery went pretty well. I chose to sleep in the recliner instead of wearing my CPAP mask. The next morning, I was so hungry. I took my medications, and swallowing was a bit more of a challenge, but not as bad as expected.

"If this keeps up, I will be doing pretty well by Monday," I thought. My mind began to plan as though it were going to be the case.

Eating Jell-O didn't do anything for my appetite, and I stayed hungry. By the evening of the second day, the pain was more pronounced, and even water was difficult to swallow.

I wanted to be ready for work the following day, so I went to bed. I thought it would be an escape from hunger and the pain. Nila stacked the pillows. I slipped on my CPAP mask and quickly fell asleep.

At midnight, I awoke to a very dry mouth and throat. I was in significant pain. I recalled the smiley face emoji and didn't want to let the pain get out of control. I grabbed a bottle of water and tried to drink.

I was immediately overcome with excruciating pain. I was in so much pain that I couldn't bear to swallow my pill or the water that would wash it down. But I had to. As I swallowed the large pills and accompanying water, the pain quickly registered as a number ten emoji.

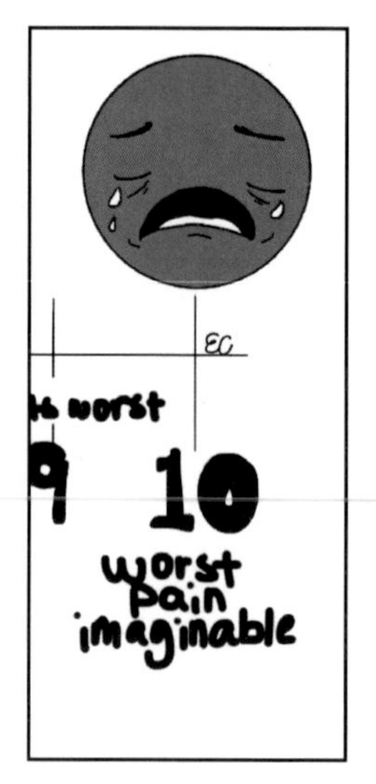

Drawing by Ezekial Cooper

I imagined the water rushing past the cauterized sores in my throat like a river, the pills bouncing around like a piece of wood or debris and hitting each of the sores on the way. I was moaning aloud and began crying.

"What have I done?" I cried aloud. "I must have ripped the scabs loose. I can feel it on the back of my tongue," I thought. "I think I can taste blood!"

The instructions said I needed to stay well hydrated to reduce the pain. I didn't understand how I could do so *because* of the pain.

I'm not sure how long the episode lasted, but after twenty minutes, the pain medication started to kick in. I was overcome with exhaustion from the experience. I found my way back to the recliner and fell asleep.

Monday came, and I found myself struggling to do the minimum amount needed to stay on top of what was going on at work. Don't misunderstand; it was never required of me from my boss. It was required of me from myself.

I was still famished by Monday afternoon and decided to "man up," although I wasn't feeling like much of a man at all.

I asked for some cream of chicken in a large coffee cup. Nila made sure it was diluted with the right amount of water for me to drink. Although the warmth of the cup felt good on my hands, the warmth of the soup was not well received by my throat.

"What are you thinking? When you burn your fingers, you know warm water only adds insult to injury," I reminded myself.

After the first try, I learned to let it cool to room temperature before taking my first sip.

As the week progressed, I found it easier to tolerate my condition throughout the day. It was difficult to talk. It was a vicious cycle. But the days were getting better. I did feel something hanging from the back of my throat, and Nila visually verified it was there. For me, it was just another annoyance in an already tough situation.

The nights were the worst. I tried sleeping in the recliner. Something about lying in the bed created a lot more pain for me. I didn't have the motivation to do any homework. But, after a few hours, I was restless. My breathing was as though the sack of gravel was still there. My hips and shoulders were getting sore. So, I headed for the bed.

I timed it to where it would be right on the cycle for taking my pain medication. I swallowed the pills and water, grimaced, and held my eyes tightly shut. After ten seconds or so, I put on my mask and got in bed.

Regardless of my routine, I was getting the same result at night when I tried to sleep. A result that was now vastly different from any other time during the day. I would wake up three hours after taking my pills. My throat and mouth would be parched. I would grab a bottle of water and try to drink. Excruciating pain! Alas, it would be another hour before I could take anything for pain. But the pain was already there. I can only describe it as a burning sensation like I had eaten some spicy Thai food and the acidic pepper juice had soaked into my throat scabs, finding refuge from the water that was trying to flush it away. My throat was still on fire, as though being cauterized without being comfortably numb, still burning, yet I was not anesthetized. Every night it was ten. Every night I cried.

Finally, toward the end of the first week following surgery, it hit me suddenly, and I understood the problem. I hadn't understood at first because of the pain throughout the day. You see, I was able to consume copious amounts of cream of chicken, with minimal pain, during the day, but it was always the night that brought on the harvester of pain.

"The CPAP is blowing so hard, and I no longer have a sack of gravel," I thought. "The heated air and the velocity are drying out my scabs. When I wake up and try to drink, I am cracking them apart. That's why I taste blood. That's what lights my wounds on fire. That's why I cry like a little girl."

The next day, one full week after surgery, I contacted the place where I had been issued my sleep machine. I explained the situation in great detail. The machine had a SIM card, and they were able to remotely see all of the data. It was how they could tell if the machine was being used as prescribed. If not, the insurance company might send out a hefty bill.

But after the explanation, I was disappointed to hear their response.

"Mr. Muse, it looks like you haven't been using your device the way you should. We show you to be at less than 50 percent usage for the week," they informed me.

"I just got another bracelet, lady. Didn't you hear a thing I said?" I thought angrily.

I calmly explained again.

"Sir, I'm having a hard time hearing you. Could you speak up?" she asked.

I maintained my composure and said, "Ma'am, I just had throat surgery. Could you please adjust the temperature and velocity of my machine down?" I calmly asked. "I no longer have a blockage, but I do have three sores, and the air is drying them out and causing so much pain that I cannot wear my mask."

"I'm sorry to hear that," replied the voice on the other end of the call. "You will have to make an appointment with the pulmonary doctor who prescribed the machine, and he will need to notify us of any changes to the machine's settings or ranges."

At that point, I was in a no-win situation. COVID made it difficult to get an appointment within a reasonable time. I still had swelling that caused some obstruction to my airway. I needed the machine but wasn't going to cry over it anymore.

I had high hopes for the second week following surgery. The first week seemed to last an eternity. However, my body had other plans.

I revisited the paperwork that Nila had been given before coming home. According to the document, "At one week following surgery, patients will often appear to relapse when their pain becomes significant again. They usually report pain in the ears, especially when they swallow. The scabs are often falling off at this time. If bleeding is going to occur, this is the most common time. This is usually the last time pain will be experienced. Overall, most patients will have recovered fully by two weeks after surgery. However, the patient will occasionally have throat tenderness with hot or spicy foods for up to six weeks postoperatively."

"ERRRRRRR," I thought as I read. "Not another week."

Then, I remembered the guy in the waiting room at "Radiation Treatment LN231." I felt guilty for complaining, knowing he had been going through esophageal cancer and radiation treatments.

"Stop whining. It's not like you have throat cancer. At least you aren't having to get very high radiation for your sack of gravel," I humbly thought.

As the scabs began to come loose, the pain and challenges mounted. Now, the tiny chunks of chicken in the soup acted as though they were made from abrasive materials sliding across the scabs and fresh surface beneath. I was hungry, but not enough to endure the pain associated with eating. I was back to Jell-O and liquids.

It constantly irritated me to feel the scabs dangling in my throat. I watched the clock and counted the hours. Meanwhile, I kept up with emails daily and sat in on conference calls from work. Since talking was a struggle, I would just text comments during the call. Everyone was quite understanding, and the system kept me involved.

By the end of the second week, Nila was taking me to work. I had retired the prescription medications several days prior. I was weak due to a lack of real food, but I was tired of riding the recliner. I needed to be at the plant, but chose not to stay long. Considering COVID, the chemicals, and my throat not being 100 percent, I had to make my visits abbreviated.

After two weeks, the scabs were gone. I had my follow-up visit with Dr. Zajonc and was released with an A+ report. He exited the room with the usual "God bless you." Then, I made my way to see Dr. Ebeo. He immediately understood my situation and ordered the needed changes to my CPAP. It is truly unfortunate that it had to be after the time I needed it most.

Prior to surgery, the velocity range on my CPAP was seven to seventeen. Nowadays it never goes above 6.5.

I survived my fifteenth surgery, but not without pain and struggle. I had several consecutive nights of living through the bright red, number ten pain emoji, and crying in the middle of the night. I lost my tonsils, adenoids, and a sack of gravel, but I got another bracelet for my collection.

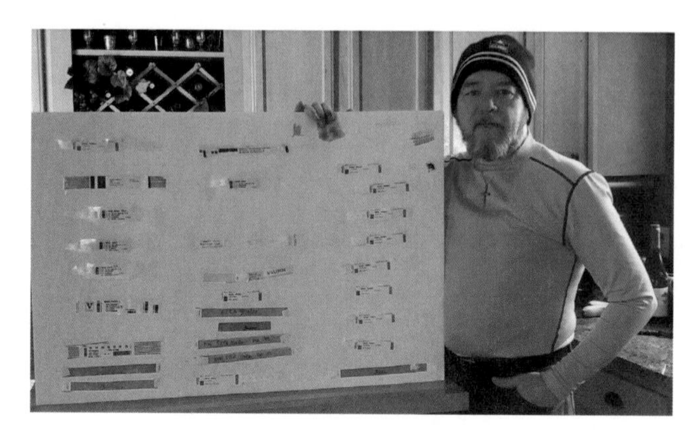

Bracelets collected as of May 2020

I fought the morbid thoughts, the negative feelings, and the negative emotions through everything in my life. Cancer was difficult to a whole new level. But I am an optimist. Lyrics like the one for this song often put me back on offense.

THE COMEBACK

Danny Gokey 2017

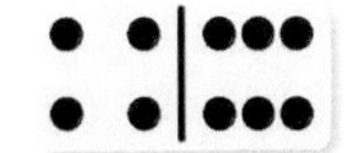 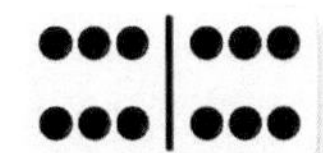

Chapter 22

THE BONUS ROUND PART I

Sagittarians are levelheaded and intelligent. They think ten steps ahead of everyone else, and that's why they are very difficult to fool.

September 10, 2020

I had been "cancer free" since June 5, 2019. Remember, that was the day Dr. Taha looked at my lab results and declared it to be so.

"Congratulations," he said, "Your PSA is <.014, which means it is undetectable. You are cancer free!"

From there he posed with me for a picture to go alongside the many on his wall. For this picture, I did not crop myself out but happily posed. I was one step closer to making the Tree of Life.

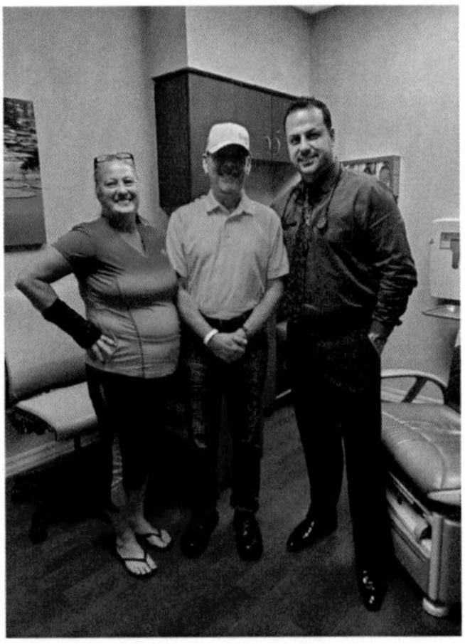

Cancer-free picture with Nila and Dr. Taha

But we all know "free doesn't always mean free." In my mind, I still struggled with the predictions from Dr. Channeler. Since that day, I had occasionally had a little too much wine and allowed my morbid thoughts to be spoken aloud.

I would mutter, "I still believe I will die from prostate cancer one day. I know that when my Lupron shots stopped, my testosterone began to rise. Once it reaches a certain point, it will begin to feed those mean cells that were immune to radiation. It will be like rain falling and seeping into the ground during a spring shower, the water feeding a dormant bulb and bringing it to life again in the flower bed."

When I first heard that I was "cancer free," I began to think of how I could do more giving. I felt like paying it forward somehow.

I was already doing a lot of visits to the VA mental health and elopement wards with Sebastian. Nila and I had sponsored a young girl from Indonesia for years. When we started, she was four, and now she was a teenager.

I wasn't sure what else I could find time to do. I just knew it was important to do more. I now knew my life was full of blessings and had always been full of blessings, yet most of my life I had been too selfish to realize that everything was a blessing from God, not something I created.

Back in October 2019, the feeling of extreme fatigue came back. The physician assistant that I saw felt it was allergies. I had some nasal drainage and fluid in my left ear.

I was prescribed Cetirizine and Flonase, medications used to relieve seasonal and year-round allergic and non-allergic nasal symptoms, such as stuffy or runny nose, itching, and sneezing. They can also help relieve allergy eye symptoms such as itchy, watery eyes.

The medications helped some of the symptoms, but after a few weeks, the fatigue was dramatically worse. It was time to see Dr. Famoyin.

He walked into the exam room.

I didn't wait for the door to close behind him.

"My iron must be low," I stated.

"Why do you feel this to be so?" asked Dr. Famoyin.

"Well, one example is an important conference call. I was the lead on the call that occurred just after lunch recently. Also on the call were our plant manager, our chemist, my boss, and the president of the company that we were trying to secure some very new business with. I was sitting at my desk at 12:53 p.m., just seven minutes before the call. During that time, I fell asleep three times and had three completely different dreams. The third and final time I awoke at 12:59 p.m., one minute before the call."

"That does sound like unusual fatigue," Dr. Famoyin said. "We will run some blood work again."

My blood work came back good on iron, so I felt something else must be going on. I was beginning to feel sure the cancer had returned with a vengeance. For once, a positive voice surfaced—prostate cancer is the slowest-developing form of cancer.

Then my negative voice piped up: "I must have developed a new cancer. This time it is stronger and already knocking me out."

I was sleeping almost any hour I wasn't working. I even had to get Nila to help me sometimes with transportation because I would be too tired to drive. I could easily sleep two to three hours after work, wake up, eat, go to bed, and sleep ten to twelve hours before getting up and starting over. I would sleep longer, but work was super important.

It was getting up and going that was nearly impossible. I was also bringing my dosage down on the prednisone, so I was losing that false energy it gave me. I got down to 3 mg a day before the inflammation returned in a way that began to limit my ROM and cause me pain. For that reason and my dire need for false energy, I went back to 5 mg.

Then, I started buying 5-Hour Energy shots again. I chose 5-Hour Energy because there was no sugar, no calories, the amount of caffeine in a single cup of coffee, and B vitamins. Nothing more. There were no jitters and no crash after having one.

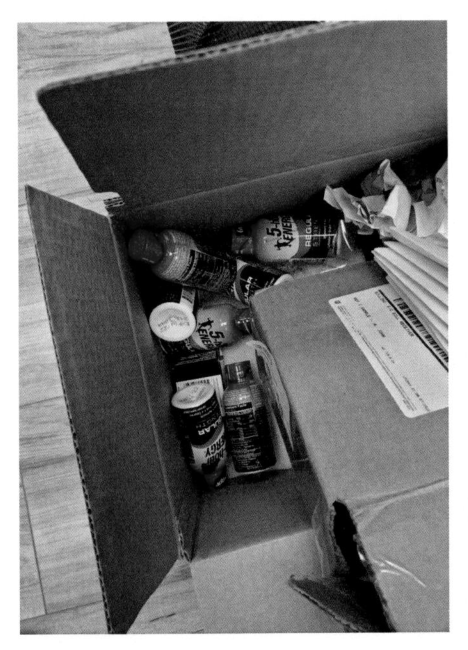

TN Office

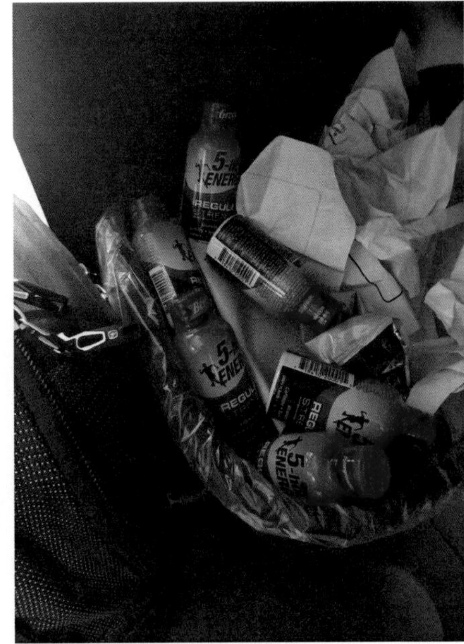

GA Office

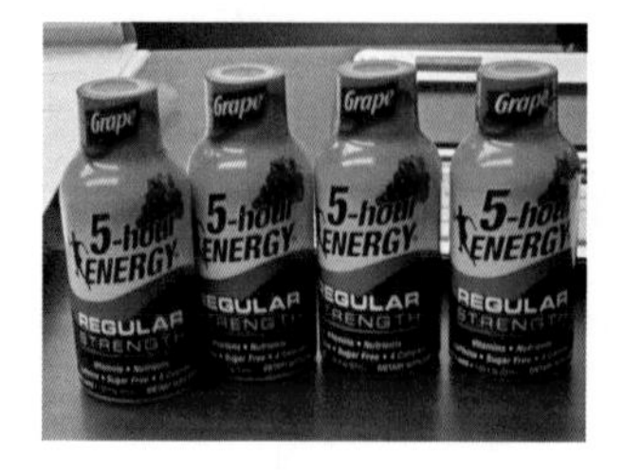

Desk

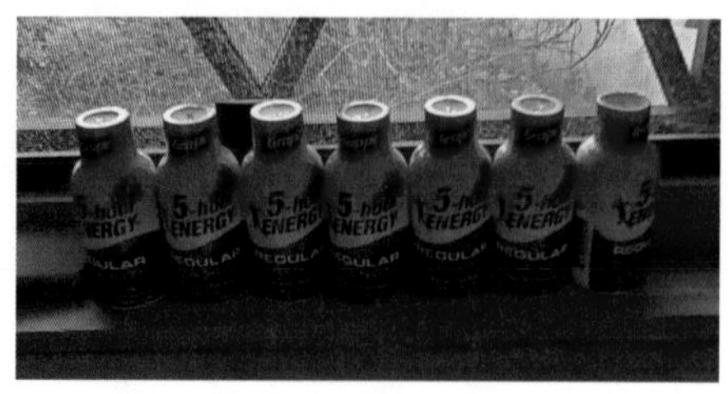

Home

It had all come back, but this time it was kicking my butt worse. I had to figure this out. If it was cancer, time was a-wasting.

"I don't feel like doing anything about it, but that's how it gets you."

Once Dr. Famoyin told me my iron was fine, he had me schedule a follow-up appointment. He told me to be sure to have him copied on the bone scan results that we scheduled. Bone scans will be a part of the routine for the rest of my life.

I went home, and over the next few days, I tried to do three things:

1. Stay awake
2. Not let FPC down
3. Not lie down (see thing number one).

I needed to have time to do research and find out what was going on.

It was a tough list to maintain. By this point, I had slept more since my cancer diagnosis than at any other time in my life. That was unacceptable. I had run out of options with doctors. No one seemed to know what was happening. I was actually told once, "You have cancer; you are always going to be tired."

But how could that be if I was "cancer free"?

I listen to all genres of music. I am always changing the channel to find something that strikes me. At this time in my life, I often listened to music to keep me going. A song caught my attention. I could have written the lyrics.

ADRENALINE

Zero 9:36

My mind was in high gear. After being told I was "cancer free," I wasn't as excited as everyone around me. I kept recalling Dr. Famoyin saying, "You will never really be cancer free. You will always have the cancer tag."

As the days went on and I fought this relentless fatigue, I thought back to my thirty-eight days of radiation. I thought of the day Nila and I sat down with Dr. Channeler, and he explained my future.

"There will be some really mean cancer cells that will be immune to the radiation. After some time, you will be taken off the Lupron, and your testosterone will come back up. Those mean cancer cells will begin to grow and spread, likely into your bones. You will experience bone pain and possibly easy fracturing. At that time, you will begin treatment for prostate cancer in your bones. I will give you a 35 percent chance of living ten more years."

"That's it," I thought. "I stopped Lupron in June, and my testosterone has started feeding those really mean cancer cells, and now it has spread. Let's think about the math. He said 35 percent chance, and it has been just over two years, which is 20 percent of ten years. That leaves me just over a year!!!"

One morning I got up and took my daily dose of supplements.

Each morning, I thought, *"Why take all of these? Your cancer is back anyway."*

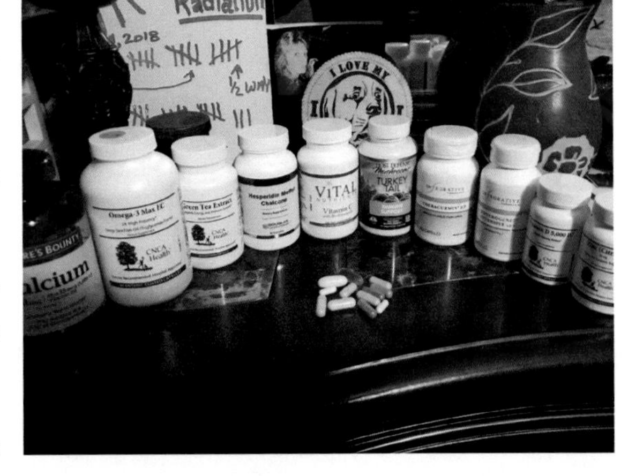

Daily supplements

But I did take them. I'm not a quitter, and the Sagittarius inside wouldn't let me. Then, I used my Flonase and started to take my allergy pill.

"Screw that. This pill hasn't done anything for me anyway," I said to myself.

Two days later I was feeling like my old self. After a week, I was over the extreme fatigue, and I was only feeling my usual tiredness from low testosterone, but that was manageable.

I wondered, was my allergy pill the cause of my extreme tiredness? I was taking cetirizine, an antihistamine that reduces the natural chemical histamine in the body. Histamines can produce symptoms of sneezing, itching, watery eyes, and a runny nose. The two most predominant side effects are unusual drowsiness and fatigue.

I went back to Dr. Famoyin and found that all of my blood lab results were in the normal range, except two items that were only out by one point. I discussed everything with the good doctor and explained how I figured out it was the cetirizine pill.

After being "cancer free" for fifteen months, all of those around me had put cancer thoughts behind them. But not me. I spent my days watching the clock, the days and weeks passing, awaiting my testosterone's rise and preparing my body for the real battle. I wouldn't say I was building a boat and preparing for the flood, but I was getting my blood, bones, and mind ready should the day arrive.

As I said before, "cancer free" is, of course, one of those psychological things one says so the patient can celebrate and stop stressing.

My last visit to SCC, just three months ago, had showed my testosterone was up to ninety. My PSA was still <.014, undetectable. I started doubting my pessimism. At ninety, I would think my PSA would have risen. Maybe those mean cells didn't exist after all.

"Could it be that I am not in the 65 percent chance of rain area? Have I spent two and a half years building a boat for nothing?"

My inflammation markers were all still elevated. I hadn't been able to see Dr. Raj, thanks to COVID and the earth standing still. I longed for the day when my PMR would vanish just as mysteriously as it had come to visit. This would be important so I could see if all three dropped back into normal range, or only my rheumatoid factor and SED rate. There is a significant difference in the outlook for a man with advanced prostate cancer if the C-reactive protein doesn't come back down. But I wouldn't know these answers until October 2020.

So, on this day, I once again made the trip down Celebration of Life Drive. My optimism was challenged by my anxiety. The days leading up to my appointments each time were very anxious, like holding a lottery ticket as the ping-pong balls labeled with numbers bounced around until, finally, one popped up. Each time the number on the ping-pong ball matched the ticket in your hand. Each time the excitement and anxiety grew.

"Five out of five so far. C'mon, give me just one more!"

I checked in as usual and made my way from Maple to the room across the hall to have blood drawn. I looked closely at my bracelet to make sure it said "Muse, Perry" and "12/19/1960." I didn't want to have Lowell Muse's bracelet on again.

"Lowell may not be on the same treatment plan as me. He may not be cancer free," I thought.

My name was called, and I went back to the private room. Once again, the nurse found everyone's favorite vein.

I had an hour to kill, so I went into the cafeteria. In the dining room, I chose a table next to a mural of a river. Mounted on the wall were plaques with names on them, the groups separated by years, starting with 2013 and through 2019. Unlike the Tree of Life, these plaques contained the names of cancer patients who had been treated for five or more years. They did not say "cancer free" as the leaves on the Tree of Life did. I wanted to be on this wall and the tree, as well.

"One year down and four to go," ran through my mind as I prepared to eat my chicken salad and fruit. The mural had replaced the Tree of Life. As I ate, I pondered the change.

"Perhaps stating 'cancer free' was rethought."

I imagined somewhere in a large boardroom was a magnificent cherry conference table, men with suits and ladies wearing dresses and high heels, conversing.

"It seems there has been some negative feedback and reaction from the families who had loved ones' names on the Tree of Life. By stating they were cancer free, it seems the shock was too great when the cancer returned, and they lost their loved one," stated the person at the head of the table. Another member, sitting farther down the table, suggested a soothing mural with plaques that replaced the words "cancer free" with the words "treated for."

I was disappointed to know I would no longer have a chance to be a leaf on the tree, celebrating being cancer free. Instead, I could only hope to live long enough to have a plaque on the wall of the lunchroom, showing how many years I fought the good fight.

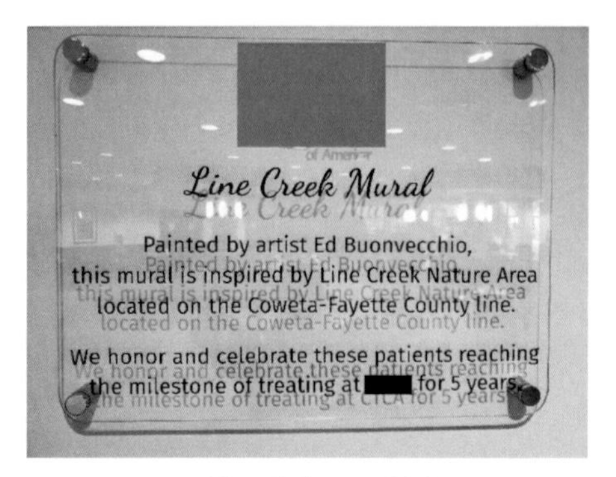

Mural plaque SCC

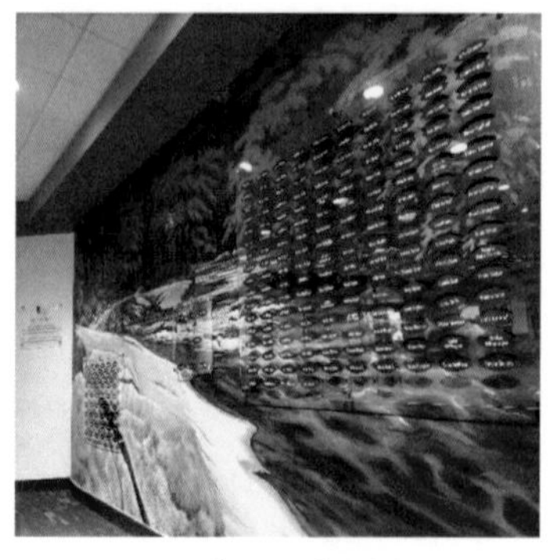

Wall mural SCC

I sat at my table and really began to miss Nila being with me even more. It's always the idle times that allow the morbid thoughts to slip in.

"If they say my cancer is back, I will just get a hotel room and go to a bar. There's no driving home alone after the 'C' bomb is dropped again."

I continued eating and looking at the names on the wall before me. The mural was probably forty feet in length. The yearly plaques were spread along its entire length. 2019 had been a good year. It had the most names of any year, by far. I was encouraged by that. The names were in alphabetical order. My eyes scrolled through the list, doubtful of seeing a name I would recognize. But I did see a familiar name. Not anyone I knew personally or had ever met. But a familiar name, nonetheless. Lowell Muse.

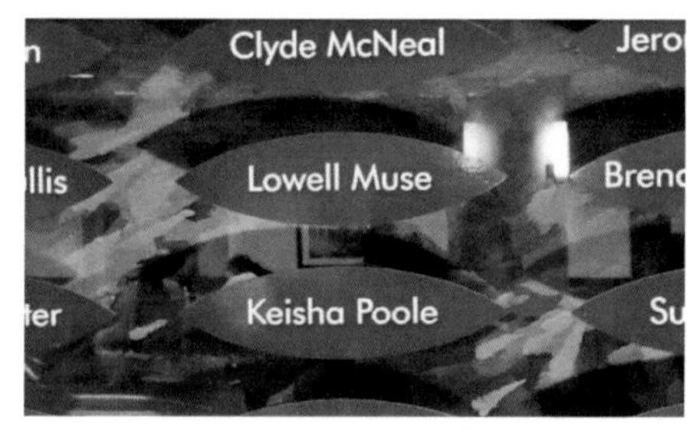

Name on mural

For whatever reason, my morbid thought turned into hope.

"What are the chances that I sat down right in front of the name of the person whose bracelet was once mistakenly given to me? Of all of the names on this wall, I sat here. Perhaps Lowell is on a good plan after all. He has already made the wall." Lowell had been fighting the good fight for over five years by then.

I finished lunch and shared the picture and story with Nila. Then, I made my way to Starbucks for my favorite: a white chocolate mocha latte. It was chilly in SCC on this day, and I needed to warm Mr. Skeleton. From there, I headed to Peaches. This was where I would find out my lab results. The closer I got, the more I missed having Nila's hand in mine and her calming voice of optimism.

Everyone sat distanced from one another, wearing their masks. It was a common sight these days. While it was difficult to read the expressions, the eyes told their story. Eyes of worry, concern, and heartfelt care for their loved ones. Eyes of fatigue and eyes of desperate hope.

My name was called, and I went back to one of the many rooms that surrounded a centralized nurse station. I looked around as I walked by, but I did not catch a glimpse of Dr. Taha. I was conflicted as to whether I wanted him to make an appearance or not.

"If Dr. Taha shows up, it will likely be bad news. News that my PSA has begun to rise. He would need to be the one to break the news, so he could answer the barrage of questions I would have," I decided.

The nurse checked my vitals and asked the routine questions. Then, she set up an iPad and said my virtual visit would start in a few minutes. As I sat in the room, I looked at each of the pictures on the wall. All of the rooms in which Dr. Taha saw patients had pictures of him and a patient that he had declared to be cancer free. I had hoped to see my picture, but it wasn't in this room.

A voice awakened me from my daydreaming-like mood. It was a physician assistant for Dr. Taha. She told me her name and welcomed me back. We went through a few questions, and then she shared my results.

"Your PSA is .054. Clinically, this is not above the level whereby cancer is scientifically considered to have returned," she reported. Then she continued, "All of your numbers look good, so keep doing what you are doing. Do you have any questions?"

"Hell, yes!" I thought. "Clinically not above? Scientifically considered? My PSA went from undetectable at <.014 to .054, and you wonder if I have questions? According to my math, that is statistically equated to a 500 percent increase!"

I immediately brought up the 500 percent increase. She did not know me well. Dr. Taha had obviously failed to tell her that I was a Sagittarius and would be well equipped to respond to the new PSA number. She had glazed over the results, but I had heard every word clearly. She wasn't aware that I had been waiting for this day to arrive since Dr. Channeler made his predictions on March 14, 2018.

"I know it's not a coincidence that my number has jumped up at the same time my testosterone has risen from <2 to one hundred and seventy," I said. "That means the testosterone is feeding some of the leftover cancer cells. What I need to know is what we do next." I was talking pretty fast, not letting her get a word in to answer my question. I just kept going. "I am writing a book on the whole experience, and I know that prostate cancer and breast cancer have a tendency to spread to the bones," I rattled off, finally out of breath with my mind still racing.

If Dr. Taha hadn't told her before, she now knew that I was a student of my condition.

She was exceedingly calm with her reply, almost clinical and detached.

"It's too soon to make those assessments. There is variation in the testing, and that is why there is a threshold number where we consider a return of cancer."

So, I stated my rebuttal: "There hasn't been any variation until now when my testosterone has risen enough to bring my cancer back to life. I am seriously concerned about my bones and, frankly, my timeline."

Once again, she replied clinically, "We can't say that has happened yet. It may not spread to your bones. It can go to your lymph nodes, for example," she explained.

Then her tone changed to a very caring and understanding one. "You need to stop worrying. That is my job. That's why they pay me the big bucks." She was kind, yet I still got the feeling she had used that line before.

"Of course, the lymph nodes," I thought. "When they removed my prostate, they removed the two closest lymph nodes. But there is a cluster of lymph nodes. The cancer may creep into a nearby lymph node before it makes its way into Mr. Skeleton."

The nurse wrapped up by telling me I would receive another shot of Prolia. As had been the case throughout my treatment at SCC, they were preparing Mr. Skeleton for a strong and painful fight. One that, if it were ever to come to fruition, he would eventually lose.

I left the room in a daze.

To be honest, I really felt as though *the* day had arrived. The day I had dreaded since early 2018. I didn't have Nurse Nila at my side, holding my hand, thanks to COVID. I would have to wait seven hours before I could get the hug that I needed now.

I went into the port room and got my shot. The staff at SCC was always upbeat and positive. I figured it was tough to face cancer patients all day, every day, and be positive. Especially when some would no longer make appointments one day. Therefore, I stuffed my feelings in my pocket, hidden, so no one could see them. When I was greeted with affirmative pleasantries, I returned them. It was the least I could do to make their jobs better.

I left the hospital and headed to my car. I couldn't begin to remember where I parked. My mind was flooded with morbid thoughts and self-pity. Once in the car, I decided that going home to get a hug from Nila was my best course. I had to spend thirty to forty-five minutes gathering myself so it would be safe for me to drive.

When I got into the car and began driving, I turned the station on Sirius XM to Tom Petty radio. It just so happened that a new Tom Petty album was going to be released in a few weeks, although he had passed away in 2017. The new album had previously unreleased songs on it. Coincidentally, the first release was making its worldwide premier. The song was called "Confusion Wheel." As I listened to the lyrics, I once again started to cry like a little girl. I pulled to the shoulder and finished listening to the song, and I cried until the tears were all used up.

We had a birthday party for one of our kids. Alanna, Cory, and a couple of their friends came by on September 13, 2020. We had to keep it small due to COVID concerns. It was that night that I pulled Alanna aside and told her the news. I didn't let the morbid guy who resides on my shoulder speak. It was upbeat, joking Dad who did the talking. But then I let down my guard and let the morbid thought slip out.

I said, "Alanna, do you remember the guy in the dream that I wrote about in my prologue?"

"Of course," she replied.

"Remember he said I was already dead, but I just hadn't finished the book yet? How dramatic of a book would it be if I finished writing it, and the dream came true?"

I immediately knew it was a mistake when I saw the scowl on her face. I had probably hurt her feelings by accident. But, like her daddy, she took a bad situation and made a great comeback.

"You promised we would go skydiving when you were one-year cancer free," she insisted.

"Well, let's book it," I said. Her eyes lit up.

"Really?" she asked in a voice that reminded me of the little girl she once was. Before we returned to the party, our skydiving was booked online.

The fact of this song playing at the time seemed more than coincidental. Tom wasn't singing to cheer me up. Instead, the lyrics were meant to tell me the truth.

CONFUSION WHEEL

Tom Petty 2020

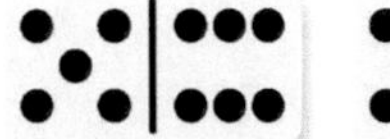 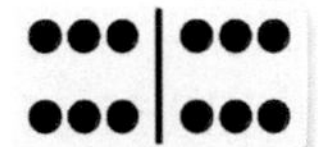

Chapter 23

THE BONUS ROUND PART II

September 13, 2020, the date of the birthday party, I made reservations to go skydiving. Seven days later, we showed up at JumpTN in Greenville, Tennessee, at the air strip. It was an exciting day. I, Alanna, and her husband, Cory, were jumping from a plane today.

I asked Nila to go with us.

Nila said, "There is no way in hell I am jumping out of a plane."

Cory's sister, Rebecca, showed up to watch.

We sat down together and watched the safety video. This amounted to the guy who invented tandem jumping talking about all of the ways you could die and how no one was responsible! It was a real morale booster.

If you don't know, tandem jumping is when an instructor wears a parachute, and a student wears a harness.

When we were there, the hangar was busy and bustling with action. Parachutes were being packed, and skydivers were falling from the sky. COVID had not slowed this business down.

Once Alanna, Cory, and I put on the harnesses, our instructors made adjustments to ensure everything was just right. My instructor took me to the back side of the hangar, where part of a cockpit sat. I followed her instructions, got in, and acclimated myself to the small area.

The videographer, whom Nila dubbed Wolverine, introduced himself, and we took pictures.

He asked, "What made you guys decide to come skydiving?"

My daughter quickly answered, "My dad has been cancer free for a year, and we are celebrating."

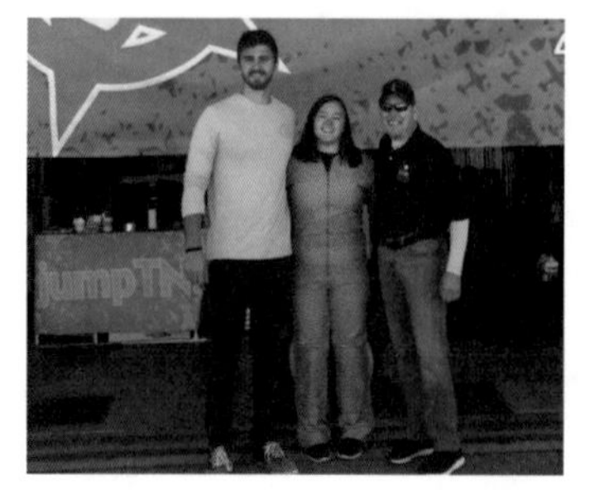

From Left: Cory Rupert, Alanna Rupert, Perry Muse

My turn finally came. Four of us loaded into the small plane. A seasoned expert was taking a free ride and sat in the open door beside the pilot. His feet were touching the back of our videographer, who was facing my instructor. I sat beside the videographer. There was no room to spare.

We took off, and I gazed outside the window. I wasn't nervous but excited. I loved the takeoff experience and being able to see the ground below in detail.

As we circled for fifteen minutes in order to get to our targeted altitude of ten thousand feet, we engaged in some small talk. I felt like I had told a little white lie about being cancer free. I struggled with it in my mind as we chatted.

The videographer pointed out various sights outside of the plane. I had taken my share of anti-inflammatory medications to ensure I would be able to function. Even so, the stiffness in my neck made it difficult to look around out of the back windows.

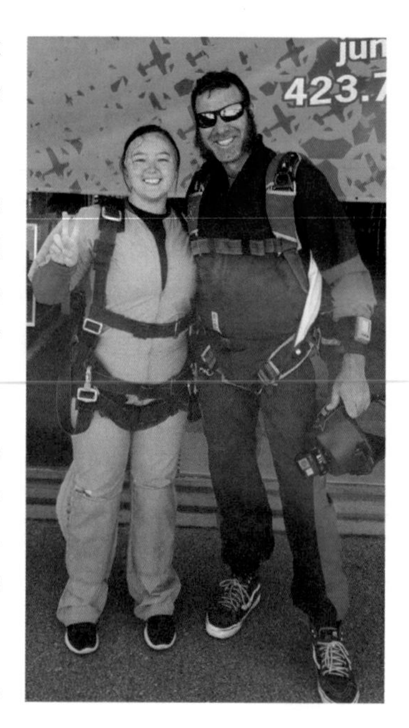

Alanna with videographer

The pilot signaled, and the door was opened. We reached altitude, and before I knew it, the seasoned hitchhiker had left the plane. The videographer slid into his spot beside the pilot. I turned and got onto my knees, facing him. It was more of a struggle than I had hoped. The ride up had been just enough time for me to rust up. The videographer was a big guy, and there wasn't much room.

The instructor proceeded to attach herself to my harness, all the while repeating the instructions from earlier.

"When he goes out of the door, walk on your knees to his spot. Once there, put your right foot out onto the step. We will rock forward and back as I count one, two, three. On three, we will jump," she instructed.

The videographer slipped out of the door. I made my way to his spot. It was awkward, being on my knees with someone attached to my back. I reached for a place to steady myself with my left hand, but I reached for the wrong place. The pilot grabbed my wrist and moved it before I latched onto some sort of lever!

Once steady, I put my right foot out, trying to place it on the small step. It was a flat silver plate that reminded me of where you place your foot when getting a shoeshine.

The wind was working against my effort.

"I don't remember it being that far away in the hangar," I thought. "I hope I don't fall out," raced through my mind. Then a little chuckle—that was exactly what I was going to do—fall out of the plane.

Once my foot was on the step, and my left knee was outside of the plane, I looked up and saw the videographer. He was horizontal to the ground, filming with one hand and hanging on to the wing's brace with the other.

Before I knew it, we were rocking. One! Two! Three! We tumbled out of the plane, and I immediately felt calm. After one or two tumbles, we were horizontal. I held my head and feet back as far as I could and formed a crescent. My arms were outstretched to each side. And there I was, flying.

The flight before the parachute opened was thirty to forty seconds. I was flying like the superhero I had pretended to be so many times as a kid living on Bluff Hill. This time, there was no towel around my neck. It was wonderful—I felt free.

Suddenly, the videographer appeared in front of us. He waved as he filmed us flying through the air. I posed for the shot, and then out came the parachute. The videographer continued his race toward the ground.

We slowly descended toward the ground. Everything was calm and quiet.

The instructor asked, "So, how was it?"

I eagerly answered, "Fantastic! I love how we tumbled and did flips coming out of the door."

With the parachute opened, we lazily floated down.

Then the instructor asked, “Do you want to control it?”

I immediately said, “Yeah!”

I took the guide cords.

The instructor said, “Pull down hard on one side if you want to do some circles.”

Um, of course I wanted to.

I pulled down on the right side, and we immediately went into a spin. It was exhilarating! After three loops, we were gliding along normally again.

The landing spot was a grassy strip between the hangar and the first runway. As we approached, I heard my number one fan cheering me.

“Legs up,” said the instructor.

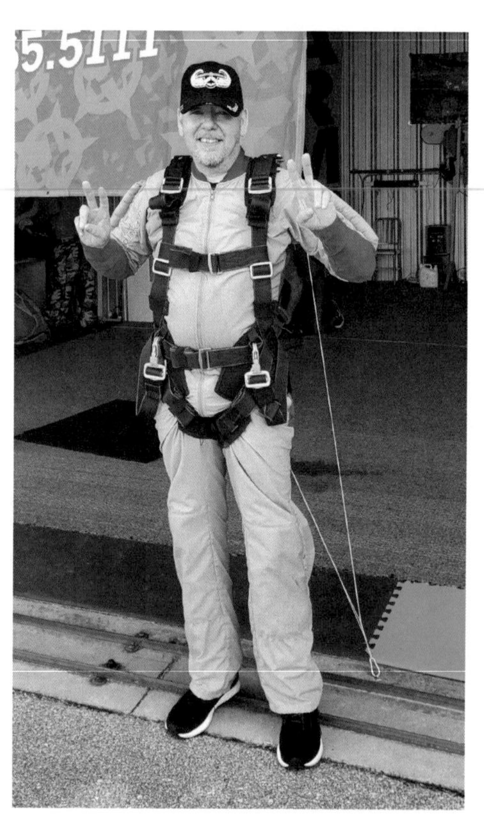

I wasn’t flexible enough to do it without grabbing my jumpsuit at the knees and pulling. My feet had to be up in the air or they would catch the ground and we would be tumbling again. I was able to get them in the correct position, and we slid on our butts to a stop.

The experience was fantastic. After watching all of us, Nila decided she wanted to try. We booked for the following weekend. When we showed up, Herb and Donna, Corey’s mom and dad, joined us as spectators. I felt humbled to have done this with my family. It meant a lot.

Perry prior to skydiving

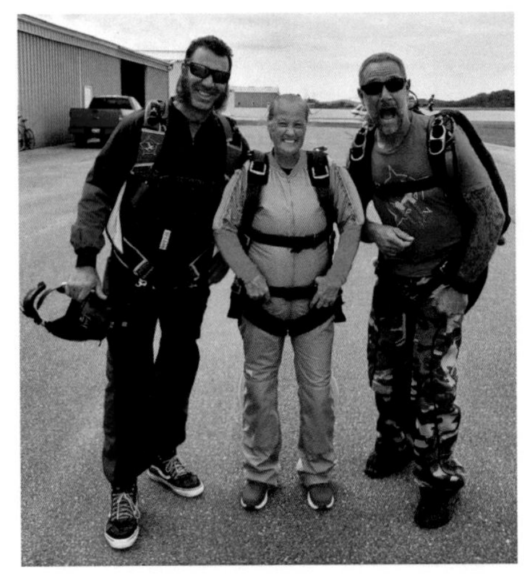

Nila prior to skydiving

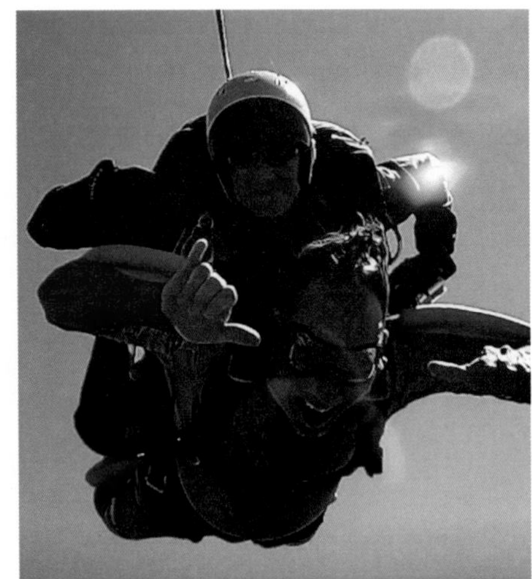

Perry flying

It was Oct 11, 2020. I had gotten blood test results from Deanna, Famoyin, and Raj. I had done so because I felt so much better in regard to inflammation. I wanted to see if all of the tests concurred with one another. They did. RF down from 200 to 3.4. SED rate down from sixty to thirty-four, with thirty being the high-end range. But CRP remained constant. This meant possible arterial issues or cancer.

Nila and I had ultrasounds at a local church (a mobile unit we had used before). All indications were good with the arteries, including the main artery running from the heart down through the abdomen. The official results would be available in another week or two, but the initial response was "no issues visible" from the technician.

I also had them check my CRP. Awaiting the results was again like holding the lottery ticket, but more like Shirley Jackson's *The Lottery*—would I be stoned to death at last? They were looking for a future heart attack in the making. But I was looking for a cancer response—still waiting for the other shoe to fall.

Once all but the aforementioned test was in (I got a call from Raj on Thursday with Labcorp results that mimicked Famoyin's), I researched everything possible about the remaining high CRP. I found it was considered an indicator of cancer that will likely be immune to chemo.

At a level of eight on the CRP lab, science says a person is 27 percent more likely not to respond to chemo. Each time that number doubles, it is another 27 percent. My number was sixty, meaning the number was doubled four times. I couldn't do radiation. Lupron, maybe. Chemo would likely be no help.

There is a test for a BRCA 1 or 2 gene mutation that supports those numbers if you test positive. To me, that would just reinforce chemo was a waste of time and money. There were experimental treatments I would be eligible for. If I were to test negative, perhaps chemo.

But my life insurance policy would run out in June 2023. I did not want to extend my "quality of life" past 2023, only to die anyway and have Nila not collect the $750,000. I believed in God. I believed suicide was a ticket to hell. So, I had a conundrum.

It had been impossible to get an estate lawyer to call me back. Evidently, the planning to die business was in high demand. I had to get this done. I had to get things in order for Nila. But they wouldn't call back, and I was feeling more like lying down to sleep than being the squeaky wheel needing grease on the attorney's voice mail.

I had been rude and angry this week. I had also been forced to do things I had no interest in my bill-paying job. For example, an important business dinner and trials. Nila got the brunt of my new test result–driven mood. I hadn't stayed home last night. I wanted to write in my book but couldn't get past the title header.

That day I went back home, skipped out on a family trip to Fenders Farm, and wrote the chapter titled "The Bonus Round." It was ironic because I had to force my way into realizing why that was still the right title.

As I worked on the chapter, I began to feel justified in writing a book called *Morbid Thoughts*. I felt like I hated Dr. Channeler although I knew he had told me the truth. If I were honest with myself, what I really hated was the cold, impersonal tone he'd used when he'd delivered his prediction. I'd accepted the news as anyone might: hurtfully. Yet I knew he didn't have doctor in his title by chance. He just had a job where he had to tell 80–90 percent of his client's good news and 10–20 percent that they were definitely going to get rain. I got it.

So I apologized to Nila and got a really, really needed hug. I sensed she was still mad, and I got that too. I explained the news to her and explained what the CRP lab results meant. Whatever I did to make up to her by apologizing was offset by my news. It was depression either way.

I remember describing to her how I had been feeling, not really trying to justify being a prick, but explaining. Pouring my heart out. Struggling to find the right words.

At one point she jumped in and said, "Depressed? It's called depression."

She was right. Sagittarians just always believe in being bigger than depression.

I texted my boss. It was the perfect time to take a couple of vacation days without letting the job slip.

When the crew returned from Fenders, I asked Nila to take me to the bar. She dropped me off, and we were all going to get together later for dinner. I needed it. I just hoped I didn't screw it all up.

That day I had felt more like I was going to die from my cancer than ever before. If only my CRP had come down. Even heart problems would have been a rosier outlook. Heart transplants, bypasses, and valve replacements were so commonplace. But curing stage IV prostate cancer with a Gleason score of eight and a CRP of sixty...not so much.

I was sitting at Cootie Browns. The bartender was one of my favorites. NFL Football was on, and I was trying hard to get out of the funk and focus on what needed to be done before I died. There was an increased intensity to finish the book. So, I drank double chilled shots of Crown, the only person at the bar, and I wrote the following in my book.

10/15/20

I was talking to Nila a couple of nights prior, on the eve of my visit to Dr. Famoyin on October 13, three long years to the day after my prostatectomy.

Without thinking too much about the way it would be received, I said, *"The day I figure out I have six months to live, I'm going to buy a carton of cigarettes, a bucket of fried chicken, and a bottle of Crown."*

It's crazy that I decided to stop smoking after my cancer diagnosis. I really never smoked routinely except in the army. Smoking relieved my anxiety and stress.

After the army, I never carried a pack of cigarettes with me. I never smoked at work. It was only those nights when the burden of work preyed upon me. Then, I sipped a chilled Crown or had some wine. The whole time, it was an exercise in problem solving. On those nights, a cigarette often cooled the engines and allowed clearer thoughts or a new strategy to prevail.

A prime example was a project with a globally known company. The battles were epic and sometimes personal, not dissimilar to politics. This company had Charlie Sheen and Michael Jordan commercials. At the time, we didn't even have much of a website. I fought this battle on behalf of my company, knowing the other company was certainly Goliath. My burden was to be David.

On the many nights that I sat at home and strategized, with Nila as my sounding board, I sipped the bourbon and indulged in Marlboro Lights. I always addressed the situation as a possible upset or bitter defeat.

In the end, we won. I often referred to the contest as the University of Alabama Crimson Tide football team (seventeen-time national champions) versus the Calhoun High School Yellow Jackets (four-time state champions).

It always concerned me the next day after having a night of partaking in the medicinal effects of a couple of cigarettes. A slight cough the following morning was a reminder that perhaps I had enjoyed more than a couple.

So, the night of October 12, 2020, I confessed to Nila, should I only have six months to live, what my wish list would include. I had decided it would no longer matter at that point. Up until the point when I had only six months to live, I reasoned, I didn't want to cause myself to have lung cancer or COPD while I was fighting to beat stage IV prostate cancer.

However, I knew if the day were to come when my time was limited, it would be because of the imperfect surgery by the imperfect doctor who left remnants of my prostate lying inside of me. Remnants that were a Gleason eight score and consumed by cancer. Left behind to fight their own battle against "very high" radiation and testosterone starvation from the Lupron shots. Fragments that were really mean and would eventually find their way into a devastating location. Perhaps even into Mr. Skeleton.

11/26/20

It was Thanksgiving morning at 4:20 a.m. We'd just had a record sales day at the grooming salon yesterday. I had taken off that week, and that night I had woken up in pain and couldn't go back to sleep. I fixed a cup of coffee and began writing.

I had an appointment with Dr. Famoyin that week. Things had looked good with my blood again since my last round of iron infusions. I felt well, except for the joint pain. I had major pain in the mid-section of my neck and back, as had been the case for a few years now. The difference was that now I could not get any ribs to pop into place after rolling on my blue cylinder. I couldn't stand the pain of a chiropractic adjustment, even though Dr. Ballard was very sensitive to my condition. When I slept on my left side, my hip woke me up, hurting after an hour or so.

The CPAP definitely helped my sleep, but the bad dreams had crept back into my life, likely spurred on by the pain during sleeping. I took two ibuprofens before bed. But over the past couple of weeks, I had been taking a naproxen in the afternoon, two ibuprofens at bedtime, and two around 4:00 a.m.

I worried about the routine dosages of the OTC meds and their long-term effect. My appointment at SCC was Monday. I would see if the PSA had risen further, as I suspected. Thankfully, Nila was coming this time.

I would see Dr. Raj on my way back. I had followed his guidance and reduced my prednisone from 10 mg to 7 mg, and now back to 5 mg. Perhaps I was becoming somewhat immune to prednisone. But why had this problem lazily hung on for so long?

We would have Thanksgiving dinner Saturday with part of the family. Shane had come to visit for a few days' prior by himself. Although it wasn't under great circumstances, it was good to spend time together. Jeremy and his family couldn't come. COVID was setting new records, and the risk was not worth traveling and staying in a hotel. That left Alanna and Cory. It would be a wonderful environment, even though we would miss everyone else.

I worried about my parents. My dad wouldn't allow us to visit. I didn't push the issue, considering the dangers of COVID at their age. His dementia condition had worsened, and my mom's memory was terrible now, too. They'd both turned eighty-seven this past October. I wondered if we would get past COVID, so I could force a visit before something terrible happened.

I was told Dad was complaining about black bugs eating them, and he routinely sprayed the house with some type of insecticide. When the bugs weren't getting them, it was the people shooting lasers and burning them or pumping gas into the house through the air vents in the floor. It was a heartbreaking situation.

I received a call one day. The caller ID said, "FBI Department of Homeland Security." When I answered, I was asked to identify myself.

"Sir, we have called to discuss a letter we received from your father," the nondescript male voice said. "He states in this letter that there is a new terror organization that can use lasers as a weapon. He further states that this new organization has mobilized."

I cut him off mid-word at this point to profusely apologize. I was stunned and feared repercussions might be in order.

"Sir, we are aware of the situation," the voice intoned. "The Federal Bureau Investigation does not wish to press charges but felt a family member should also be aware of the situation." Then, a click and the dial tone. I placed the phone back into the receiver. Things were getting worse for my dad.

Yet, for me, the upcoming visit to SCC was at the forefront of my thoughts. Dr. Taha had left SCC since my last visit. I planned on taking the opportunity to have a detailed question-and-answer session on this visit with whomever his replacement was. Dr. Taha would be sorely missed.

I also had an appointment with my urologist at SCC. I hadn't seen him since 2018. I wanted to talk about options for me to have a chance to be intimate with Nila again. I loved her dearly and missed our intimacy.

I am a lifelong Rush fan. As I sat and listened to the lyrics of this song, I knew exactly how the writer felt. If only we could command it to be so.

TIME STAND STILL

Rush 1987

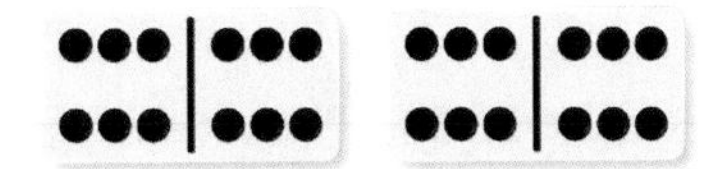

Chapter 24

BUILDING A BOAT PART I

The Sagittarian man is intensely devoted and hardworking. He comes with a commanding attitude of finishing a task on time. He doesn't have a problem when it comes to solving daunting issues.

Unlucky thirteen. Whether you believe in superstition or you see it as only coincidence, the number thirteen has been remarkably commonplace after my cancer diagnosis. Looking back, there were several events that involved unlucky thirteen. For instance, my prostatectomy was on Friday the thirteenth. My thirteenth radiation treatment was on the thirteenth. I returned to work on the thirteenth day after my shoulder surgery. My rheumatoid factor was thirteen times above the upper limit. The fluoroscopy and pulmonary test were scheduled on the thirteenth. My first rheumatology appointment was on the thirteenth. The plaques on the Wall of Life at SCC started with 2013 (the first year I failed to get my annual blood test). September 13 was the birthday party when we made our reservations to go skydiving. As I pondered, the list went on.

Nila and I found out my PSA had risen again on December 3, 2020, so I started back on the Lupron shots. Cancer had reared its ugly head again. A full-body check was in order—where was cancer? I was scheduled for a full skeletal X-ray, an upper CT scan to check all of my vital organs, and a CT bone scan.

"I'm pretty sure I know where," I thought. "Mr. Skeleton, of course."

I had been concerned for years. After all of my research and morbid thoughts, I had concluded that bone cancer was my fate. In fact, I had predicted it many times as I wrote pages of my book.

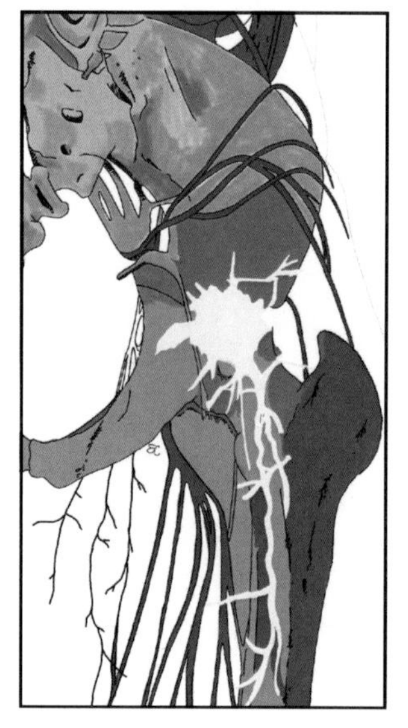

My left hip had been hurting worse. Over the past two months, I hadn't been able to sleep on my left side for more than an hour. Lately, not at all. But I wasn't sure it was cancer. It often felt like a muscular problem or perhaps even an irritated sciatic nerve.

Sciatic nerve pain radiates along the path of the nerve, starting in the lower back and running through the hips and buttocks and down each leg. Pain or discomfort can be felt almost anywhere along the nerve's path. The pain can vary from mild discomfort to a sharp burning sensation to even excruciating pain. At times, it can even feel like a jolt of electricity.

Drawing of sciatic nerve pain by Ezekial Cooper

Over the past ten years, I had gone to my chiropractors for relief. Dr. Kind and Dr. Ballard had been incredibly wonderful to us. Not only had they provided much-needed chiropractic care, but we had used their guidance for pillows and beds. They always took time to discuss my medical treatments and offered smart advice. I wouldn't hesitate to call them friends. For them to take such a caring interest in our lives had been incredible. I could never say enough. They had been a blessing to us.

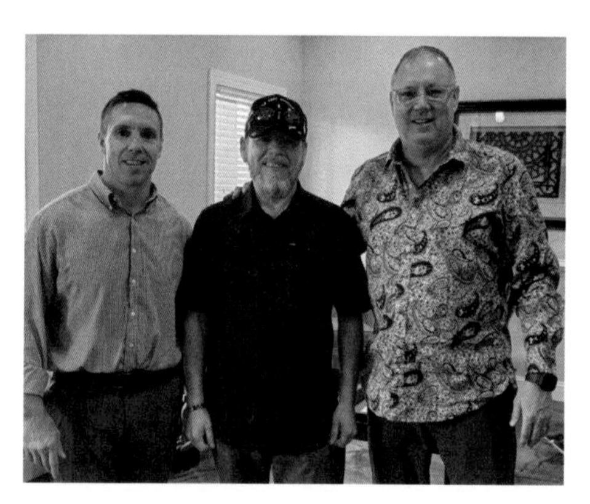

From left: Dr. Ballard, Perry Muse, Dr. Kind

Even though there were whispers in my ear about the impending outcome of my scans, I remained positive. I felt great. I had an increased amount of fatigue, but I knew the Lupron would create that when my testosterone was knocked back down. The hot flashes were back in full force, coming every two to three hours around the clock. I was emotional at times, but I really felt well. I was active on my job and at the salon during my off time. I cooked and helped with housework. Perhaps my morbid thoughts were off base. Otherwise, how could I feel this well?

On January 12, 2021, we trekked along Celebration of Life Drive to SCC.

Upon entering, we went through COVID protocol. Once complete, Nila and I stepped over to our normal spot for a picture.

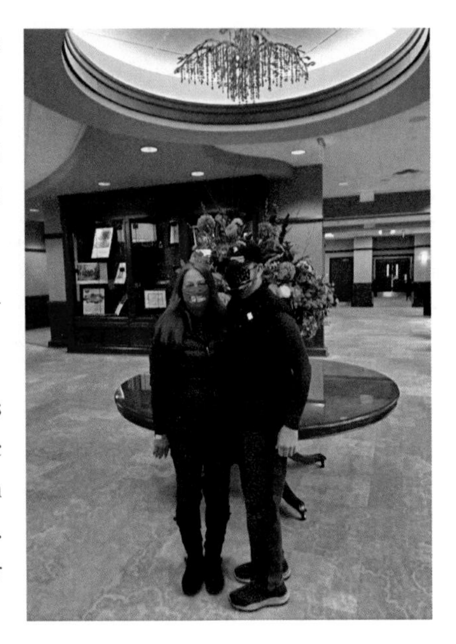

Perry and Nila at SCC during COVID

From there, it was the routine check-in at Maple. However, this time I wasn't directed across the hall for my lab draw. We ventured further down the hallway.

All of my tests took place in the imaging department. I had two CT scans scheduled.

Nila and I sat in the waiting room. It was obvious that COVID had diminished the traffic at SCC. The hallway that had once bustled with people was now nearly vacant by comparison. The waiting area was marked to ensure proper social distancing. Even so, it was not full.

A nurse walked through the door and came over to greet me. I thought it was a nice touch that they knew who the patient was, rather than just calling my name. I was sure it was just a photo taken at check-in to allow them to find the right person. Either way, it seemed more personal.

I followed along until we came to the room. I thought I was getting my first CT scan of the day, but that wasn't the reason for me being taken back.

Later in the day, I would have a bone scan. This required a shot of a very small amount of a radioactive drug called a radiopharmaceutical. It was dispensed through a device and into my IV port. I had never seen such a device before.

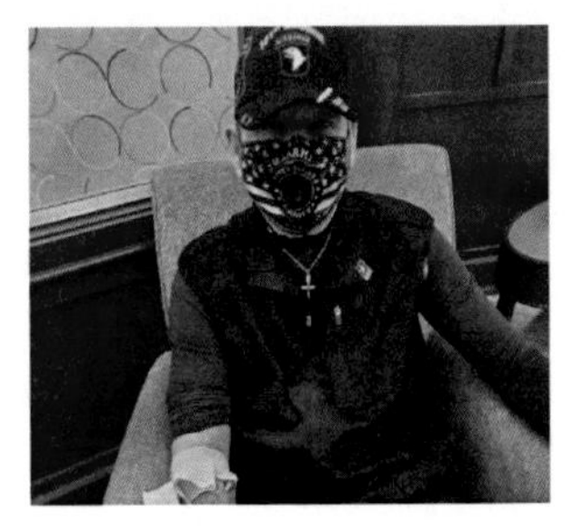

Perry at SCC, awaiting radiopharmaceutical

Following the injection, I was escorted back to the waiting area.

"Nila, why don't you go back to the hotel room?" Her eyes were weighed heavily with the fatigue of our long trip down from Tennessee in the rain. Plus, the impend-

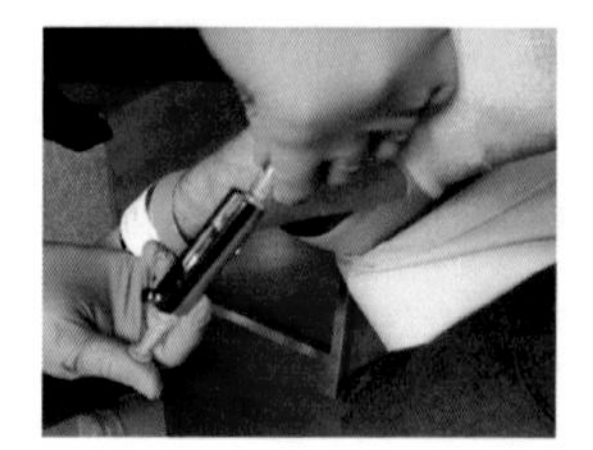

ing stress of the day was already hanging on her. I felt there was no reason for her to sit in the waiting area all day. She argued a bit, but finally conceded that there was little she could do there.

Radiopharmaceutical syringe

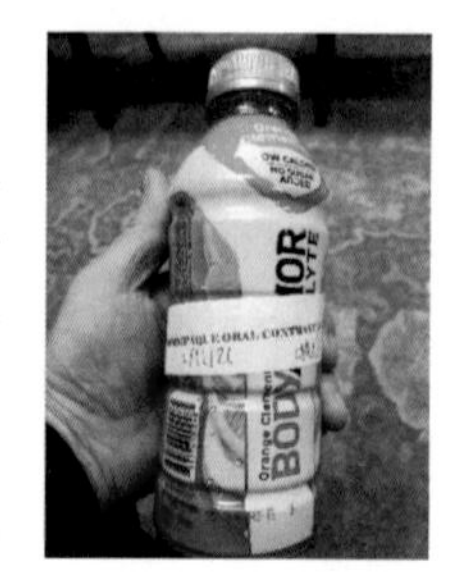

After Nila left, a different nurse came through the door and walked to where I was sitting. I was asked to identify myself and show my bracelet. Then she handed me a drink. This was for the CT of my chest, abdomen, and pelvis, with contrast.

Contrast with electrolyte beverage

As I walked around, drinking my contrast liquid, I passed a large sign on the wall. It read: "Cancer Fighters." This was a room where people met to discuss and learn about their cancer. That is, they had met prior to COVID.

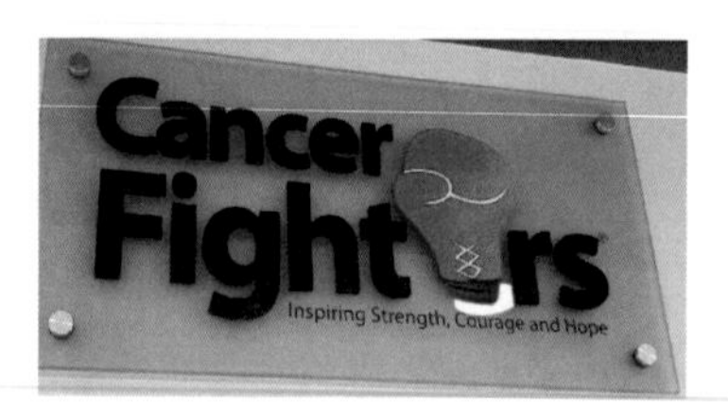

Cancer fighters sign

As I looked at the sign and drank the contrast, I pondered.

"I never was a fighter. I still don't feel so much like a cancer fighter. But tomorrow I may become one."

After lunch, the tests began. The first of my two tests was the CT with contrast. Another nurse greeted me. I walked through the door at imaging, surgery, and radiation for the fourth time. The sign on the door read "Radiation Area." I was thankful not to see "Very High Radiation," although my mind did wander back to my thirty-eight days of radiation treatments in early 2018. The sign on the wall read "MRI Zone 2." From there we made our way to IM189. This was where I would have my CT scan.

Once in the room, it was an all-too-familiar routine. I had prepared myself for the hard, painful table, but, to my surprise, this table was cushioned and immediately felt better than previous tables when I lay back on it; however, there was still some discomfort.

"Are you in any pain?" asked the radiology technician.

"Yes, some," I gritted out, as I felt my bones creak into place on the table. My mouth said "some," but I think my body was telling him a different story.

"Let me help," he said, grabbing a wedge-shaped cushion that he slid under my knees. Welcome relief flooded my lower back and hips immediately, and I took my first deep breath since lying down. It was a simple thing, the cushion, but it made all of the difference.

I closed my eyes and relaxed, thinking of Nila and looking forward to dinner with her later that evening. I knew the tension would be eased with laughter and perhaps a sip of chilled Crown.

The table slid into the donut ring, and my thoughts made the time slip by quickly. When the test was over, I was challenged to get up.

I was able to rise up, but not without some help from the technician. I picked up my crucifix necklace and strained to reach behind my neck to fasten it. I gave up and placed it in my pocket, knowing it would have to be removed again for the next test anyway.

The technician escorted me back to the waiting room, where I had spent most of my day.

"One down, one to go," I thought. I waited and waited with nothing but my thoughts and my phone for more than an hour before a nurse came through the door to greet me for the last time.

Finally, I thought, the time had come for my last scan. I walked, accompanied by the nurse, through the familiar doorways from earlier. This time we would go into M130.

I removed the crucifix from my pocket, gave it a kiss, and got onto the table. Unlike the previous table, this one was not cushioned. I really needed it to be, from the hours of waiting, plus my prednisone was starting to weaken. I didn't get any questions from this technician about my comfort.

Once I was settled, lying down on the table, the technician had me move slightly and then used a large wrap to hold my body in place. Once the Velcro was secured, he walked away.

This time I didn't daydream about Nila and laughing. I said a prayer and thought about what was happening.

"Is this the test?" I thought. "Is this where they see the impact from some of those really mean cells in Mr. Skeleton?"

I opened my eyes and forced myself to think of something else. I don't remember what I thought of, but my eyes remained open for the rest of the scan.

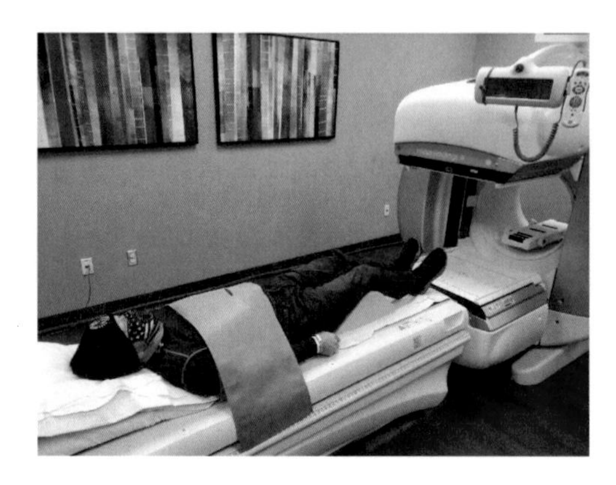

Perry strapped into place

As soon as I was finished, I called Nila to pick me up. She arrived with a hug and a helpful hand, getting my crucifix back around my neck. From there we headed to dinner. We wanted to arrive early and avoid having to be around too many people dining.

Our dinner was at a nearby grill and tavern. When we were ready to check out, I looked at the receipt. Nothing jumped out at me. I calculated the 20 percent tip, which came to $12.72. Without a thought, I rounded up. When I added up the total and wrote it down, it surprised me.

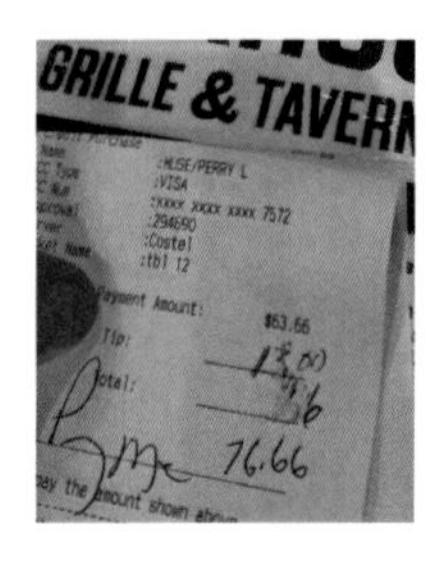

The bill was $63.66. The tip rounded up to $13.00. I didn't like seeing the three sixes, and I immediately regretted rounding to $13. But then there was the total. $76.66. The first two numbers, seven and six, equaled thirteen when added together. The last three numbers were 666.

Receipt from dinner

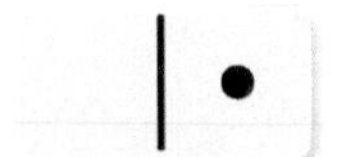 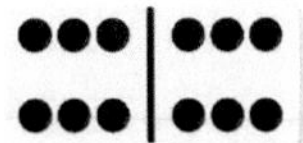 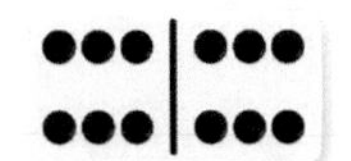

Chapter 25

BUILDING A BOAT PART II

I had never seriously believed in being jinxed or bad luck from walking under a ladder or breaking a mirror. But then again, I made sure never to walk under ladders, mainly due to safety!

The number thirteen became very prevalent after my cancer diagnosis. It didn't occur to me until writing this book. As I pointed out, my prostatectomy was on Friday the thirteenth. My thirteenth radiation treatment was on the thirteenth. The number thirteen shows up all too often for me.

One of my favorite bands is Black Sabbath. As a young teenager, my mom would hide my albums because she didn't like the band's name or the picture on the cover.

In June 2013, Black Sabbath released their thirteenth studio album, titled "13." My favorite song on the album was "Damaged Soul." One particular lyric that resonated with me said, "Dying is easy; it's living that's hard." When I first heard the song played, I felt sad for whomever it was written for, fictitious or not. I loved life. Life was a challenge, but Sagittarians thrive on challenges. People likely wondered why someone in my situation would enjoy this music with such lyrics. But for me, it was oddly cathartic.

"2013 was also the first of five consecutive years that I would fail to get my annual blood test. I was somehow too busy working and loving life to take a few minutes off for the simple blood draw. Perhaps the day will come when I understand the lyrics from a new perspective," I recently contemplated as I considered the importance of thirteen.

As we sat in the room awaiting the oncologist, I had decided the test would be in my favor. I was...cautiously optimistic. I still believed I knew my destiny with cancer, but I felt too good for it to be bad news today.

"If only we were sitting here on another day and not the thirteenth of January. I hope I don't regret not rescheduling," I thought on a loop.

The oncologist walked in and greeted us. As with many of the doctors I encountered, I couldn't read his face or tone. There was no hint of bad news, and maybe for obvious reasons.

The reports read as follows:

CT Chest: No significant axillary, mediastinal or hilar adenopathy is seen. **Axillary refers to lymph nodes in the armpits. Mediastinal and hilar refer to lymph nodes between the lungs, in the region of the heart and esophagus. Adenopathy refers to swelling.** *No suspicious lung nodules are detected.* **A nodule refers to a spot on the lungs.** *The heart is normal in size and shows no significant coronary plaque with no pericardial effusion.* **Pericardial effusion refers to fluid buildup between doubled-layered sacs around the heart.** *No significant infiltrates or edema noted and no pleural effusion.* **Edema refers to fluid and infiltrates refers to fluid seeping through pores to cause buildup.** *No chest wall abnormalities. The pancreas and adrenals are normal in size and configuration. No renal masses, stones, or obstructive changes are seen.* **A renal mass refers to a tumor.** *No significant paraaortic or pericaval adenopathy and no evidence of mesenteric mass.* **Paraaortic or paracaval refers to lymph node masses located in front of the lumbar and near the aorta. Mesenteric mass refers to a tumor or lesion.** *No evidence of bowel obstruction, or focal wall thickening. No suspicious pelvic masses, adenopathy, or fluid collections are seen.*

Skeletal structures: There are stable sclerotic lesions demonstrated in the iliac bones unchanged from previous exam. **Sclerotic lesions are often seen in the long bones and refer to an unusual thickening of the bone.** *No evidence of pathologic fracture or new bony lesion.*

So far, so good. The word "no" was used frequently in the report. Actually, thirteen times. This was verbatim from my report. However, it was the lack of the word "no" that would indicate trouble.

The bone scan report reads as follows:

Comparison is made with prior bone scan performed at an outside institution on 8/24/2017.

There is no pathologic uptake of the radionuclide within the cervical, thoracic, or lumbar spine. **Radionuclide is the chemical, or isotope, used and pathologic uptake refers to a gathering of that chemical in a location.** *No abnormal uptake of the radionuclide is* *associated with the pelvis or either hip. The lower extremity long bones are entirely normal. There is uptake of the radionuclide at the sternomanubrial joint and at both medial clavicular heads.* **Sternomanubrial refers to where the upper parts of the sternum meet. Medial clavicle heads refer to the upper third of the clavicle.** *There is uptake of the radionuclide overlying the anterior aspect of the right third rib. A CT scan done on this day demonstrates a small punctate sclerotic area within the rib at that site.* **Punctate refers to tiny holes or dots.**

Impression: Positive bone scan demonstrating uptake within the anterior aspect of the right third rib where there is a corresponding tiny sclerotic area within the rib on same day CT scan. This abnormality is ***consistent with a small metastasis.***

"You now have prostate cancer that has metastasized into your bones. Your cancer is now incurable," stated Dr. Taha's replacement. "Now we need to talk about treatment options," he continued. "We will continue the Lupron shots and Prolia. I recommend an oral chemotherapy treatment called Xtandi. You have the choice if you want to start it immediately or wait until after the next scan in three months."

"I will start the chemo immediately," I responded. Nila began to cry.

"Why would I want to wait three more months and let the cancer get ahead of me?" I thought. "I'm not ready to die yet. I still have much to do."

And so, the long-anticipated day had finally arrived. Cancer had invaded Mr. Skeleton. Nila and I heard the words loud and clear. "Your cancer is now incurable."

My heart broke for Nila. I couldn't imagine if the situation was reversed. In June 2019, I had been proclaimed "cancer free." Nineteen months later, my cancer was "incurable." In truth, I had been preparing for this day for three years, yet Nila had hoped I was wrong while she dealt with my morbid thoughts, morbid thoughts that came free with a cancer diagnosis.

The rain inside of our lives grew stronger. I had definitely found my way into the 100 percent chance of rain region, with no end to the storm in sight. During all of this time since I had been diagnosed with cancer and "cancer free," I had often recalled Dr. Famoyin telling me about a storm that might occur in ten years, or it might never metastasize. His point was that it would be a waste of life to spend all of my days building a boat for that storm that might never occur. Try as I might, I had not been able to completely stop working on mine.

On unlucky January 13, 2021, I began spending much of the day building my boat. This time I knew the flood would come. The rain had already begun.

My cancer fight was officially on. Everything prior to January 13, 2021, had been mental and physical preparedness. It was a warm-up to the real battle.

On the way home from SCC, Nila and I met my boss Erik in Calhoun. I had kept him abreast of everything prior. This conversation would need to be face to face, and so, we sat on his front porch.

I was relieved to get the visit out of the way. I needed to be sure he could see and hear that it wasn't over yet. I needed him to know the fire was still there to be productive for Foam Products. I also needed him to know that I needed to work.

Two days after the diagnosis, I began taking four chemotherapy pills per day. They were each about the size of an omega vitamin, with a slick coating and shaped like a football. The bottle read Xtandi.

DAY ONE:

I waited until 7:00 p.m. to take the pills. The instructions warned not to touch the pills and to wash anything that came in contact with them.

"The pills can't touch the outside of your body, but it's all right for me to swallow them?" I thought as I read along.

We had just finished supper when I took the first four doses. I wanted plenty of time for any side effects to wear off before I had to be at work the following morning.

About thirty to forty-five minutes later, I began to feel...high. It was similar to the feeling of intoxication when the first shot went into the IV before going to the operating room.

As time went on, the feeling increased. I felt somewhat out of body, sitting in my living room. Talking to Nila felt like she was far away from me. I began to panic and asked her to put me in bed.

Simple things confused me, like taking out my contacts. I had a reading contact in one eye and a distance contact in the other. It was never good when they got switched!

I took my nighttime anxiety pill, slipped on my CPAP mask, and crawled into bed.

As I lay in bed, my muscles began to sporadically spasm. I felt tense and continuously had to force myself to relax. However, each time I would relax, it would only be a minute later, and I would realize I was tense again.

I told Nila that it felt as though my bones should be glowing beneath the covers.

As I lay under the covers, the feeling running through my bones was incredibly uncomfortable. It felt as though an electrical plug had been slipped into an outlet on my heel, providing a constant source of low-level electricity. Waaaaaahooooowww. Waaaaaaahoooowww. I could almost hear the low humming.

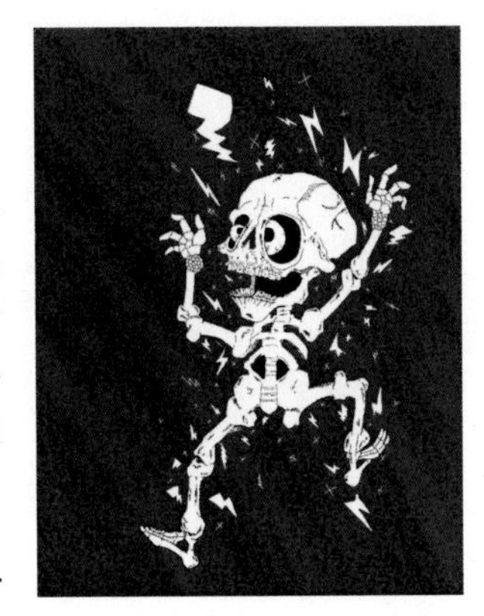

Drawing of electrocuted skeleton by Ezekial Cooper

The next morning, I awoke and struggled to get out of bed. It felt similar to a hangover. After an hour or so, I managed to make it to the kitchen and get the coffee maker going. Meanwhile, I put in my contacts and jumped on the daily production conference call at 9:00 a.m.

I muted my phone, afraid of trying to say too much. The coffee was ready, and I was anxious to drink it. I needed a pick-me-up. While waiting for it to cool and listening in on the call, I took my morning pills.

"Surely the prednisone and coffee will snap me out of whatever this is," I thought. "I had better add a couple of milligrams to the prednisone dose if I am going to be productive at work."

But after day one of taking the new pills, I was not feeling productive. I was a little confused and lightheaded. When I tried to talk, my words were slurring.

"How can I work like this? I can't drive. I heard myself speaking to you. Anyone who didn't know would think I was drunk," I said to Nila. "Is this the end of my job? How can I possibly live this way until the end?" ran through my mind.

DAY TWO:

Day two was a repeat of day one. I took my pills around the same time and got the same result. It reminded me of what I had been told in statistics class by a professor back in the nineties.

He would say, “If you keep doing what you’ve done, you will keep getting what you got.”

He meant that I needed to find a plan B for day three.

After reading through the Xtandi literature repeatedly, I called my oldest son, Shane. Even though he didn’t have experience treating cancer, he had medical training from the army. His wife Monica was also in the medical field.

One thing that stood out to me in the list of side effects was “electrolytes imbalance.” As a former athlete, I was aware of electrolytes. What I didn’t know was whether or not I could add this to my water intake without consequence.

Shane did some quick research and recommended that I drink some Powerade or Gatorade before taking my next dose. By creating an electrolyte imbalance, this medicine was most likely lowering my potassium or sodium. We both agreed it couldn’t hurt, so I added it to my regimen.

DAY 3:

I stocked up on Powerade Zero. I also bought the equipment to check and monitor my sugar. I had experience being around someone who is diabetic and had witnessed firsthand how they behaved when it was too low or too high. My symptoms were similar to when a person’s sugar drops. I had confusion, dizziness, and slurred speech.

On the third evening of taking Xtandi, I did so while consuming a full bottle of the drink. I had also studied up on sugar levels, glucose, and how a person’s numbers could fluctuate, or what normal levels could be. For the first time, I was able to stay up for three hours until bedtime after consuming the Powerade. This was encouraging.

From there, I eliminated all drinks from my diet except water and Powerade Zero. After checking my sugar multiple times, I crossed it off my list of potential problems. I couldn’t be exactly sure how much of the boost came from counteracting electrolytes and how much was just hydration. It was likely a combination of both.

WEEK 1:

At the end of week one, I had made progress offsetting some of the side effects of the Xtandi. But the medication further added to my fatigue. It was truly a battle getting out of bed and getting to work. Once I got going, it was easier. It was like trying to move a huge boulder alone, pushing and straining with all of my mental fortitude to get it to budge. Once it began to roll, the battle became easier. But it was still a boulder. Each day, the boulder sat idle, awaiting my test of strength to get it moving again.

Newton's first law, or the law of inertia states, "An object at rest will stay at rest, and an object in motion will stay in motion unless acted on by an external force." I felt like this law applied to me if I rewrote it just a little.

My version would read, "A Perry in bed will stay in bed unless acted upon by determination and strength. A Perry in motion could easily become at rest without grit and staying power."

At the end of only one week, I had amassed quite the collection of empty water and Powerade Zero bottles. I was unsure about my ability to keep up the pace. Making it to the restroom on time was critical. My office at work was located upstairs and halfway between the two men's rooms.

One week's worth of empty Powerade and water bottles

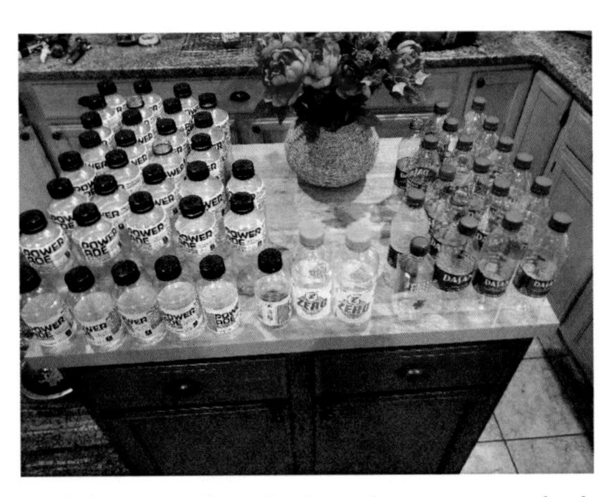

On the eighth day following the start of Xtandi, I was struggling with a lot of things. I wanted to write in my book after work but found myself in bed again. It appeared to me that stress increased tension in my body and started to wreak havoc on my muscles. The muscles in my back seemed to be affected the most. The pain throughout my upper back was compounded by ribs that had popped out again, but this time, neither Dr. Kind nor Dr. Ballard were able to get them to pop back in. Using my TENS unit became a daily routine. Sometimes that wasn't even enough.

"Remember, you will have bone pain, followed by easy fracturing," I reminded myself. "Is this the bone pain? If so, I don't need to get my ribs adjusted and cause a fracture. I don't need any more domino effects."

I continued this part of the battle for a month. Some days were better than others. Despite my insistent efforts to figure out this puzzle, I was unable to find consistency in the way I felt. But one thing was consistent—taking my four pills and having the feeling of being plugged into a low-level electrical source. Each night I would lie down to the hum of waaaaaaahooooowww running through my bones.

Every evening, my day would end not long after taking my oral chemo. Every night, I lay in bed for an hour or better, trying to force my body to relax and my mind to clear. I was starting to understand the lyrics a little more than before: "Dying is easy; it's living that's hard." What's more, I was certain I would have a full understanding of how much harder living could be before my life was all over.

One day, I was listening to a guest DJ on the radio while driving home from work. A song came on that I loved from 1975. One I'd never heard played on the radio. In a flash, I could see myself: fifteen years old, listening to this song at a low volume in my room, hoping my mom wouldn't catch me because she had already confiscated this record, forcing me to rescue it and hide it in my rarely used bottom clothes drawer.

Forty-six years later, the lyrics reached out and grabbed me. It had a totally different meaning to me than in 1975, or in any of the years since. I listened to the words, sure that nobody else in the world derived this same new meaning I had just conjured.

I often lay in bed and recited the words of the song quietly in my head as I struggled to go to sleep. It was my mantra. My bones humming, my muscles randomly spasming, my mind racing. Lying there, trying to sleep, unable to sleep, I routinely caught myself planning my funeral, or envisioning other events. I was doing what a true Sagittarius does: planning. But for what future, I wondered?

"Open your eyes and stop the planning nonsense," I thought morbidly. "You don't have to do that anymore. The cancer is incurable, and you won't be here anyway."

If cancer was a woman, this song would be about her. Although the lyrics are not about cancer, I often made them so.

MISS MISERY

Nazareth 1975

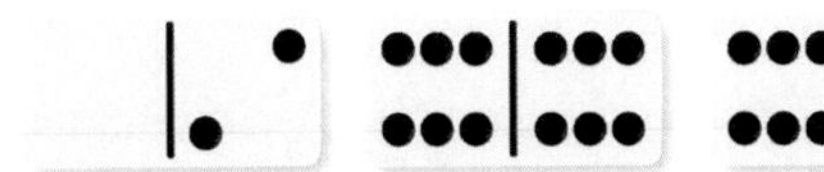

Chapter 26

BUILDING A BOAT PART III

Over the past three and a half years, I had managed to work, take some exciting vacation trips, open a new business, and write this book.

Life has a way of introducing us to stress and challenges, apart from having cancer. I can certainly share some examples.

We were blessed to have some of our family come to live with us. It was such a welcome event. So many wonderful things were made possible. It was quite medicinal and strengthening for our family.

The family members had a dog. The introduction of the new family members into our house and lives also impacted our dogs. Thor, Hooch, and Sparky hit it off immediately with their dog, but it is a difficult task to maintain order when there are four male dogs.

Sparky and Thor had already had their clash. It was really out of the blue and over something insignificant. The main problem was that Sparky ended up with stitches. From that day forth, we couldn't allow them to be together. However, one day Sparky darted out of the door, and the fight was on.

Thor outweighed Sparky by at least one hundred and twenty pounds. Sparky didn't care. He was fearless. But this time it resulted in far more serious injuries to Sparky. Thor's move was to pin the other dog to prevent it from hurting him. Sparky being inside of his mouth was like trying to hold a squirrel. The more he squirmed for freedom, the more Thor's teeth did their damage.

We all thought Thor and the new dog were great playing together. They both played exhaustively and rough. What we failed to realize was that the competition was slowly escalating. This was when Thor and the new dog ended up in a fight two times within a week. I was the one who ended up with stitches. The other family members had a badly wounded foot from being barefooted while wrestling Thor away from their dog, and some huge contusions, thanks to Thor stepping on their foot during the first altercation.

I believe we all developed PTSD as a result. We had bad dreams and panicked at the sound of a door opening. We even started a system of texting to make sure we were all on board.

"Thor is locked up," I would text.

"OK, letting Rover out," they would text back.

"Rover is back in," they would text again.

"OK, letting Sparky and Hooch out," I would text. "Sparky and Hooch are back in and letting Thor back out," I would text.

"OK, Rover is still in," they would text.

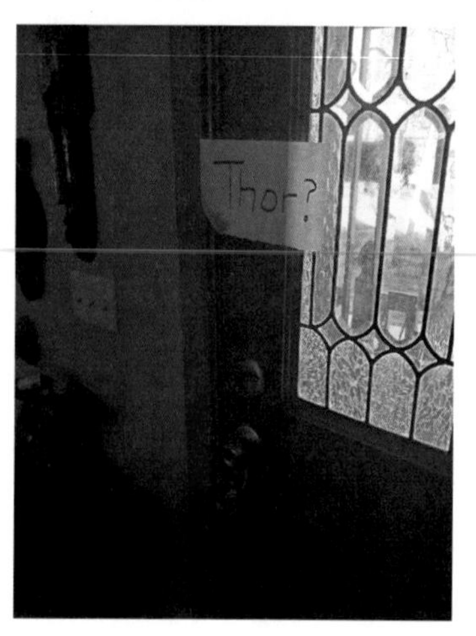

"Thor is definitely back out now," I would text.

"OK," they would text. And this would go on throughout the day.

As time passed, and especially after starting my Xtandi, I needed reassurance that I hadn't made a mistake and created another dog fight. So, I had to put a sign on the door to remind me. Even then, my PTSD from the dog fights made me double check before letting any other dog out.

Sign on inside of front door

Within one week's time, our grooming salon went from being profitable to losing three of the four groomers. What was supposed to be a career for Nila when I was gone instantly became debt-ridden stress and anger.

All of the normal stresses of life, like running a first-year business, my normal job, the issues with the dogs, etc., just compounded my life's struggle with cancer, especially once I knew I was going to die. Living had gotten very hard.

One day, I passed a nearby church and read the sign. It was speaking to me, I thought.

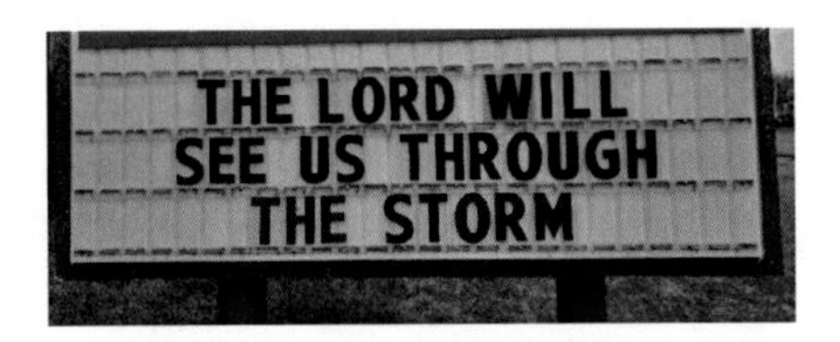

Local church sign

On January 23, 2021, I had an appointment with Dr. Famoyin. When he arrived in the room, it was a welcome sight. We exchanged the initial pleasantries without the handshakes due to COVID.

"How are you doing on Xtandi?" he asked,

I told him about my symptoms and issues and ended by telling him that I had replaced Powerade with a product called DayLyte.

"So DayLyte is recommended for cancer patients on chemo, as well as athletes. I did the research. It must be better than Powerade because just 1 ml in a bottle of water replaced several of the Powerade drinks I was drinking, and the change made a significant difference in my trips to the men's room."

"You need to be cautious about drinking DayLyte or Powerade," he said.

"I brought the box from the DayLyte product for you to read," I said, handing him the broken-down cardboard box from the floor. "I am wondering about my potassium because it has routinely tested high, and there are copious amounts of potassium in Dayyte and Powerade." I waited while he looked at the box.

As I had thought, potassium was a concern.

"The potassium here is a problem." Dr. Famoyin explained, "Too much potassium can cause heart problems. Too little potassium can cause heart problems."

We further discussed the chemo pills. He explained that I could cut back if it was too much for me. Sagittarius wasn't about to do that. Cutting back on the pills—wouldn't that let those mean cancer cells invade Mr. Skeleton easier?

Dr. Famoyin got up to escort me to the lab.

I said, "Doc, every time I wake up, I think of dying. I think of how I will die, how it will feel. I find myself planning my funeral and trying to think of everything that needs to be done to make sure Foam Products and, most importantly, Nila and my family are taken care of."

Dr. Famoyin placed my file back on the desk and sat back down. The look of caring in his eyes showed above his mask, and I could see it was genuine.

"Mr. Perry," he began. "Prostate cancer is the slowest-growing form of cancer." He paused here to let that sink in, staring into my eyes. "Sometimes, depending on age, we don't even treat it. Do you understand? It means that something else will get prostate cancer patients before the cancer. It is very possible to live ten or more years with this cancer, IF you do all of the right things."

"But not after it has metastasized, right?" I interrupted.

"Yes. Even after it has metastasized." Again, he paused for it to sink in. "You are doing all of the things you need to do. We must treat the cancer without killing the patient."

Unexpectedly, he laughed. "Do you hear me?" he asked rhetorically. "We can't kill the patient while we are trying to treat the cancer. What you need to understand is that you must learn to live with cancer. If a treatment isn't working for you, we will find another one. Learn to live with cancer."

"Living is hard; it's dying that's easy," I thought.

I followed the good doctor to the lab and had my blood drawn. I had shared with him that I didn't plan to return to SCC on Celebration of Life Drive. He would now be the sole proprietor of my oncology needs.

At 5:30 p.m. the following day, my phone rang. It was Dr. Famoyin. My iron had trickled down, and I was in need of some infusions.

The next Monday, I showed up for my infusions. I made my way back to the familiar room and found a recliner. I took my pillow and faithful American flag blanket for comfort and hoped to catch a nap.

The blanket was to be put under my left leg to relieve pressure on my hip. I had been to see Dr. Kind and Ballard about my hip a couple of weeks earlier. They set me up with an in-house appointment for a deep massage. The pain was lessened on the same day and even more the day after. By day two after the massage, the pain was gone. I actually slept for extended times on my left side for the first time in weeks.

Unfortunately, I bent down the wrong way, something made a slight pop, and I was back in pain.

I made myself comfortable, pulled my hat over my eyes, and tried to relax and go to sleep, but the prednisone and Xtandi pills made sure I didn't sleep. I lifted my cap from over my eyes, and I glanced around the room.

"So, does anyone notice that I have become the grape slowly dying on the vine?" I wondered. No matter. I knew that I was.

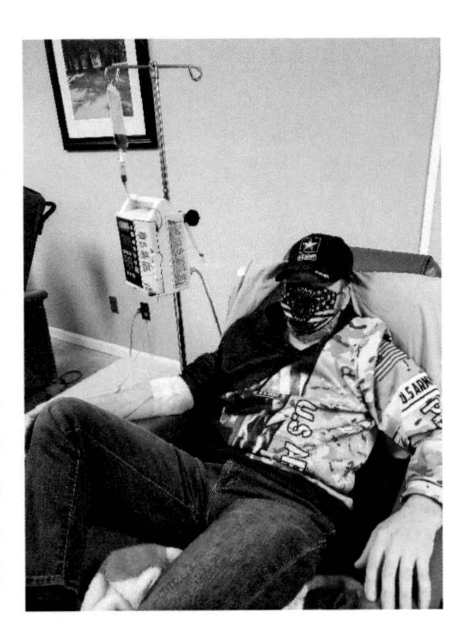

Perry receiving iron infusion

As I was leaving, I passed Dr. Famoyin at the workstation. He stopped me with some excitement in his voice.

"Mr. Perry, I am so glad to see you. I was going to call," he said.

Then he got close and began to speak quietly, like two young boys secretly talking about a cute girl and not wanting her to hear. I knew it was confidentiality, but it was even better than the personal treatment at SCC when they knew I was Perry Muse without asking.

He explained that my skeletal X-rays looked very good. A bit of straightening of the spine, a bit of arthritis. I wondered why he sounded excited.

"There is nothing here that shows me problems. Your pain is not from bone cancer," he said in a low but enthusiastic tone. "You do have a lot of inflammation and muscle spasms, especially in your back, but not from bone cancer."

We began to exchange thoughts. I caught him up on my motorcycle accident.

"I flipped and rolled a hundred and ninety-two feet on the asphalt," I explained. I continued to tell him how my upper back had plagued me for a few years. "If I didn't have that pain, I would feel so much better. In the late afternoon or early evening, I have to stop all activity," I explained.

As we wound up the conversation, I asked him if a muscle relaxer would be possible. He proceeded to write a prescription for Flexeril.

I left with a renewed sense of living, albeit living with cancer. I was again uplifted by the "Famoyinisms" and laughter. I drove to the salon and tried to do the same for Nila.

The next day, I couldn't wait until I got home. My back was so angry and inflamed. I couldn't stand for anything to touch my back, including a chair or a bed. I had been sitting at my desk for most of the day and sitting on the edge of my chair. Couple that with the Xtandi and the prednisone making me tense.

Tense, relax, tense, relax, tense, relax. This was the pattern all day. It was like having an all-day workout!

By the time I went to bed every evening, my back muscles were incredibly angry. It was extremely frustrating to be in so much pain that I couldn't lie down without the bed causing me to cry out. At the same time, I was so tired all day long and looked forward to the time for sleep. It was a frustrating combination that I had lived with for years.

I took half of one Flexeril pill as a precautionary measure. Twenty minutes later, the pain had subsided. I took advantage of the time to prepare dinner. Nila had put in a hard day at the salon, and I wanted to have dinner ready. Afterward, it was time to take the other half.

But twenty minutes later, I was out of control again. I stumbled when I walked and felt lightheaded. I asked Nila to put me to bed. It was only 8:00 p.m.

I slept through the night. The next morning, I struggled to get out of bed. This time it was the effects of the muscle relaxer and the Xtandi. I made it to work, but by lunchtime, I was struggling to stay awake. I let my boss know, drove home, and crawled back into bed.

After two hours of hard sleeping, I woke up feeling great. I hurried out of bed and immediately plugged back into work.

That evening I skipped the Flexeril. I couldn't afford to miss work again, even if it was only a couple of hours. I needed to stay engaged.

After that, I began a new routine. Sagittarius wasn't about to give up on finding a solution.

During the workday, I sat back in my chair when at my desk. In the army they had taught us to relax, slow our breathing, and lower our heart rate. I put this into practice. The more I could keep myself in a relaxed posture, the less I aggravated the muscles in my upper back.

I also made sure to get up and walk through the plant. I had always loved to engage with the people and processes happening throughout. This also provided me with the much-needed restroom break from all of the water I consumed.

The weekend arrived, and it gave me an opportunity to experiment. I needed to find the boundaries of my tolerance to the various medications. And that was exactly what I did.

My autoimmune condition, which was another domino effect of my cancer, was the culprit behind the muscle inflammation and spasms. I learned this from studying about my condition. I felt as though it may be myositis.

Myositis refers to any condition causing inflammation in muscles. Weakness, swelling, and pain are the most common myositis symptoms. Conditions causing inflammation throughout the body may affect the muscles, causing myositis. Many of these causes are autoimmune conditions in which the body attacks its own tissues.

I would need to wait for a doctor's diagnosis to be sure, but, at this point, I felt like it properly depicted what I had been experiencing for almost three years.

"The cancer got my immune system into fight mode," I thought. "Then, lucky me, I got polymyalgia rheumatica. All of the inflammation has likely created another domino. Myositis. Cancer keeps lining up the dominos and knocking them down. I just have to stay ahead of the fall."

By the end of the weekend, it felt as though I had solved the complex medicine problem.

My solution: In the morning, I took all of my first round of supplements and prednisone. No more coffee, as it only encouraged the tension. After lunch, I took my second round of supplements, along with a naproxen, but only if I felt the upper back was hinting at being aggravated. In the evening, I ate supper around 6:00 p.m. By 7:30–8:00 p.m., it was time to take my Xtandi. By 9:30–10:00 p.m., I took a low dose of Xanax and one-quarter of a Flexeril. The next morning, I repeated.

This routine had a significant impact on the way I felt. I was sleeping better and waking up feeling pain free. Living wasn't as hard.

I was thankful for the relief. I now felt as though I had something to help keep me from the debilitating pain, even if just for a while, although the consequence was feeling hungover. It caused my memory to slip and my sharpness to dull. But being pain free, even for a short time, was wonderful. I know, free isn't really free. But I didn't care. I was grateful. As with everything these days, I said a prayer and gave thanks for relief and life.

Meanwhile, my daily routine continued. Every evening I made my way down into the dimly lit, cool basement. There I sat with Nila, my American flag blanket covering me, with the lights off and the television on. I watched the clock constantly, waiting on the time to take my chemo pills and for my night to end. I often told those closest to me that I was down in a hole. I meant that literally (the basement), mentally, and figuratively.

Lately at night I would lie in bed and sing a different song in my mind to distract myself from the discomfort and low voltage humming in Mr. Skeleton. The morbid thoughts no longer ever left me. The song that popped into my head most often was certainly inspired by the shadowy figures on my shoulder. I didn't even realize it at the time. I know now that I was lost and beginning to lose the fight.

The lyrics to this song have long been memorized. At this time in my life, I often described my situation to people as being down in a hole. I was struggling to get out, but unsure how. The lyrics said it best.

DOWN IN A HOLE

Alice in Chains 1992

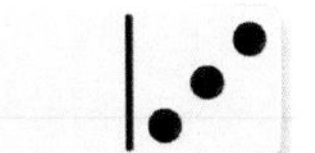
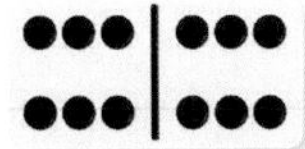
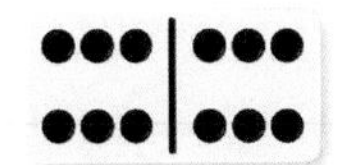

Chapter 27

LIVING IN BLUE

Sagittarians love to get to know other people, as this is another way of learning new things. They have a bunch of friends from all sorts of social and cultural backgrounds.

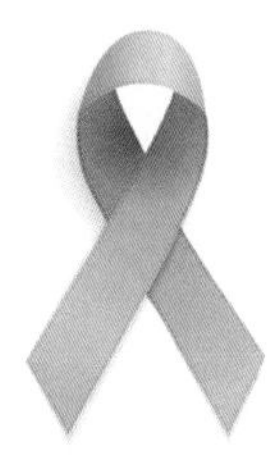
PROSTATE CANCER

As I said before, there were many days that I picked up my phone, opened the daily horoscope app, and tapped Sagittarius. But make no mistake, I put my faith in God and not an app on my phone.

Could God speak to me through an app? Absolutely! Because He is the creator of everything. Would He? Who knows...but on days like today, I liked to think the answer was yes.

Courage is defined in various ways, depending on the person or circumstance. One person might say, "Hey, that was courageous!" while another says, "No, just stupid." For example, there is one instance that my wife referred to as courageous, yet, looking back on it, I might call it a momentary lapse of reason.

It was 1990. Nila and I were visiting a good friend of hers named Marty. Nila and I were only dating at the time, and I was just getting to know some of her friends.

Marty was a special person. He was smart, caring, and sometimes generous to a fault.

At this particular time, in 1990, Marty found himself associating with some bad people. It was obvious that these people were way out of place at Marty's house. I wasn't exactly sure where they came from, why they were there, or what their connection was to Marty.

Marty had a very nice Carolina Panthers jacket with patches and the works, just like a letterman jacket from high school. It came in handy on crisp, cool Georgia nights in the late fall and winter. Marty loved to have close friends over, build a fire, and pitch horseshoes.

One evening, we were at Marty's, pitching horseshoes and having fun. Then, these people who looked out of place showed up. Before long, they were gone again. A little bit later, Marty noticed his Carolina Panthers jacket was missing. The only people that were at his house were trusted friends, except for the standouts.

As soon as I heard what happened, I joined in the conversation and wanted to know where they lived.

"I know where they live," said Jeff.

"Let's go get it," I said to Jeff. I didn't think twice. If I had, I feel certain I would have kept throwing horseshoes with Nila by the fire.

Jeff and I drove to the location.

As we drove, Jeff said, "By the way, these guys are drug dealers."

"Oh..." What should I have said to that? "Can we go back to the house now?"

Then we pulled up in front of a house with one broken shutter and a worn-out paint job. There was green algae growing on the siding. It needed a pressure washing and a paint job. There was a cardboard box on the front stoop with bags of trash piled in it. That didn't worry me as much as the three guys waiting outside the house. It seemed like they were waiting on people. And we weren't expected.

The whole place screamed "wrong, keep moving," but I felt compelled to park. I was going to walk into a crack cocaine house. We would likely be the only two white people there.

I did not care at the time. It was wrong to steal, and I wanted the jacket back. So, I walked past the three guys waiting by the road, tipping my head at them in the universal sign of greeting, then straight up to the door where I knocked and prepared to wait.

However, I hadn't even finished my knock when the door swung open. Three black men stood there.

"What the f**k do you want, and why are you standing at my door?" the man on the left said. His voice was loud and drew attention from inside. I was caught glancing past the three men into the living area, so the greeting was repeated.

"I said, what the f**k do you want?"

This time it was louder. The other two men gathered closer to the door to obscure the view. The smell of marijuana and crack burning slipped by the three men and out onto the porch.

I looked at the man and said, "Look, I don't want any trouble. I am a friend of Marty's, and I was at his house when you and your friends stopped by earlier. One of your friends stole Marty's Carolina Panthers jacket, and we came to get it."

"Hold up," the man said and turned away to walk into the house. The other two men filled the gap and positioned themselves as guards. I was hoping he wasn't going to retrieve a gun, but something told me the guns were already at the door.

A minute later (it felt like a long time), the man returned with the jacket and handed it to me.

"Tell Marty I'm sorry," he said. "I ain't no thief. Evidently, I associate with one, but I will handle that."

"Thank you," I said, "I appreciate that." Then I turned and got in the car.

When we got back to Marty's house, he was impressed.

"I can't believe two white boys went to that house, got this jacket, and lived to talk about it," Marty exclaimed.

That is how our friendship, spanning decades, began. I still wonder about the feat that began our friendship so many years ago. What do you think? Courageous or careless?

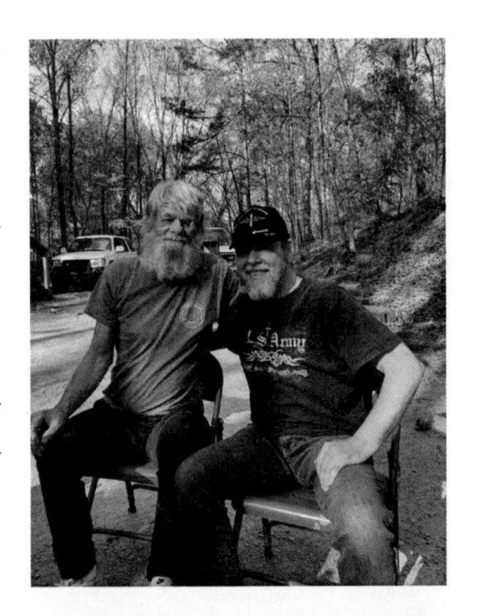

From left: Marty Campbell and Perry Muse 2021

Nila and I had decided, long before cancer, that we would renew our vows to celebrate our thirtieth anniversary. We had originally planned to do so on one of our annual trips to Las Vegas. But that was before cancer found its way into Mr. Skeleton and before COVID caused the world to stand still. So, we devised a plan B.

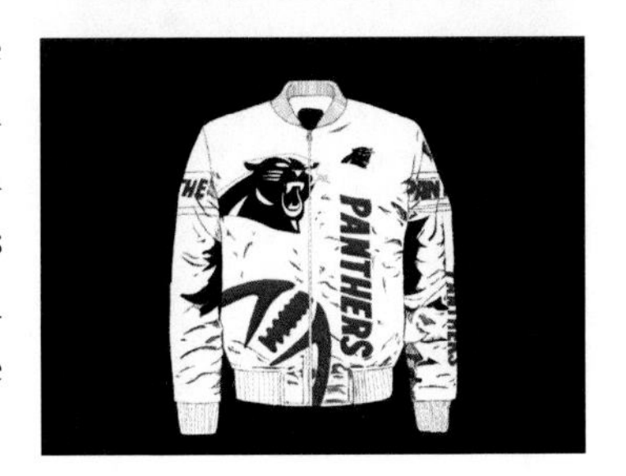

We decided instead to have the ceremony on the thirtieth anniversary of the day we met. So, Saturday, May 8, 2021, would be the big day.

Things were more upbeat these days. Planning the ceremony was energizing. I had so much I wanted to say to Nila. It is unfortunate that so many people do not really know the Nila Muse that I do.

Nila married me when I was broke and starting completely over in life. I was fresh out of the army, divorced, and recently homeless. I never stopped working, but I was aimless. I just went from friend to friend for a while, drinking myself to sleep on various couches.

One of those couches belonged to Steve and Paula Keylon. They took me in and allowed me the opportunity to get back on my feet. It was such a gracious thing they did for me. I had only known Steve a short time at work. I will never understand how they could be so kind to me. It taught me what kindness really looked like.

For me, getting back on my feet meant renting a furnished 1950s trailer with a fenced-in yard at the end of Sanford Street. That was where I lived when I started making life memories with Nila and our three boys, only three, four, and five years old at the time. Steve and Paula are still like family to me, some thirty-plus years later.

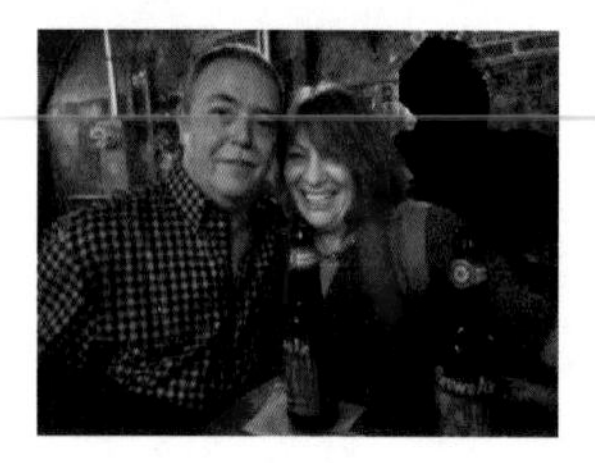

Steve and Paula Keylon

As Nila and I made preparations for our vow renewal, we often reminisced about the days on Sanford Street and how much we were in love in those hard early days. Over thirty years later, we may have more, but our love for each other is still exciting, yet it is deeper and stronger after thirty years of tempering. We wanted the world to know. We planned a testament to our partnership.

We were also planning a family celebration on the weekend after the wedding. Family only. All the kids, spouses, grandkids, etc., would be there. This time I was praying for no Family Feud.

However, before all of the celebrations, it was time for my quarterly Lupron shot and CT scans.

March 10, 2021, I was scheduled to be at Mountain Forest Hospital. This was the familiar hospital I'd visited when the sack of gravel caused excessive swelling in my throat.

"They solved the swelling in my throat from that sack of gravel, so I hope they can give me a good report on Mr. Skeleton and my organs," I thought. "I can't look like I'm dying on the vine at my wedding."

I was grateful that neither the scans nor the results would be on the thirteenth. I felt like no one could blame me for being superstitious at this point.

I had a grasp of my medicine, dosages, and routine. The chronic fatigue was there all of the time, of course. Although I was managing the pain in my upper back muscles, it was discouraging how little I was physically able to do without making my upper back muscles angry. I spent my days trying not to feel blue: not the color of my cancer, but the color of misery and despair.

Nila was doing more than ever, especially with the salon. Her hair was a solid blue color these days, the color of my cancer ribbon. Words can't describe how wonderful it made me feel every time I looked at it.

It was starting to sink in that I might never be able to work in the yard again, or build anything, or do any of the tasks that I had always loved. And if not me, then who? We had a big house and yard. For the moment, I just prayed about it and gave thanks for all of my blessings, for feeling well, for being able to work, and for Nila and me being so happy. I also prayed for courage.

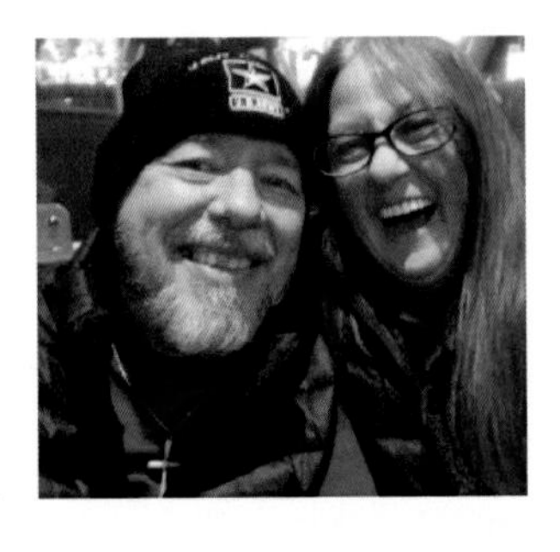

Perry and Nila, February 2021

On the Saturday before my scans, it appeared we were going to close the salon. We had three groomers that had walked out, and the fourth was scheduled to leave at the end of the month. I had been praying so hard for God to send us a seasoned groomer because this would allow us to keep the salon open. Yet it appeared that wasn't what God had planned for us.

Then, at the last minute, we had an applicant. The résumé said she had been to grooming school and had five years' experience. Hallelujah! She was scheduled to come in and groom as part of the interview process.

Monday afternoon, the grooming applicant showed up at the shop. I was stunned to find out that she, too, had blue hair! I couldn't be at the interview because I was having an iron infusion. Nila sent me a text. It read, "She starts on Wednesday!"

The other stunning aspect of this was that I had gone to see the landlord on two separate occasions to tell him I was going to close the salon. Each time, he had a phone call and had to leave. By the time he caught back up with me, we had hired the groomer I had prayed so hard for.

I lay in the recliner getting my iron infusion and just repeatedly said a prayer giving thanks. It was all so surreal. Not being able to pin down the landlord to tell him the bad news. The new groomer having blue hair like Nila. It just felt like a sign.

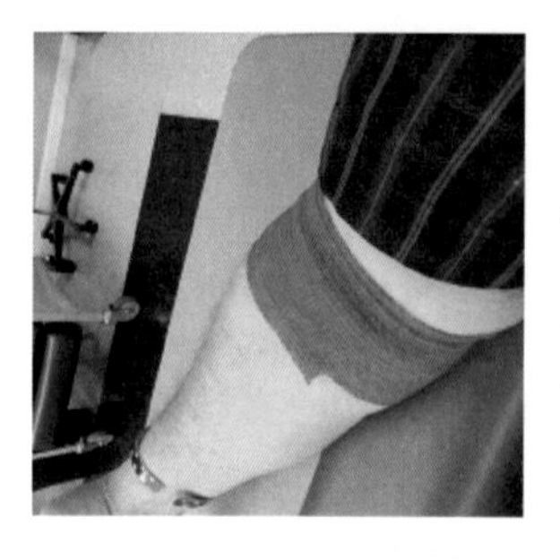

But then, my infusion was over. When the nurse removed the needle and wrapped my arm with the medical tape, I just looked skyward, laughed, and said, "Of course."

For the first time ever, it was blue, the color that represented my cancer. I felt as though I was living in the color blue.

Perry with a blue wrap

Of course, on Tuesday I had to open my horoscope app.

Daily / Weekly / Monthly
Sagitarrius
11/22 to 12/21
Alias: The Archer
March 9, 2020

You may be coming close to the end of something that has not been going well. It may seem obvious that this cannot work out, Sagittarius, but it can. If you try for a moment to defy your natural logical approach to life, you will see that sometimes things are possible that seem impossible. Just as there are racehorses that win in the last lengths of a race, you can pull off a major feat if you believe you can. It certainly can't hurt to try.

On Wednesday, March 10, 2021, I arrived at Mountain Forest Hospital. I checked in and went through the routine COVID protocol of having my temperature checked and answering some questions.

From there I went to finance/check-in window number one. I took care of payment and electronically signed some documents. Before going to the next check station, I was given yet another bracelet. This would be number twenty-nine to add to my collection since October 2017.

I made my way past the coffee shop and gift shop before making a left down a short hallway to my third check-in station. Once checked in, I had a seat in the waiting area and caught up on work emails.

After about forty-five minutes, my name was called by a nurse at the door beside the check-in. Unlike SCC, she did not know what Perry Muse looked like. As we walked along the hallway, she verified my name and birth date.

We entered a room, and I sat down in a chair that was made for lab draws.

"That is everyone's favorite vein," I said, pointing it out on my right arm.

"That one looks pretty good," she said, tapping it after she had wrapped my arm with the band and asked me to make a fist. Then she pulled out the needle and tried to slip it into the vein.

Fail.

"Ooow," she said. "Well, that didn't work? Did it? I'll just try again."

She tried unsuccessfully to put in the IV eight times: pushing and pulling the needle in and out of my arm, trying to get a successful stick.

From there we went to my left forearm on the outside of the bend. For me, it was a more painful location, but I had become a master of dealing with pain at this stage.

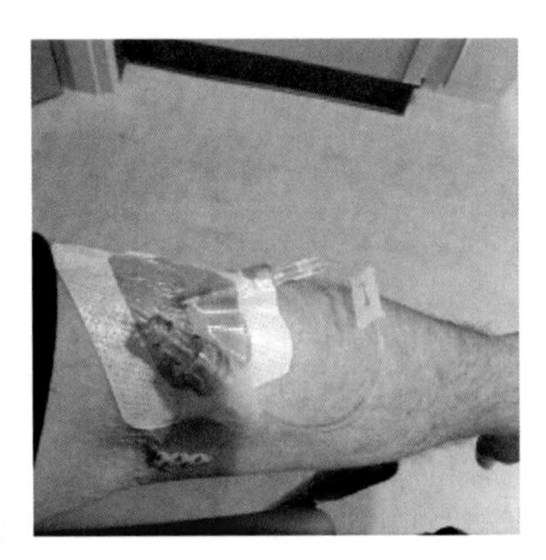

IV in forearm

Next, I had to lie down on the familiar-looking table that extended from the donut ring. At this point, I asked the nurse for a picture, and she hesitated but took my phone to take the photo. I explained to her that I was writing a book, and the pictures would be helpful for the reader.

We started the process, which was a scan of my upper abdomen without contrast. Although the table wasn't painful, I knew it would only be a matter of time.

With the first scan complete, the technician explained she would be injecting contrast into my IV. There was a large tube protruding from the machine on the left and above me. There was a coiled tube attached that reminded me of a spring. The technician attached the other end of the tube to my IV port.

"So, tell me about this book...and why are we doing this scan today?" the technician, dressed all in blue scrubs, asked as she efficiently moved hoses and hooked my IV to something on the machine.

I told her that I had already written over two hundred and fifty pages about my cancer journey and that I had recently found that cancer was in my bones.

"I am so sorry," she said.

Quickly, she was ready for the test to start. The contrast rushed into my bloodstream and through my body. First was the taste and smell. Then a warming sensation in my chest. Finally, the slow warmth in my pelvis area that felt like I was accidentally urinating on myself.

When the second scan was finished, the technician asked if she could take the pictures for me. I was perplexed as to why she would want to take more, but then she explained in an apologetic tone.

"Since we were taken over by a new company, we aren't supposed to take any pictures in the hospital. I didn't really take one the first time," she confessed.

The whole experience was so different from any of my other scans. The IV being put into my arm in the scan room was different. The device with the protruding tube that delivered contrast into the IV port, rather than drinking the contrast, or the contrast being delivered via syringe.

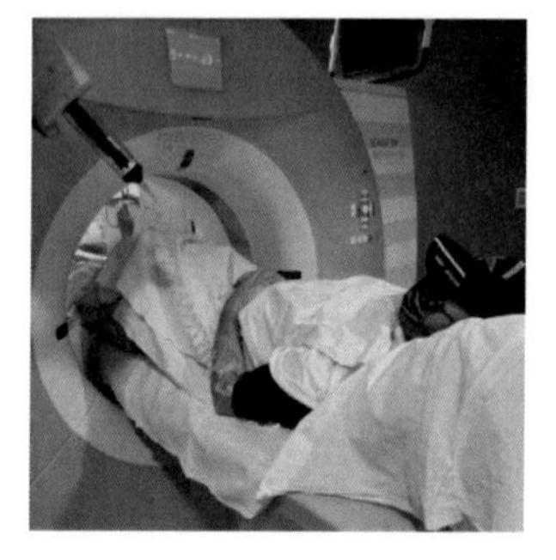

On CT table

Once the test was finished, I needed help from the technician to get up. I had rusted up again and had gotten a little sore in a short time. Then it was back to the waiting area, where *Rosanne* was still on the television.

A few minutes later, it was a different nurse who opened the door and called my name. This time we made a few turns along the hallway to a room with a familiar sign on the door. I was instructed to sit down as the nurse left through the door.

With nobody around, I took a couple of more pictures.

The nurse returned, holding a tray. A large blue capsule was the only thing in the middle of the tray.

"What is that?" I asked.

"It's called a blue pig," she said. "It's a lead containment capsule to limit our exposure," she explained. She told me that the odd-looking syringe that was used at SCC was a lead shield. It was for the same purpose.

She removed the syringe from the blue pig that weighed about five pounds and screwed it into my port. One slow squeeze, and the radiopharmaceutical was pushed into a vein on my left forearm.

"Now you can go eat lunch and come back at 1:15 for your last scans," she told me.

As we walked back to the waiting room, I explained about my book and why I had asked for a picture of the blue pig. I thought it was more than coincidental that it was blue.

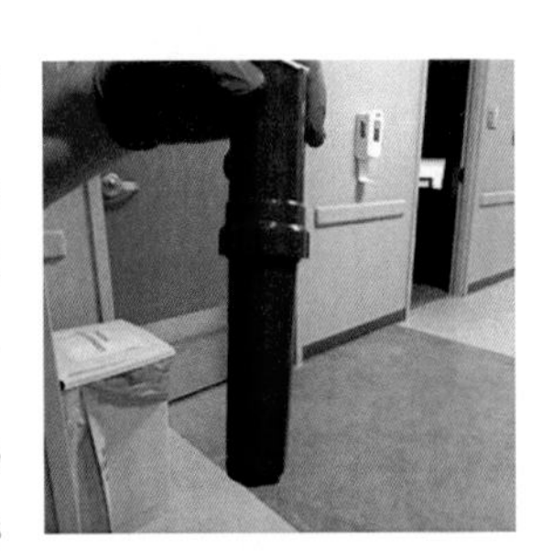

Blue pig

While looking for a place I could have lunch and catch up on emails, I kept thinking of the nurse and the five-pound blue pig that was used to protect the workers from exposure.

"The blue pig, made of lead, is to limit their exposure to the liquid that is injected into my body," I thought. "This is a quarterly routine, plus I am taking four pills of Xtandi each night that can't be handled, especially by anyone who is pregnant. How long can Mr. Skeleton hold up? I hope they aren't killing me, trying to treat the cancer."

At 1:15 p.m., the same nurse that had introduced me to the blue pig opened the door. This time, she did recognize me.

"Mr. Muse, come on back," she said in a friendly voice.

We walked down the hall to a new destination. The room was dimly lit, and music was playing, but too softly for me to make out what it was. I removed my belt, hat, and crucifix. I gave the crucifix a kiss and laid it on the table. I laid down on the table, and a triangle-shaped foam was placed under my knees. The nurse covered me in a sheet-like fabric with Velcro to hold it in place, and then she asked me to pull my pants down to my knees. For the first time ever, a large rubber band was put around my feet to keep them in place. It felt very comfortable. I knew that would change by the time the scans were complete

"Please put your hands by your sides, not across your pelvis," said the technician. "We don't want any bones crossing over bones."

There were four sets of scans in total. Then the table slipped out of the ring, and it was time to get up.

Again, I asked for a picture. The technician knew my story from our chitchat while I was getting situated on the table. I heard her make a call to get permission.

The phone was on speaker, and I heard the response.

"So, he is writing a book about cancer and wants you to use his phone to take a picture?" said the ambiguous voice coming out of the phone stuck to the wall.

"Yes," answered the technician.

"Let me call you back," stated the voice on the other end of the call.

I lay on the table for another ten minutes. Patiently.

I imagined the call going up to the fifth-floor boardroom where men and women in suits and dresses pondered the request for an exception to the rule.

"So, I have a motion to put before the board right now to allow a patient an exception for a picture," said the suit at the end of the table. "The patient is writing a book about his own cancer, and he wants a picture of his procedure. Do I hear a motion?"

"I don't know, Cal," said another suit, "It does set a precedent."

"I'll make a motion," said a dress.

I could see them going back and forth while the muscles in my upper back started to warn me that a picture might not be worth waiting on.

As I lay there quietly, the music became clearer to me. I could now tell it was Christian music. Through the speakers, a soft voice sang, "Come to Jesus. Come to Jesus. Sing to Jesus."

I wanted to tell the singer, "I am trying to come to Jesus."

Just before I called out to say I didn't need the picture, another technician came through the door to tell me it was approved.

I was mesmerized by his mask. It was a medical mask, but the center was open and had a clear plastic cover on it. His mouth was visible as he spoke and explained the "no pictures" policy. It was the fourth time I had heard it, and I let him know I understood and was grateful for the exception.

Strapped in for CT scan

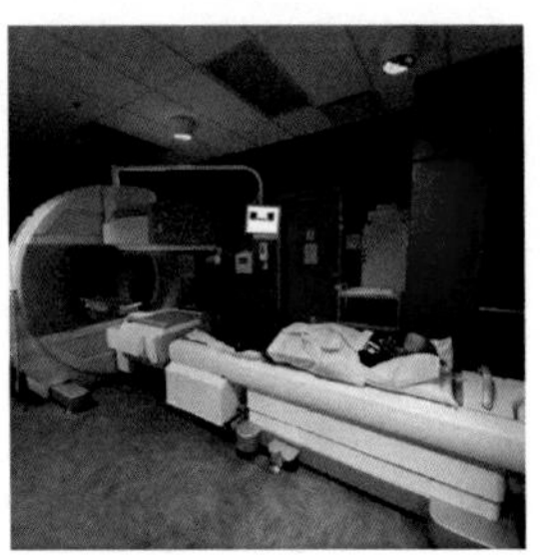

This time, getting up was more challenging. When I tried holding one of the technician's arms and pulling up, it was too painful.

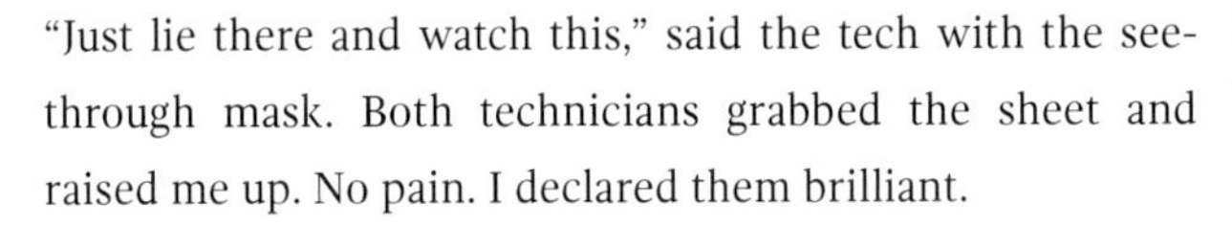

"Just lie there and watch this," said the tech with the see-through mask. Both technicians grabbed the sheet and raised me up. No pain. I declared them brilliant.

I left the hospital and drove back home. The day was all but over, but the sun was shining, and the temperature was close to seventy degrees.

Once home, I got myself a comfortable chair and sat in the sun in my yard. I watched Hooch and Sparky play and hunt while I caught up on emails and made a couple of work phone calls. It was a beautiful day, and I was grateful to be able to enjoy it. The only thing missing was my blue-haired wife Nila.

On Friday, following my scans, I received a call from a restricted number. After a moment's hesitation, I answered.

"Hi, Perry. It's Sara Hammons from Dr. Famoyin's office," was the familiar voice on the other end. "We got your scan results back and thought you would like to know that the report says there is no indication of bone metastasis."

I was temporarily stunned and in disbelief of what I had heard.

"No bone metastasis?" I asked.

Sara repeated, "That's right, no bone metastasis. We thought you would want to know."

I ended the call in a daze, like a dream. I could not believe what I had heard, and suddenly questions flooded my thoughts.

"Did the Xtandi kill it?" I wondered. "Was SCC too aggressive in the diagnosis? After all, it was a tiny sclerotic lesion that anyone could have. Does this mean I can stop the awful chemo pills? Is the cancer still there, waiting until a later day to slip into Mr. Skeleton?"

All these questions would have to wait until I saw Dr. Famoyin again on Monday before my next iron infusion. Meanwhile, I talked to Nila and made the executive decision to stop taking the Xtandi. It was an easy choice. The pills had robbed me of my evenings with Nila. The Saturday nights of listening to music, playing Angry Birds, and getting lost slow dancing had all been absent since I started the medication.

I skipped my Xtandi on the Friday night that I received the call from Sara. I wasn't sure it was the right thing, but I needed a break.

On Saturday I woke up feeling great. I felt like the old Perry was back. I do not mean to imply that I was healed. I knew that too much work would bring the pain back in my upper back and hip. I just felt generally like my old self.

That night Nila and I made time to do what we loved most: listen to music, play Angry Birds, and get lost slow dancing with the lights dimmed. It was wonderful. I missed those nights so much. We held one another extra close, knowing now how special the moment was. Our favorite song to dance to was by Tesla and called "What You Give." I wanted it to last forever.

On Monday, Nila joined me at Dr. Famoyin's office. We both needed to hear his assessment. Before he entered the room, I asked Nila to remember to get a picture of us together for the book. I realized I did not have one after all this time.

The good doctor entered the room in his typical jovial mood. He had not seen Nila in a while, thanks to COVID and the salon, and he immediately took the opportunity to have some fun with her.

He looked through my report.

"This all looks really, really good," he said. "Just keep doing what you are doing."

That was when I had to break the news.

"Dr. Famoyin, you are probably going to get on to me, but when Sara called and said there was no indication of bone metastasis on Friday, I stopped taking the Xtandi."

It was at that point that Dr. Famoyin did what I always respected. He told me the whole truth.

"You know we talked about how it seemed very aggressive of SCC to start the Lupron and then to pronounce the bone metastasis," he began. "But once they make that determination, we typically don't go against their judgment. This is why I told you to stay the course. However, you are in a very gray area now," he continued. "The question becomes whether there was bone metastasis and the Xtandi worked, or whether there never was."

I voiced my opinion: "The report from January 13 said I had a tiny sclerotic lesion on my third rib. We know that anyone can have the same thing, and it could not be cancer related."

Dr. Famoyin agreed with my remarks.

"So, it becomes your choice. You have always been very aggressive with your treatment to stay ahead," Dr. Famoyin said. "You can start back on the Xtandi or not. If not, we will continue to monitor your PSA."

"If it were to start rising," I interrupted, "would it become castration resistant?"

"Yes," he replied. "If it becomes castration resistant, it means the cancer will have evolved and found other testosterone or estrogen to feed it." He paused for a moment to let that sink in. "At that time, we have other treatments to knock it back down. If it were to metastasize into your bones or soft tissue, you would go back to chemo."

"To be honest, Doc, before Friday, I felt like a cancer patient all day, every day. Once I stopped the Xtandi, I felt great. I didn't think I could ever feel this good again," I explained.

"So, I agree with you about stopping the Xtandi. Who knows, if the time comes when you may need to start chemo again, there may be new medications available. There are new ones coming out all the time. If needed, we will do something besides Xtandi. It shouldn't make you feel that bad anyway," he concluded.

Nila and I were beyond thrilled. I was given a new lease on life. I was not cancer free, but I was free of Ms. Misery.

I stood up to have Nila take our picture.

Before heading out to get my infusion, I realized Dr. Famoyin was wearing a blue shirt. Coincidence? I think not.

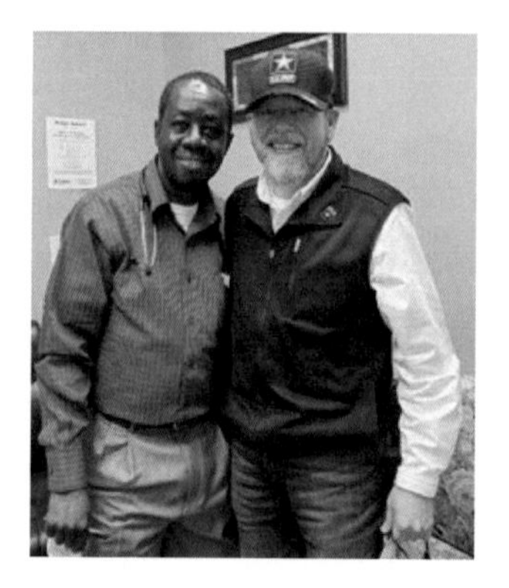

From left: Dr. Famoyin, Perry Muse

Blue is the color of my cancer ribbon. Appropriate since blue is often how I felt. But the lyrics to this song told me how to deal with feeling blue.

SONG SUNG BLUE

Neil Diamond 1972

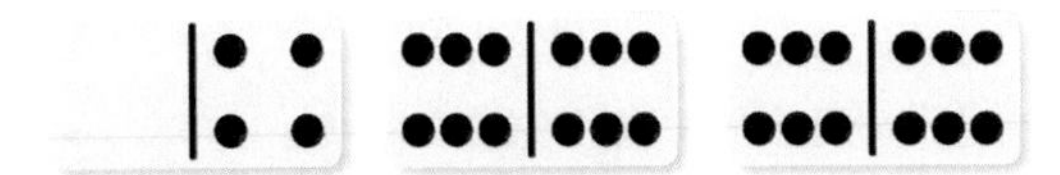

Chapter 28

MOVING FORWARD IN REVERSE PART I

Sagittarians never give up when things get tough. They are experts at moving on, and they can rebuild themselves time and time again whenever things turn sour.

My internal dialogue was very active after meeting with Dr. Famoyin: "Can this be real? Is it possible my cancer hasn't metastasized after all? Is it just another case like hepatitis C where I got a false positive?" said the optimistic voice that ran through my mind. But my negative shouter wanted to be heard as well, and most times, he was the most persistent. "You will know in three months when they bring out the blue pig again," whispered the pessimistic shadow on my shoulder.

The questions circulated in my head often, especially when I laid down to sleep. I never wanted to think about it. But the devil was always there, perched closely to my ear, encouraging me to keep building my boat.

I believe that only God can cure cancer. I will not engage in the philosophical debate as to why He does not if He can. It is just my belief.

Imagine if you dedicated your life to curing cancer, and finally, after years and years of work, you broke the code. You unlocked the door to cure cancer and save millions of people worldwide. The ultimate reward for your life's work.

But then Big Brother said, "We are sorry, but you can't tell anyone about this. It will economically ruin the medical industry and cost Big Pharma billions of dollars." I do not see how that could be kept a secret. Big Brother cannot pay more than the cure is worth. Even if he did, how do you keep it quiet? And if the bribe were offered, wouldn't you just write a best-selling book and tell the world? So, if man hasn't been able to cure cancer, then it stands to reason, in my mind, that only God can.

I do not think I am "cancer free." But I can't explain why I suddenly felt so well. I cannot explain why Mountain Forest Hospital did not detect the tiny sclerotic lesion on my right third rib. And, if they did detect it, why didn't they report it as being consistent with bone metastasis?

"Perhaps they did see the lesion but thought it normal for me when they compared it to my previous scan from January 13," I considered.

In the past three and a half years, I had been through a lot. The first eighteen months, I had four major surgeries, radiation, and a minor surgery that included a cuss, a fart, and a scalpel lying on the table. Who would feel good after all that? But even after I was pronounced "cancer free" and my testosterone began to rise, I had not felt this good.

I knew I was not nearly as strong as I was before the "C" bomb was dropped in July 2017. I had been in a perpetual state of recovery; thanks to cancer and chemo, my body had been fighting itself. Plus, the Lupron had caused all the muscles in my body to wither away and shrink. However, when spring came in March 2021, and I quit the chemo pills, I felt rejuvenated. I fully understood the positive mental impact of finding out cancer might not have metastasized, but what about the pain and misery?

On March 20, 2021, the weather app had forecast sunshine. The weather was beautiful, and it was time for yard work. The temperature was near freezing at sunrise. I waited until around 11:00 a.m. for it to warm up. The high was forecast to be seventy degrees, perfect for yard work.

My first order of business was to pick up the debris from a prior night's wind, and there was a lot.

"It's all a part of living in the forest," I thought. I was sure bending and picking up limbs would set off the pain in my upper back or my left hip.

Once all the limbs were put in the firepit, I began cleaning up the patio, partly from the wind knocking over the trash cans, and partly from leftover tables and coolers from a get-together last fall. Uncharacteristically, I had often seen the clutter but never quite felt up to doing anything about it until now.

Next order of business was the firewood. We had several ricks, or cords, of wood for inside and outside burning. Half of them had toppled over thanks to the wooden support shelf collapsing from the weight and the high winds testing the strength of the interlocking split wood. I had known for days that this would be the true test of my strength and physical limits.

I managed through the chore of restacking the wood and found myself still able to work further down my spring to-do list.

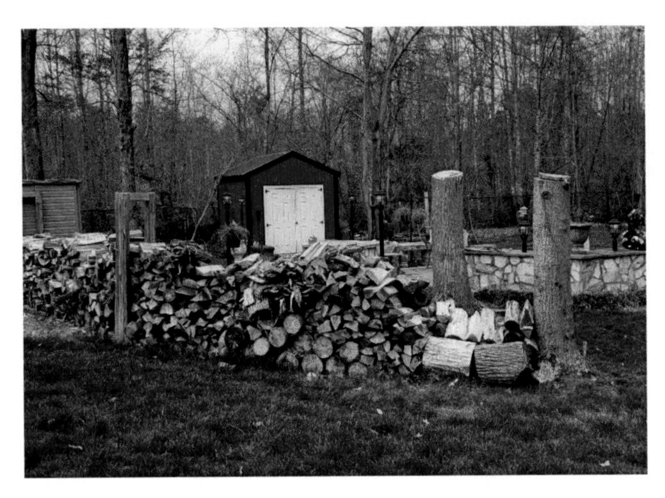

Ricks of firewood stacked

I opened the red and white outbuilding that contained everything for yard work in it. After dragging the picnic table to the patio from its storage spot, I gassed up the riding lawn mower. I took my position on the seat and turned the key.

The mower's engine churned over and over, but at last, it fired up. The sound and feel as I backed out of the building were deeply satisfying. Still, I wondered if the constant demand of pressing the clutch with my left foot while steering would ignite the pain in my hip and back.

As I finished mowing the lawn, my son-in-law Cory pulled in. I had rented a walk-behind aerator, and we were going to share the use of it. We had a deal. I would pay for the rental, and he would do a large patch in my yard before taking it to do his own yard.

Shortly after he arrived, the job was finished, and Cory was headed out. I retrieved the bag of grass seed and the spreader from the outbuilding.

The boxes on my list were getting checked off, and the day had moved into the late afternoon. It was still going to be a while until Nila was home from the salon, so I grabbed the string trimmer to cut back the monkey grass before the new sprouts were too tall.

The string mower revved in my hands as I moved around the yard. Halfway through my monkey grass job, the battery died. It was time to call it a day. But what a day it had been. I had done a tremendous amount of work, some of it physically demanding, and I was not anything more than tired and a little achy. I cannot imagine any sixty-year-old man being as out of shape as me and not feeling the same.

I walked over and sat down on the swing near the patio. The sun was behind me, and I looked back on my busy day. As I gently swayed back and forth, I said a little prayer. "Lord, thank you for this beautiful day that you made. Thank you for allowing me to feel so well."

When I got the news from Dr. Famoyin about my bone scan, I had to share the news with the handful of people I had talked to previously about the scan results from January 13. I was thankful I had not made a full-blown announcement and told the whole world. It would have been awkward to undo that announcement.

One of those few people was a friend and coworker named Rick. This was the same Rick that I had gone flying over Fremont Street with on our last business trip to Las Vegas.

Rick was elated with the news and made the comment, "You are invincible!" I was humbled to hear such a thing and found myself struggling for a response.

"People don't realize that to be invincible means you are made of scars," I thought.

The following weekend I had planned for more yard work. But first, I needed to do my part on the inside since Nila was working at the salon and making late-night trips to care for our boarding guests.

I spent some five hours on Friday cleaning and organizing. We had wooden floors throughout most of the main floor of the house. I swept, vacuumed, and used a Swiffer to finish off the floors.

When Nila walked into the house, it was filled with the aroma of Hawaiian plug-ins and supper.

While cleaning the house doesn't seem like such a monumental task (everyone has housekeeping chores), it was a big deal for me. Just a few weeks prior, I would not have been able to do the floors. The constant pushing and pulling of the Swiffer would have wreaked havoc on me.

That night, I was unable to sleep. I felt energized and awake. Not the way it felt when the low-level electricity was running through my bones, but like I was alive. At 1:00 a.m., I gave up on sleeping and decided to write in my book.

"I can sleep when I'm dead" passed through my mind once again.

I crawled back in bed at 2:45 a.m., knowing I needed to sleep if I was going to have another big day on Saturday. It was 3:30 a.m. the last time I looked at the clock. Sometime shortly after that, I fell asleep.

I woke up and jumped out of bed at 8:00 a.m., ready to pick up where I had left off on my to-do list in the yard. I gave Nila a hug as she left to work in the salon. Saturdays are always busy for dog grooming salons.

I wondered how long this could last, how long until the pain returned and the rust started forming again in my joints. I decided to open my horoscope app and sit down with my cup of coffee before heading out to begin the day's to-do list.

I revisited the weather app and was disappointed to see rain in the forecast. This forced me to find some new tasks. So, I got up from my coffee break, got dressed, grabbed some laundry to wash, and loaded Thor up to take to the salon.

I found myself still amazed at how I felt. My sister Gail would say she was not amazed at all. We spent almost two hours on the phone when I told her the news.

"I have been waiting on this phone call, Perry," she said. "You don't realize how many people are praying for you. There are people as far away as California who ask about you and tell me that you are on their prayer list at church."

Daily / Weekly / Monthly
Sagitarrius
11/22 to 12/21
Alias: The Archer
March 27, 2020

A person who worries frequently can find something to worry about in even the most seemingly insignificant situation. And the keyword here, Sagittarius, is "find." When a worrier, or anyone else for that matter, goes on the search for something to worry about, they will surely find it. You are not typically a big worrier, but you may be ultra-concerned about something now where a lot is at stake. Don't start looking for something to worry about. Start looking for something to celebrate!

I did not want to get overly excited just yet. But it felt as though I had topped the mountain and was headed back down. Maybe as though this had all come full circle, and I was

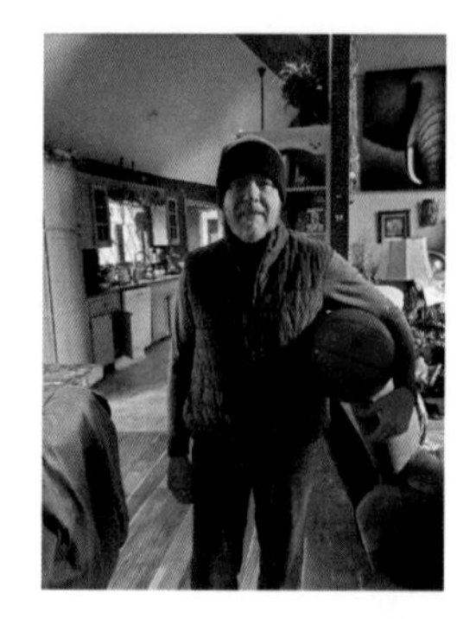

back to normal. I had gone from needing Nila to help me get out of a chair or bed, to doing so with ease. Getting into bed or rolling over did not make me cry out in pain. My energy was good. Not normal, but good. I couldn't recall the last 5-Hour Energy drink I'd had. My appetite was good. The other day I'd picked up the basketball Nila got me for Christmas and shot the ball in the cul-de-sac.

Perry ready for basketball

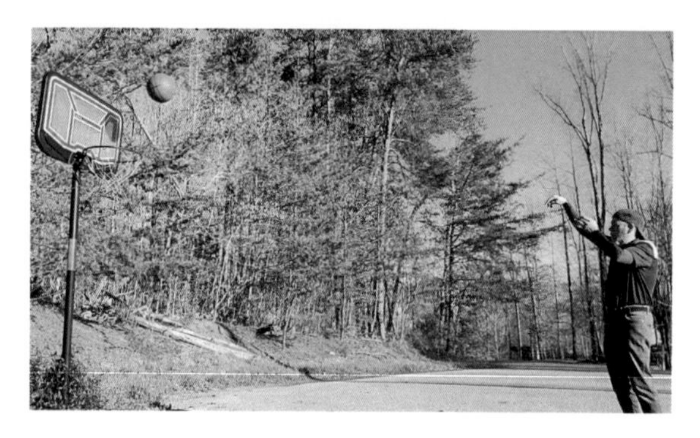

Perry shooting basketball in cul de sac

In two weeks, we were finally getting to go on vacation to Myrtle Beach. It would just be the two of us, and we needed the getaway. Nila had been working six days every week at the salon, plus going in after-hours for boarding dogs. This after not working a job for twenty years!

I had not been to the Calhoun plant in a long time. I hadn't been sure I would ever feel like making the trip on my own again. But now I felt ready.

I crammed a lot into the few weeks leading up to vacation. We were planning the start of the new coater that had been built and installed at the Calhoun plant. There were trials for new customers that I wanted to be a part of. It was one of the most enjoyable parts of my job. It was always so rewarding to create something new.

I made the four-and-a-half-hour trip to Calhoun three times in the weeks leading up to vacation time. All the trips were very productive and busy, just the way I liked it. On one of the trips, we had our quarterly executive meeting. This meeting lasted for hours and covered all the business of Foam Products. This meeting was a good gauge of my body and energy.

I was again amazed at how well I felt after the long drive. Unlike in the past, I did not take any naproxen or pain relievers. I did not feel the need to drink a 5-Hour Energy. I felt normal. My hips did not hurt from sitting. My joints did not rust up on me.

"How are you feeling these days?" a member of the executive team asked me after the meeting. I was excited to answer honestly and explain how well I really felt.

"You have to understand," I began explaining to the group, "a couple of months ago, I was down in a hole. The chemo pills wiped me out every night, and I struggled to get over the effects the following day. I was told my cancer was incurable, and that may still be true, but something has changed, and I feel incredible. I am not exaggerating when I say I was down in a hole. I can only explain the turnaround as divine intervention."

The expressions were of surprise.

"Very good, Sagittarius. You have hidden your struggles well," I thought as I gauged their expressions.

On Tuesday, April 13, I had my follow-up appointment with Dr. Famoyin. On a previous visit, he had discovered SCC had been giving me Prolia for over two years. He was perplexed and explained that Prolia is for patients with osteoporosis, and it would not benefit my condition, in his opinion.

I originally had high hopes for SCC. I was impressed with many things about the facility and personnel, like Dr. Taha. But, looking back on it, I see some things I question. The prefix of my name is not doctor. However, it is my opinion that SCC's modus operandi is to test, test, test and treat, treat, treat. This is an aggressive method of treating the patient's condition, but it also costs a great deal of money. In my case, I would say it is not necessarily in the best interest of the patient.

On my April 13 appointment (again with the number 13), Dr. Famoyin was happy and surprised to hear my report.

I said, "Doc, you don't understand how great I feel. I feel better than I have in years. And consider that a couple of months ago, I was on chemo and down in a hole. I believe God had another plan for me."

Dr. Famoyin remarked on the crucifix that I wore around my neck: "I see you have a crucifix on today."

"I wear it every day and night. I have for years," I responded. He explained that he grew up Catholic and that he kept a rosary with him.

"Then you understand that we are here for God and not ourselves," he said. I did know, more so now than ever before.

Before ending our visit, he recommended I get Zometa. He reaffirmed that Prolia was not for me but felt Zometa was the right treatment.

Without hesitation, I said, "I trust you, Doc. You are my primary medical caregiver."

I made my way back to the infusion unit. Zometa is given intravenously. I would also have my quarterly Lupron shot.

Once I was hooked up to the IV, the medication was injected. Unlike the iron infusions that took a few hours, this would only take about fifteen minutes.

As the injection was given, I took the opportunity to ask the technician a question: "Why am I getting this?"

The answer caught me off guard. In my mind, it was being administered to strengthen my bones, to protect Mr. Skeleton in the event the cancer was to metastasize, but that wasn't the reason, according to the tech.

"You are getting this because of high calcium in your blood," she explained.

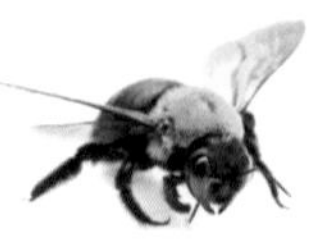

Through all my research, I had learned about high calcium levels in the blood. When cancer metastasizes into the bones, it attacks the bones and deposits calcium into the bloodstream. I always thought of it as a carpenter bee. Carpenter bees look similar to bumblebees but have shiny backs, whereas bumblebees have hairy backs. Carpenter bees bore holes in wood to lay their eggs.

The idea had haunted me..."Once the cancer is in Mr. Skeleton, it will begin boring into the bones like a carpenter bee. Instead of a pile of wood dust, I will just have calcium ground away and deposited into my blood. My bones can only handle so much grinding before they begin to break."

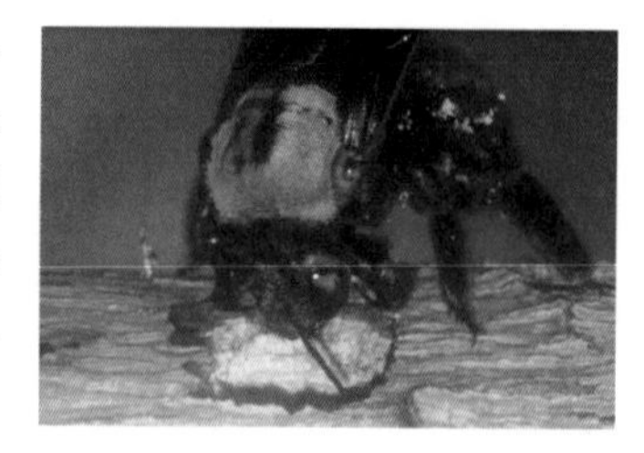

The images of carpenter bees boring away inside my bones haunted me even before I learned that there was a high calcium level in my blood. As I sat watching the Zometa trickle into my vein, I decided to read more about it. Here is what I learned.

- Zometa is a prescription drug used to treat hypercalcemia due to cancer. Hypercalcemia is a high level of calcium in your blood. In this situation, it is caused by cancer.
- Zometa contains the active drug zoledronic acid. It belongs to a class of drugs called bisphosphonates. Bisphosphonates help prevent the breakdown of bone.
- The typical Zometa dosage for adults with hypercalcemia from cancer is 4 mg, *given as a single dose*. This should be infused over at least fifteen minutes. If your blood calcium level doesn't fall to a normal level within seven days, you may need a second dose of Zometa.
- The typical Zometa dosage for adults with multiple myeloma or bone metastases from solid tumors is 4 mg, given *every three to four weeks*. Each infusion should be given over at least fifteen minutes.

The list of possible side effects was the longest I had ever read. I say this having had a lot of experience with studying medications. The side effects for Zometa were three pages long!

Suddenly, my heart sank. I had thought this was something in addition to the vitamin D3 and calcium to strengthen my bones. But if my calcium level was already too high, it meant something more dreadful.

"Could it be that the nurse was just telling me what Zometa is typically for? Perhaps Dr. Famoyin is just being proactive. Could the 1,200 mg of calcium I take daily be the reason my test was high, or was it even high at all? How can I feel so well if cancer is grinding away inside of my bones? How long until the pain and fractures begin? How long before the storm returns? How long until I'm down in a hole again?"

The morbid thoughts washed over me like a summer rain shower. A little voice on my shoulder screamed that I needed to take up building my boat again.

This time I did not listen to the voice. I did not begin working on my boat again. I felt great. I couldn't imagine the worst-case scenario was true.

I took some time to analyze the whole situation. The facts were overwhelming. I was experiencing the least amount of pain I had had in years. I was able to shoot a basketball. I was sleeping great. I had plenty of energy at work. I was doing yard work again. We had a vacation planned to Myrtle Beach at the end of April. In just over a month, a week after returning from vacation, I was going to marry my soul mate again. I could not wrap my mind around the feeling of stepping back in time, as if I had teleported back to an earlier period in my life and been given another chance at living. It was as though I was moving forward in reverse.

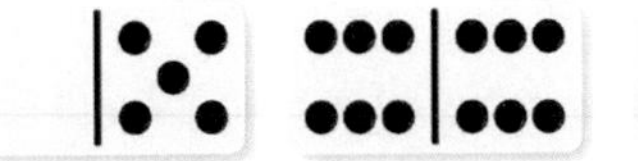

Chapter 29

MOVING FORWARD IN REVERSE PART II

After running through the facts in my mind a hundred times, I decided that I no longer cared. Why drag myself and my morale down when there was so much to be grateful for?

And so, I put the morbid thoughts away in my pocket (they would always remain close by). I began to live life like I never had before.

My goal was to cherish each minute. To recognize everything as a blessing and be grateful. To be humble and to be a positive influence. To talk to my children and grandchildren routinely. To thank God each day for allowing me to feel well and for all our blessings. To love Nila and not let anything petty cause us a moment's grief. And, most of all, to celebrate life.

I reminded myself that God would not give me more than I could handle. That had certainly been proven time and again in my lifetime. Although there would always be rain, I must not focus on the storm, but I should recognize the strength and wisdom I gained from it.

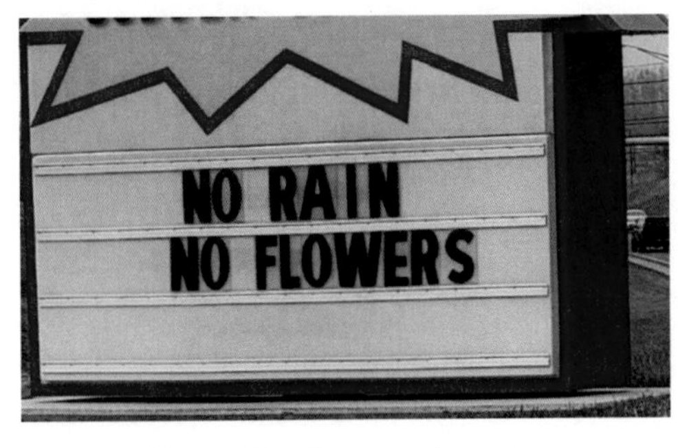

Sign at Pals by grooming salon

On my way to the grooming salon one day, I passed the nearby Pal's restaurant. Anyone familiar with the chain knows they post new sayings on their roadside sign daily. This particular day it seemed as though the sign was meant for me. It affirmed the mindset I had recently adopted.

On April 23, 2021, Nila and I loaded up to head for Myrtle Beach. We would make it halfway and spend the night in Columbia, SC. I wanted to be sure I could handle the trip. I had just returned from Calhoun, GA, and this would be the most riding I had done in a very long time. Although I had mentally embraced the new outlook, I was still guarded about the reality of my abilities.

The drive was great. Nila spent a lot of the time napping, and I listened to CDs and sang (terribly) along with my favorite parts.

The next morning, I got up early and was feeling great. My tummy rumbled, and so I set out walking to find coffee and some breakfast. I left Nila sleeping peacefully in the dark, cool room.

I walked to a nearby Shoney's, where Nila later joined me. After breakfast we loaded up and headed for our final destination.

Our vacation together went splendidly. I didn't experience pain from the drive or from the beds. We stayed at a great condo on the beach, compliments of a dear friend. We spent time on the beach during the day, with Nila critter hunting as she always did. In the evening we checked out various local restaurants.

One evening, we walked along the boardwalk and the main street lined with shops, restaurants, and bars.

"Look, Nila! It is a tiki bar!" I said. Right there in our path was the 8th Ave Tiki Bar. This was important because our living room was decorated with elephants and tiki masks that we had collected from our travels. This place had more tiki masks than anywhere we had ever visited.

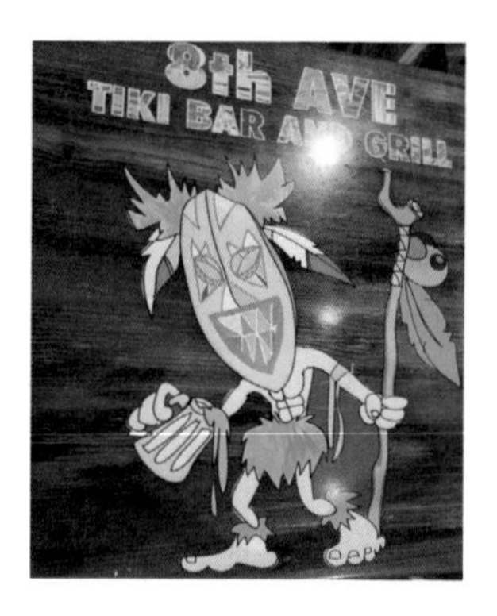

8th Ave Tiki Bar

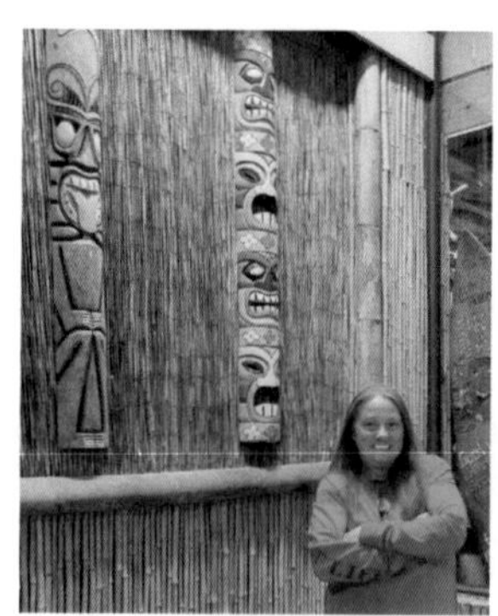

Nila at 8th Ave Tiki Bar

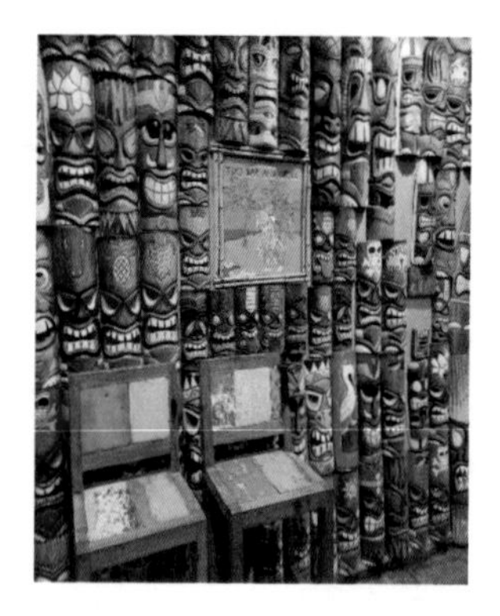

Inside at 8th Ave Tiki Bar

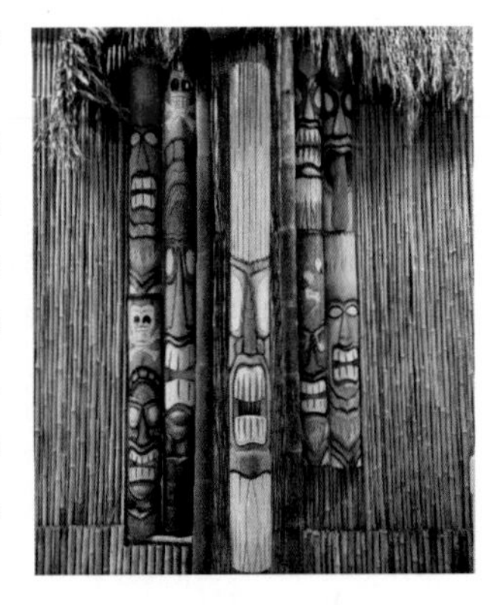

8th Ave Tiki Bar

The owner was also a collector of tiki masks. Before leaving, I was able to find a really unique mask. This one had burlap around the edges that gave it the appearance of hair. It was in an obscure location and behind some other signs. To me, it appeared to have been forgotten. By the time we left, I had negotiated a deal to buy it. Nila used it to stand on the busy roadside and scare people. It was absolutely hilarious and freaky at the same time.

Nila had bought a shovel for her critter hunting on the beach. Holding the bag with the shovel only added to the effect.

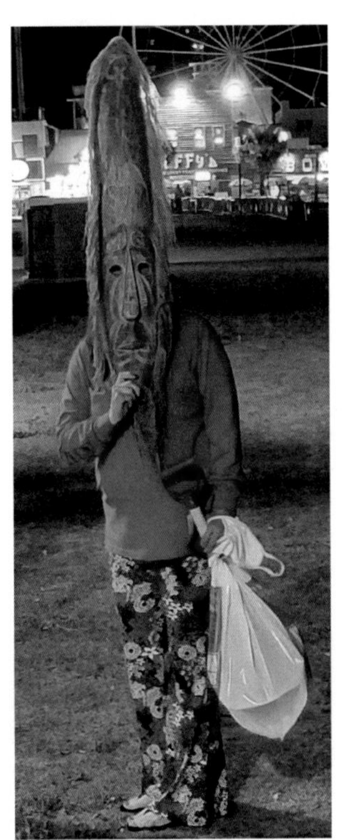

Nila wearing tiki mask

Tuesday, April 27, was Nila's birthday. I got up early and made my way to the local Publix grocery store. My first order of business was to buy three red roses. Next, I had to find the perfect card, with the perfect writing. Lastly, I had to buy some things to decorate the envelope. For thirty years, I had bought or made cards for Nila throughout the year. For each and every card or letter, I took great pride in writing, drawing, or presenting her name in a way that was unique and completely different from any other card. As the years passed, I often thought of *The Simpsons.*

The Simpsons is an animated series that started in 1989. At the end of the intro for each show, the animators find a way to show the Simpsons family gathering together in a unique way. I always wondered how difficult it was to find something new after thirty years, but they did. And so, I was inspired to do the same.

For this particular birthday card, I just used some peel and stick bedazzles. Normally I would have used crayons, markers, and colored pens to create a drawing.

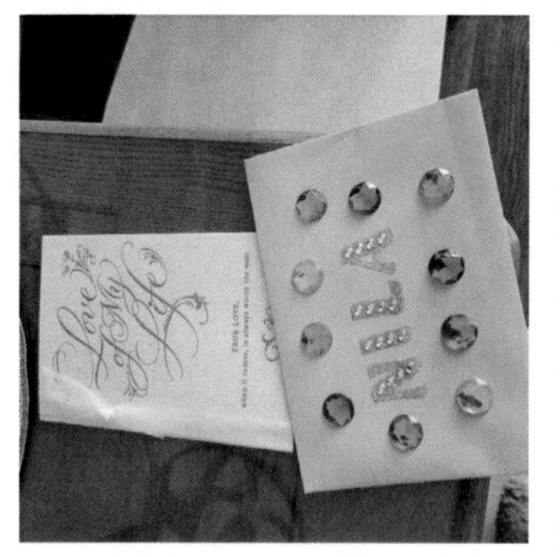

Nila's birthday card

We had a busy day. I took her out to breakfast, shopping, and then down to the beach. We spent the day listening to music and critter hunting (of course). We topped the night off with an elegant dinner and went back to the condo to watch a movie.

Slowly but surely, I stopped expecting things to turn for the worse. As each day passed, and I realized I was continuing to feel great, my mindset became more normal. I was achieving my goals. Every day was a celebration for me.

At the end of the day, Nila asked what my horoscope said for the day. I opened the app and read it to her.

Daily / Weekly / Monthly

Sagitarrius

11/22 to 12/21

Alias: The Archer

April 27, 2021

The more you fantasize about a dream coming true, the more excited you get. And the more excited you get, the more you realize just how much there is to lose. And when you start to think about losing, the idea of being disappointed may become unbearable. This is not a required pattern, Sagittarius, but it may be one that you are allowing right now. Break that pattern by staying in the initial state of fantasy and excitement as you work through your goal. Then you can celebrate!

The following day, we went to the Grand Prix go-kart track. There were six tracks to race on and Putt-Putt golf courses, as well. We parked and were able to see a nearby business that gave helicopter rides. We spent thirty minutes watching the helicopters take off and land.

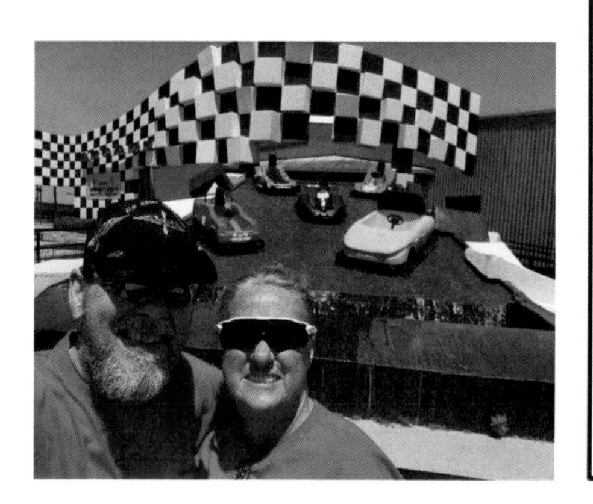

Nila and Perry in front of Grand Prix go-kart, Myrtle Beach

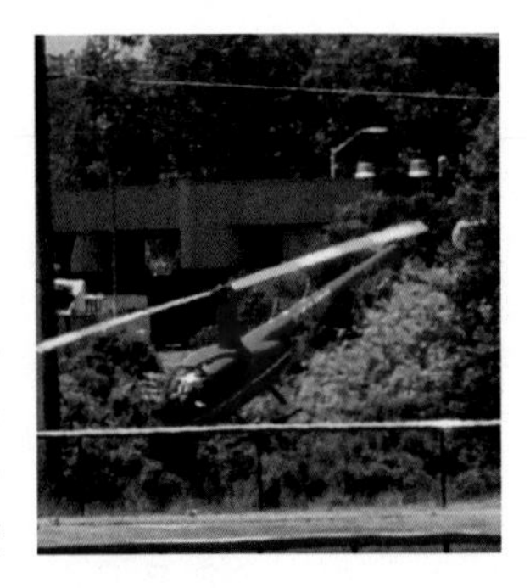

Watching helicopter rides

When night came, we sat on the balcony and watched for the pink moon to rise. We had never heard of a pink moon.

The name pink moon comes from one of the first spring flowers, wild ground phlox, as they cover the ground like a pink blanket. These brightly colored flowers are native to North America, and they often bloom around the time of April's full moon.

We were not disappointed. Once the full moon was high in the sky, it lit up the beach. Nila and I took the iPod and portable speaker and walked down to the beach. We had the whole beach to ourselves. I set the speaker on the lifeguard stand. In the background were the calming sounds of the ocean, and I located our favorite dance songs.

First, we slowly danced to "Harvest Moon" by Neil Young. Then we boogied to "What?" and "Werewolf Women of the SS" by Rob Zombie. It was so incredibly wonderful, dancing on the beach together. We wrapped up the evening sitting on the balcony, listening to music, and playing Angry Birds.

We have always loved to go out at night with flashlights and look for crabs when at the beach. When we were in Cape Santa Maria, Bahamas, we made friends with the bartender at the resort. We went out with him, and he taught me the proper technique for catching crabs without getting injured. Learning the proper technique was important. I had one bad experience with a crab as a young boy and definitely did not want to repeat getting injured by one.

When I was young, probably less than ten years old, we took a family vacation to Florida. One day, while walking around in the ocean, I stepped on a blue crab. In self-defense, the crab planted one of its claws firmly into my foot. The pincher went deep into the top and bottom of my right foot, about midway down the right side and on the meaty edge. Anyone close by might have thought I had been attacked by a shark when they heard my scream.

I walked gingerly out of the water, the blue crab in tow, as my dad hurried to get to me. He was unable to get the crab to release its hold. My foot was bleeding, and I remember hoping the crab wouldn't decide to use the other pincher too.

By the time I made it to the house we were staying in, the pain had started to kick in. Dad grabbed a utensil and was able to pry the claw apart and out of the top and bottom of my foot.

We used a water hose to rinse the wounds. The two wounds would eventually become scars to remember the crab by. Meanwhile, my dad put the crab in a bucket and cooked it later that day.

After the ordeal was over, I made my way back to the ocean. This time I chose shallower water and watched closely for what might be lurking.

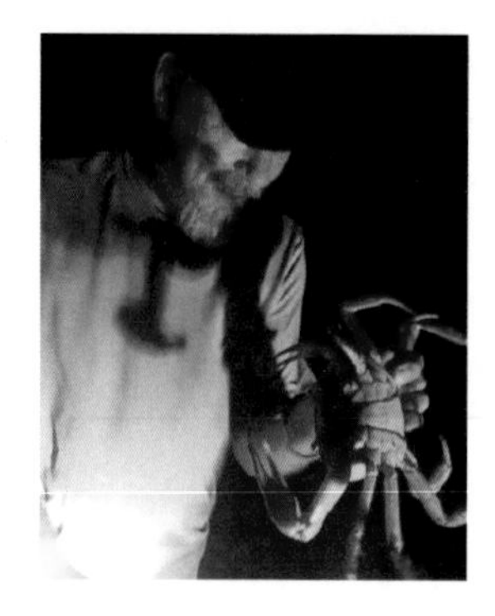

But the ordeal was not over. The saltwater was now able to find its way into the wounds. The pain was immediate and long-lasting. I left the water and tried rinsing it again, but to no avail. That night I lay in bed with my foot throbbing. The pain had made its way up my leg. I tossed and turned most of the night in agony. At some point I exhausted myself from the pain and fell asleep.

Perry catching crab, Cape Santa Maria

Vacation came to an end, and we loaded up to head home. Along the way we would make a slight detour, so I could stop in and visit a new customer. It was close to the halfway point of the trip and would give us a short break. This time I intended to make the seven-plus-hour trip all in one day.

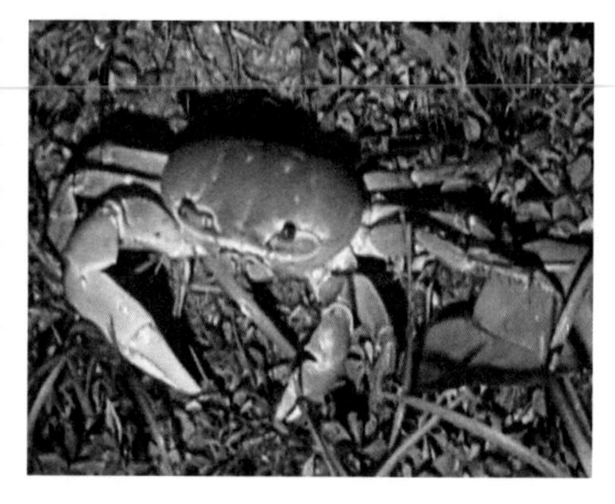

Blue crab, Cape Santa Maria

The trip went well, and we were finally back home. Nila spent the next day working at the salon. But I was feeling the impact of the long drive.

My left shoulder was incredibly sore. This was the shoulder that I had the rotator cuff surgery on. I equated the pain to the type of soreness one might feel after starting a workout regimen. Working the steering wheel was that workout.

I also felt fatigued. Maybe even jet-lagged. While I had high hopes for another busy Saturday, checking off to-do boxes, I gave in to the fatigue and rested.

The following week I made another trip to the Calhoun, GA, plant. It felt rewarding to be able to travel again and be productive. This trip was an especially rewarding one. Foam Products had started a new program called the "milestone celebration." This was where we recognized employees for their time with the company and awarded them $500 for every five years of employment. I was thrilled to be a part of it. Two days later we would do the same at the Erwin, TN, plant.

This took me through Thursday, May 6. In just two short days, Nila and I would celebrate the thirtieth anniversary of the day we met. We would have close friends and family attend, and we would share heartfelt words in place of vows. But my hip pain had returned. This time it was impeding my ability to walk upstairs or to squat and stand back up without a struggle. The pain had begun disrupting my sleep again. Following the celebration in Erwin, I decided to visit the orthopedic walk-in clinic.

The pain in my hip had come and gone for a long time. I honestly expected to have learned months ago that my hip showed signs of bone metastasis. I was thankful it had not been mentioned on two consecutive scans.

My plan was to get through the wedding celebration and family reunion before going to see an orthopedic doctor about my hip. I was concerned about what might be uncovered and did not want it to rain on my special day with Nila.

The pain quickly escalated to a point that forced me to the walk-in orthopedic ahead of schedule.

I explained why I was there and was asked to change into a blue pair of paper shorts for an X-ray.

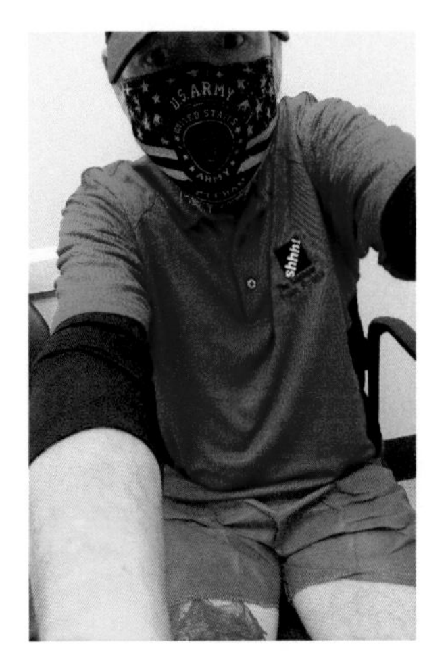

Perry awaiting X-ray in blue paper shorts

Shortly after the X-ray, I was joined in the room by a physician assistant. She was a very cordial young lady who was extremely attentive to what I had to say.

"I was diagnosed with stage IV, Gleason eight prostate cancer that spread beyond my prostate," I began explaining. "I am an excellent student of my condition and have reason for concern about my hip," I continued. "I have quarterly bone scans. On January 13 of this year, I was told the cancer had metastasized. Three months later, I had a scan that said otherwise. I am hoping that my hip condition is bursitis, but I am aware of the other possibilities."

I closely watched her eyes over her mask as I talked. The expression went from upbeat and positive to concerned. "Considering your situation, I am going to go back and review your X-ray again."

She left and returned shortly after. "We reviewed your X-rays again and did not find any sign of fractures. That is important," she started to explain. At that point, I jumped in and finished her explanation.

"I understand that taking prednisone, even at a low dose, thins out my bones. If the cancer has metastasized, it will start to eat away at the bone and deposit the calcium into my bloodstream. I will know when that happens because an elevated calcium level will show up in my routine blood labs. As the cancer eats away at the bones, they will be weakened and develop stress fractures or may easily break from a bump or fall," I rattled off.

The physician assistant looked at me and said, "Wow. You are exactly right. You don't even really need me! Let us get you scheduled for an MRI and focus the attention on that hip. If it were not for your cancer history, I would also have said it was bursitis."

Nila did not take the news well. The day before our celebration was hard for her. There were tears and anger. I understood. I had witnessed the impact of this kind of potentially bad news before. I was thankful for the peace I felt inside, so I could be there for her. This may sound confusing since it is my issue. But that is just how it works when you love someone.

May 8 was a beautiful Saturday. We would have the initial ceremony outside on the terrace at the beautiful Carnegie hotel. Steve Keylon was my best man, and our daughter Alanna was the bridesmaid. Our granddaughter was the flower girl and sprinkled blue flower petals along the path. Alanna's father-in-law Herb was there to marry us.

When it was my turn to take the microphone and speak to Nila, I said to myself, "Don't cry, don't cry, don't cry..." I had thought about and practiced what I wanted to say to her for months.

“There were many times in my life that I thought I was in love. The first time was my third-grade teacher, Ms. Thompson.” I talked about all of the women in my life that I'd “loved” and explained how each time I found out it was not really love at all.

At the end of my talk, I looked deep into her eyes and said, “The first time we married, we said for better or worse, for richer or poorer, in sickness and in health. We have experienced all of those. At sixty years old, I now know you are the only girl I have ever really loved.”

I almost made it all the way to the end, maintaining my composure. But as I spoke that final sentence to her, I began to cry like a little girl. Then, I placed the bubblegum machine ring on her finger, just as I had done thirty years prior.

Inside the reception area, I had placed a folder at each seat. I had pictures of our life together scattered on each table. At each place setting, along with the folder, was a plastic ring inside of a plastic container, each of them sealed with a blue cap (of course it was blue). Inside the folder was the two-page summary of our thirty years together. This is the letter.

> *NILA & PERRY MUSE*
> *30 years*
>
> *1990 was a tough year for me. I had gotten out of the army a few years prior because of my two very young children. But I found myself divorced and homeless.*
>
> *After spending countless nights bouncing from one person's house to another, drinking myself to sleep on their couch, I met Steve Keylon. Steve took me home and gave me an opportunity to reboot. I still do not know why. He had one child in diapers and another on the way. But that is just the kind of people Steve and Paula are. Today, thirty years later, we are like family, and he is my best man.*
>
> *On May 10, 1991, I walked to a coworker's house. I had rented a 1950s trailer but had lost my car. While there, a beautiful young lady came in. She was petite and definitely had the vibe of someone who was not going to be pushed around. It was my coworker's little sister.*
>
> *We spent most of the first two hours not speaking. She thought I was a narc, and I thought she was a bitch. Later, her brother told her, “If I were ever going to pick out a man for you, it would be Perry.”*

I was sitting at the dining room table, doodling a unicorn on a napkin, when Nila stopped by to look. It opened the door for conversation, and before we knew it, the house was empty.

Nila and I spent hours talking before she seduced me. She had just recently become homeless, so we had plenty to talk about. I became mesmerized looking at her and listening.

The next day, I was at work when a dozen red roses arrived for me. She had walked five and a half miles and spent all her money on flowers for me.

She came by the trailer when I got off work and never left.

She had a son, and I had two sons. It is tough raising a family, but especially when you are poor and mixing a family from broken homes. They just do not have a manual for that. It was quite the challenge. We failed often but kept working at it.

We spent the summer laughing, talking, and slow dancing. One of our favorite songs was "Wish You Were Here" by Pink Floyd. I filled the yard with flowers so she could have a different flower every day. Both still remain true, even today.

We never celebrate Valentine's Day. Instead, we surprise one another with gifts or cards throughout the year. Love is something to be celebrated three hundred and sixty-five days a year. Not just on the 14th of February.

On September 28, 1991, we got married. Nila borrowed a wedding dress from her best friend, Lisa. I could not afford a ring, so Nila got one from a bubble gum machine.

Today we are celebrating the thirtieth anniversary of the day we met. Our children have grown up, and we added one together, this time a girl. We have two granddaughters, as well. The car I lost back in 1990, a 1985 Monte Carlo SS, has been 90 percent restored and is primer yellow. It is parked in our garage today. It was our family car for many years.

Thank you for taking time to celebrate this wonderful day with us. We can honestly say we are even more in love today than back in 1991. Your presence makes it even more wonderful.

Sincerely,

Written by Perry Muse

The reception was wonderful. Nila and I danced to "Harvest Moon," just as we had done on the beach and hundreds of times before that. I found myself lost again as she sang to me, just as I had for thirty years.

We opened gifts, and I took the microphone again to introduce everyone present, one by one. They all had special places in our life together.

After the formalities were behind us, it was time to dance and celebrate. It was so incredibly fun to dance with Nila and all of the others on the dance floor. Alanna's mother-in-law Donna was right there with us. Dancing is in her soul, and she could not sit out if she wanted to.

Table with pictures and blue rings

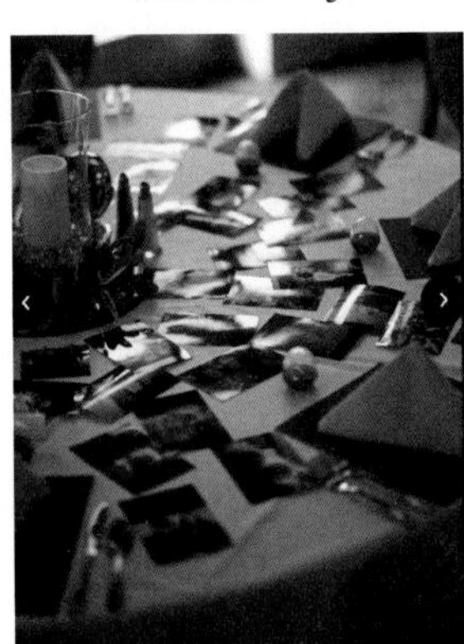

Nila Muse

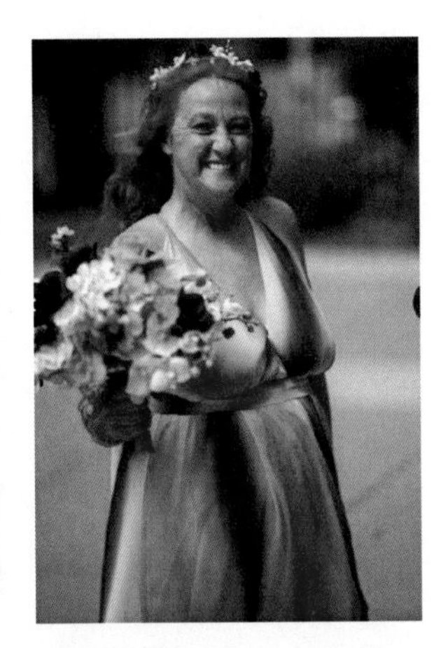

Perry and Nila dancing

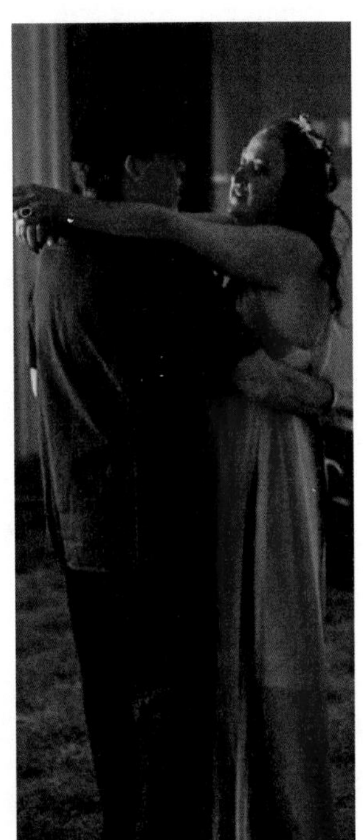

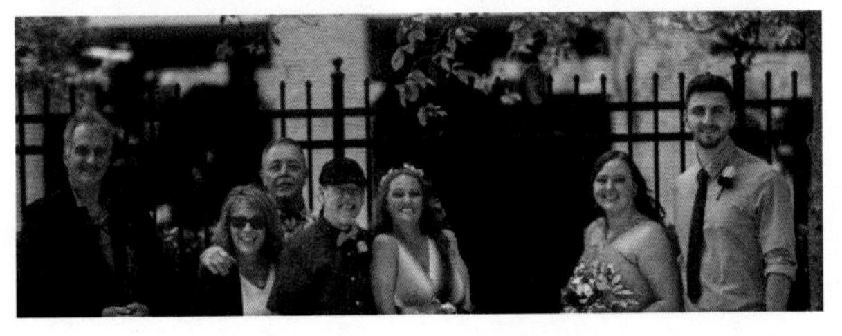

From left: Herb Rupert, Paula and Steve Keylon, Perry, Nila, Alanna and Cory Rupert

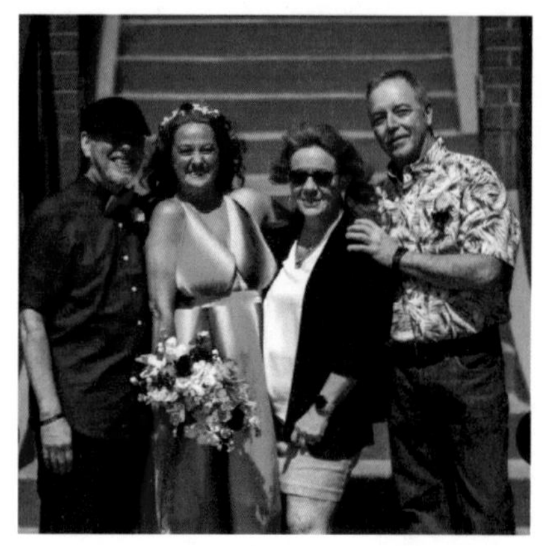

Perry and Nila, Paula and Steve Keylon

The celebration of our thirty years together was remarkable. Most of those in attendance knew it was more than just an anniversary. It was a celebration of our life, just like the name of the road leading to SCC, Celebration of Life Drive. It isn't often in life that one gets the opportunity to do something amazing twice. But there I was, married to my soul mate again. Unlike thirty years prior, we knew what we had in each other. There was no guessing or hoping. There were no false expectations. We certainly knew it was "until death do us part." I felt so incredibly blessed to be moving forward in reverse.

The lyrics to this song are just another love letter from me to my wife, Nila. No matter what was going on in our world, we could always turn this song on, dim the lights, hold each other close, and get lost in our love.

"WHAT YOU GIVE"

Tesla 2012

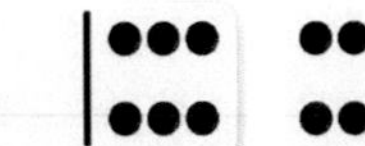 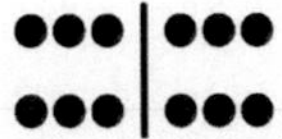 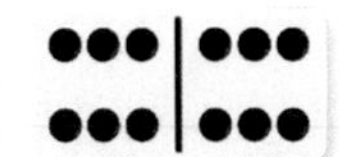

Chapter 30

MADE OF SCARS PART I

Sagittarians love life, adore laughing, and are always eager to undertake funny and crazy things.

I went to Mountain Forest Hospital on May 10 for my hip MRI. This was a familiar routine at a familiar place for me. After checking in with the nurse at the entrance, another bracelet was placed on my right wrist. I then made my way past the coffee and gift shop to check in for the procedure.

I sat down facing the television that had been showing a rerun of *Roseanne* the last time I visited. I was quickly called back and taken to the room, where an IV was placed in my arm.

The MRI was performed with an injection into my IV port to provide contrast. The scan took about twenty minutes, and I was finished.

My follow-up appointment with the orthopedic office was scheduled for May 13, of all days. It would be three days of waiting and wondering. Although my spirits were optimistic, the date of the thirteenth showing up again made the morbid thoughts audible in the back of my mind.

Despite the time dragging by, the day finally arrived, and I went in to find out the results from my MRI. Even though I gave my best effort to paint a pretty face on the situation, I had continually found myself concerned about the pending results in the past three days. After all, it had been in my thoughts for six months or more that the hip pain was cancer related.

When I got the results, I was surprised. I had a trochanteric fracture, a torn gluteus medius, and bursitis—not what I was expecting at all.

The trochanter (**trō-kăn'tər**) is the top portion of the femur, the largest and strongest bone in the body, located between the pelvis and knee.

On the outermost portion of the trochanter is the bursa. A bursa is a sac-like cavity containing a viscous lubricating fluid. It pads the bone over the greater trochanter. It is located between a tendon and a bone at points of friction between moving structures. Bursitis (**bər-sī'tĭs**) is an inflammation of the bursa. It is common to inject steroids into the bursa to reduce the inflammation and alleviate the pain.

The gluteus medius muscle is fan-shaped and starts at the greater trochanter, where it looks a bit like a stem and widens up and out to cover the side of the hip bone. The function of the gluteus medius muscle is to work with other muscles on the side of your hip to help pull your thigh out to the side in a motion called hip abduction. It also serves to rotate your thigh. According to my research, injury to the gluteus medius is rare, but it can happen. Tears of this muscle can occur after injury or with long-term wear and tear.

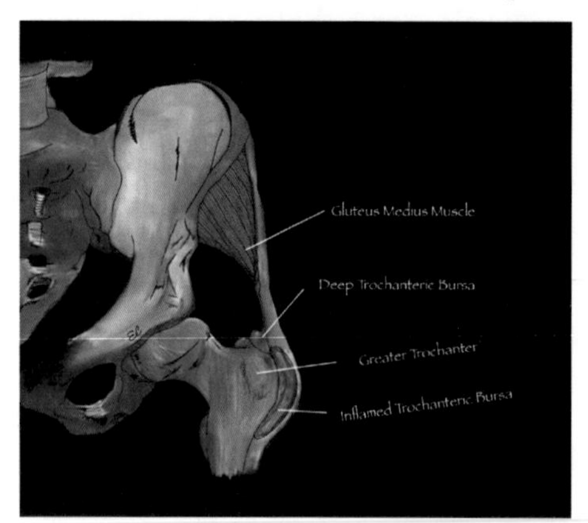

Drawing of hip by Ezekial Cooper

This meant another surgery (number 16), another bracelet, and another scar. But it also meant cancer was not a factor, something I wanted to celebrate.

Meanwhile, I had an appointment with Dr. Famoyin. My quarterly bone scan was scheduled for May 18, but I felt as though my iron was low. I was determined not to let it sink too low this time. I was sure that my iron had been so low before that my recent infusions had only brought it up to the low end of normal.

Nila went to the appointment with me. Dr. Famoyin made us feel like we were more than just patient and spouse. He entered the room and was in a jovial mood, laughing and cutting up with Nila and me.

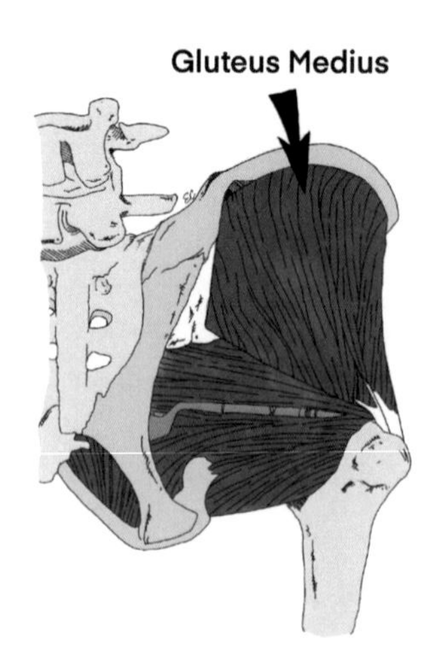

Drawing of gluteus medius by Ezekial Cooper

I took the opportunity to ask about the Zometa. I needed to know if he had noticed a rise in my calcium or if he was being proactive. He explained it was only being proactive. But then Dr. Famoyin surprised us with a bombshell comment.

"The cancer is likely already in your bones. It is just that the test can only detect down to a certain level, and the level has not risen to detection yet," he remarked.

Nila and I were caught so unsuspectingly that neither of us had a comment. This was a revelation we would have to deal with later when it fully sunk in.

COVID had hit the lab personnel at Quality of Life, and I had to be sent to get lab work at my normal medical care facility. Nila and I left the doctor's office separately and did not speak of the doctor's surprise remark. I went to the medical care facility for my blood draw, and she returned to the salon.

I called for the results the following day and found out they had not been sent to Dr. Famoyin. I picked them up myself and noticed they'd failed to test for iron. I was frustrated. I knew my iron was low. I could feel it. My ferritin said one thousand fifty-six. Normal high range is three hundred and fifty. We knew it was likely a false number, but at that level, it showed I had recently received the iron infusions. I dropped by Quality of Life, and they drew blood for my iron test. The next day I was called and scheduled for another iron infusion. It would be May 18, the same day as my bone scan.

On the morning of May 18, I steered into the familiar parking lot at a local medical center. Almost every day, I drove by this medical center and usually could not resist looking over to see the entrance of Radiology- Oncology. I did not know why I looked. I knew what feeling came with the memory of my radiation treatments. But I looked anyway.

This was my first bone scan at this facility and my third different location in as many tests. I checked in with the nurse at the entrance, and like all medical facilities, I answered "no" to the five questions from the COVID screening. I collected another bracelet from them, and I made my way to the waiting room.

It was somewhat of a lengthy wait on this day, unlike my experience at Mountain Forest Hospital. As I sat waiting, I remembered the dream from the night before.

It was all related—my trip today to this medical facility and my most recent nightmare. You see, this place would forever be remembered as the place where Dr. Channeler gave us his grim prediction of my future with cancer. I guess the thought of returning for my bone scan was on my mind more than I realized. It had been a long time since my last nightmare, especially one related to having cancer. But the bone scan scheduled at this facility changed that.

In my dream, I remember passing Dr. Channeler in the hallway. I did not speak, partly because I did not want to hear what forbidding words he might have to say, and partly because I doubted he would even recognize me. After all, he had not even taken the time to sign my radiation graduation certificate. However, in my dream, he did recognize me and spoke. He said, "Hey, Perry. Sorry about not signing that certificate. I really did not expect to ever see you again, but I do see the dark storm that's following you."

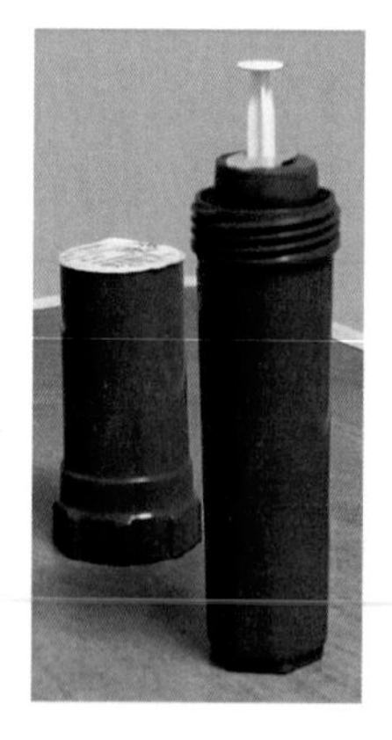

"Perry Muse," called a nurse, interrupting my recollection. I was happy to change the focus in my mind, so I quickly got up to make the dreaded trip down the all too familiar hallway. As we walked along, I do not recall much of the chitchat with the technician. I kept returning to the dream and hoping not to see anyone I recognized.

I asked the nurse if the blue pig would make an appearance. Shortly after asking, there it was.

Blue pig

The IV was placed in the normal spot in the bend of my right arm, which was bruised from all the recent traffic visiting everyone's favorite vein.

Meanwhile, I had been staying especially hydrated, as I always did when getting radiopharmaceuticals injected into my body. This was important to ensure they could quickly be flushed out of my system after the procedure. Flushing was done by drinking more water. The syringe containing the radiopharmaceutical was removed from the blue pig and dispensed into the IV port. I was escorted out and told to come back in three hours.

"Well, great. That means I get to experience the emotions from visiting this place again later today," I thought.

I left and ran by the salon while killing off a couple of bottles of water. I returned at 12:15 and went straight back to where the scan was to be performed. My hip and back were incredibly sensitive and sore. The torn gluteus medius caused swelling and pain in all directions. Lying on the table was an eight emoji.

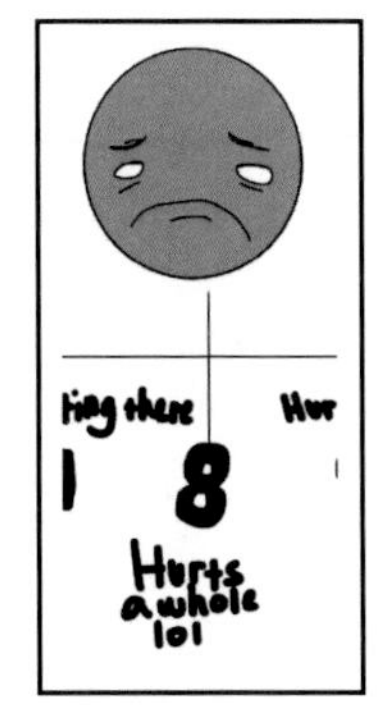

Drawing of pain emoji by Ezekial Cooper

I lay on the table and shifted my thoughts to what was at hand. The technician wrapped me tightly around my torso and banded my feet together. On this day, I was not motivated to ask for a picture. I just wanted to be finished.

I closed my eyes and said a prayer. I tried to relax and send the machine positive vibes. The scan lasted thirty minutes. Once finished, I found it fairly easy to get up. Perhaps part of it was simply feeling better. Most likely it was being so anxious to leave.

I left the facility and headed straight to Quality of Life for my iron infusion. I looked forward to getting the iron because I knew it meant feeling better and having more energy.

I grabbed my pillow and blanket from the car and went inside. The last iron infusion I'd received was hard on my hip and back. Sitting for three and a half hours was not something I was able to do comfortably. I rolled my trusty American flag blanket into a cylinder and placed it under my knees. The pillow went behind my back to give me something comfortable to lay my head back on without causing neck pain.

"No Benadryl," I reminded Connie.

"I remember, Perry," she replied.

The IV needle struggled to find its way into the vein in the bend of my right arm, which wasn't surprising given the number of times it had been used. This was the fifth time in just over a week.

I was exhausted and looking forward to a nap. I took four ibuprofens to alleviate the pain that would come from sitting in the recliner for so long. Then, I watched the steady dripping of the saline with Zofran (for nausea). Once it was gone, it was time for the iron. When the iron began to drip into my bloodstream, I fell asleep.

Thirty minutes later, I was awakened with pain in my bones. It was mainly my arms, shoulders, and chest. I felt extremely anxious, and my first thought was to pull the needle out and get outside where I could breathe better. But there was nothing wrong with the air inside. The pain in my bones felt like a cross between a frozen chill and high-voltage electricity. It radiated from deep inside of Mr. Skeleton.

Connie quickly came over and stopped the iron flow.

"I just had a bone scan with contrast earlier," I explained. "I've never felt like this before, like I'm freezing and being shocked with electricity at the same time. I've never felt like this before." I know I must have sounded a bit manic, my words tripping over each other as I tried to breathe through the pain.

"Why don't you sit here for several minutes, and we will see if we can start again after you feel better?" Connie suggested.

I nodded. I had had many iron infusions and no issues, ever. But this was a major issue, and it took a lot of effort to maintain my composure. After about fifteen minutes, I felt minimally better. I just wanted to get it over and leave, so I asked them to try again.

Within ten minutes of starting the iron, it hit me again. It was definitely related to the iron going into my bloodstream. But why? The only thing I could think of was that the radiopharmaceutical from my bone scan and the iron were clashing deep inside of me.

The iron was cut off again. This time they checked my blood pressure. One twenty-five over seventy. Near perfect for me. Yet, the aching pain emitted through my arms and shoulder, as if electrical currents were shooting directly into my bones, was not going away. Dr. Famoyin was consulted, and they chose to give me Decadron and Ativan.

Decadron is a steroid that prevents the release of substances in the body that cause inflammation. It can also be used to treat allergic reactions. In my situation, it was being used to treat a possible allergic reaction. That is also why they typically put Benadryl in the iron cocktail.

Ativan is used to treat many different conditions, such as anxiety, chemotherapy-related nausea, or insomnia.

In five minutes, I was asleep. Shortly after 5:00 p.m., the technician woke me to remove the needle from my arm. The iron infusion was over, and I had been asleep for four hours without moving. She was the only person left in the infusion room.

I made my way to the restroom and then weaved through the building toward the front door. The lights were out, and I saw the silhouette of a sole figure standing at the desk along the hallway. It was Dr. Famoyin. Unlike all of the other times, I just wanted to leave and get home. I had no desire to strike up a conversation. I was foggy and in a state of numbness, so I kept putting one foot purposefully in front of the other, passing by him on my way to the lit exit sign.

Dr. Famoyin caught up to me and said something about the Decadron. I responded, but I'm not sure what I said. I got into the car and drove to Food City. I went inside and picked up a few things to take home for supper. Once home, I spoke to Nila and lay on the couch, where I fell fast asleep.

I do not remember most of anything that happened after I got in my car at Quality of Life—actually, I do not remember much after waking up in the infusion room. Sometime later that evening, I woke up on the couch, ate, and watched television with Nila until she had to run to the salon to take care of a boarding dog.

I could not stay awake. I stumbled to the bedroom and fell onto the bed, immediately asleep. Nila came home and helped undress me, took my contacts out, and tucked me back into bed, where, in a matter of a couple of minutes, I was again fast asleep. At 3:00 a.m., I woke up. I have a clock that projects the time on the ceiling. Within a few minutes, I realized two things: I was still too tired to get up, and I had urinated on myself. I woke Nila and embarrassingly asked for help.

The next day I felt hungover. I had plenty to do at work and, thanks to an extra cup of coffee, made it in on time. After lunch I had to dig into my backpack and find a 5-Hour Energy. That would get me through the rest of the day and my dinner date with the boss at six thirty. All day my face felt as though a heat lamp were in front of it. In the mirror, I noticed how red it appeared. My temperature was normal, but not everything had returned to normal. Note to self: no Ativan in the future because it had knocked me out just like Benadryl. Also, no more getting radiopharmaceuticals and iron on the same day. That really made Mr. Skeleton angry.

My scan results were supposed to be ready on May 19 or 20. I was waiting for a call from Dr. Famoyin's office and finally got it.

Before I answered, thoughts raced through my mind.

"If it is good news, they will be happy to tell me. If it is bad news, it may be the good doctor who calls. If not, they may likely just say I need to come to the office."

But then a new thought: What if I was asked to come into the office so Dr. Famoyin could tell me the news face to face? I answered the phone in anticipation.

The lady on the other end said, "Perry, Dr. Famoyin would like for you to come back into the office next Tuesday."

My heart sank, and my stomach became nauseated.

"I don't need to come to the office," I wanted to say but didn't. "I already know what the good doctor needs to tell me...I wonder what chemo treatment he will recommend?"

Then she continued, "He said you need another iron infusion. Can you be here at ten thirty?"

Wow, what a relief! My body slumped over as the tension left it like a balloon with a pin hole in it.

As the day progressed, my hip pain slowly returned and, with it, my slight limp. The distraction of work and my negative reaction to my latest iron infusion occupied my thoughts for the day. But as the hip pain returned in the late afternoon, the morbid thoughts slipped out of my pocket and into my mind.

The PA at Watauga Orthopedic, Alvin, said it might be July or August before my surgery got scheduled because COVID had caused everything to get backlogged.

"If my bone scan comes back with bad results, I will be faced with chemo again. I will also have to deal with limited activity and pain from my hip. A positive bone scan means one to two years to live, most likely, and I will have this hip pain and surgery just before the real pain comes."

By Friday, May 21, I was at the end of my rope, awaiting the bone scan results. I picked up my phone and called to find out if they had forgotten me. But Quality of Life was closed on Friday. This meant waiting through the weekend.

Nila kept telling me, "No news is good news. If it were bad news, they would have called right away." I needed constant reassurance from her to keep my composure through the weekend.

On Monday, I called the office first thing. I explained to Tony about the bone scan results.

"Please have someone call me back. I have been waiting for days and need to know the results," I pleaded.

Within the hour, my phone rang. The caller ID read: "Quality of Life." This was what I had been waiting for. I ran through the scenarios again to be able to read between the lines.

"Is this Mr. Muse?" the voice asked.

"Yes, this is him," I responded. And then there was silence that just seemed to drag on and on. I caught myself wanting to say, "Just spit it out already!" An unfair response by me again.

Then Tony continued slowly, "You had requested the results of your bone scan. And so, I spoke to Sara and explained your request. Sara reviewed your bone scan results and wanted me to share with you the report summary. She said to tell you that the report states there is no sign of bone metastasis."

I said, "Thank you so much," and hung up. I was with Nila and everyone at the salon when the call came. The phone was on speaker for all to hear. Cheers rang out, and Nila gave me a big hug.

"Thank you, Lord. Thank you for all of my blessings and allowing me to feel well" was my silent prayer.

I now had had two consecutive negative scans since the positive scan on January 13. I was not sure why I had been blessed with this fortune, but I was beyond grateful.

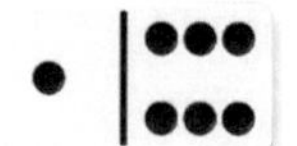 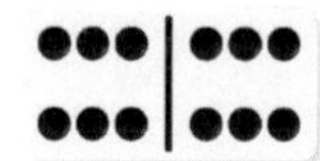 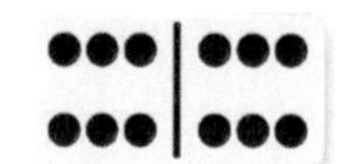

Chapter 31

MADE OF SCARS PART II

Everyone is familiar with the story of Frankenstein. The original novel was written in 1818 by Mary Shelley. The novel tells the story of Victor Frankenstein, a young scientist who creates a creature and brings it to life.

When you mention Frankenstein, most people think of the creature, not the scientist. However, Frankenstein's creature was never given a name.

Dr. Frankenstein used fresh body parts from deceased individuals and stitched them together to form a single individual. With the use of embryonic fluid and electricity, he was able to bring the creature to life.

The creature was loving and kind. Unfortunately, his scars were how people judged him first.

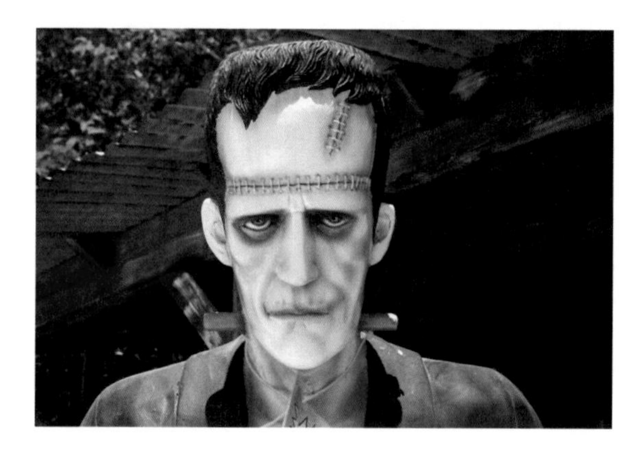

We all have scars. Each scar has a story behind it. Each scar was created with some level of pain and perhaps stitches or staples. Scars can result from accidents, diseases, skin conditions, or surgeries.

My scars all have a story, many of which you have read about here. Scars teach us and remind us of accidents, or perhaps careless behavior. Scars may be visible or not. Some scars may be on the inside or out of sight. Scars are a reminder of the miracle that is the human body.

Scars form when the dermis (deep, thick layer of skin) is damaged. The body forms new collagen fibers (a naturally occurring protein in the body) to mend the damage, resulting in a scar. There are many, many treatments, creams, vitamins, and even surgeries to improve the appearance of scars.

But scars should not be something to be ashamed of or to judge a person by, at least not to judge their appearance, as was the case of Frankenstein's creation.

I sometimes think of my friend Rick calling me invincible. I still submit that to be invincible, you must be made of scars.

I wear my scars with pride, like battle wounds. The installation of the plate and ten screws that created the scar on my left wrist reminds me every day that I should have died in August 2009 when my bike left that curvy road and headed for the telephone pole at over 110 mph. It makes me shiver and wonder why I am still here. My mom would tell me it is because I have not fulfilled my purpose in God's eyes.

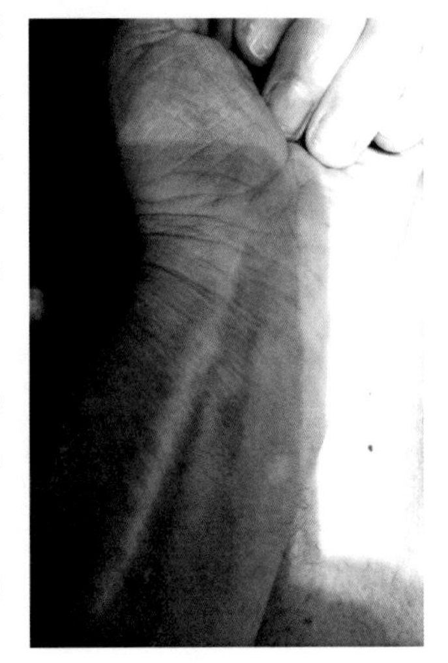

Scar on left wrist from motorcycle wreck

I knew the next scar for me would be my hip surgery. I called and pleaded to be put on a call list in case of any cancellations. I selfishly did not want to be in pain for two months, limited in what I was able to do, and then go through the lengthy recovery process on top of that.

"You have to get this surgery and PT behind you as soon as possible," I constantly thought. "Eventually, Mr. Skeleton is likely to get a bad report."

I was thrilled to receive a call from the lady who did surgery scheduling for Dr. Stewart.

"Mr. Muse, I wanted to let you know we have a cancellation and can do your surgery next Thursday. Will that work?" she asked.

"Yes, absolutely! Put me down. I am fed up with this pain and would come today if you told me to," I enthusiastically responded.

And so, it was done. I was getting in early, just as I had hoped for. Next Thursday, May 27, I would get another bracelet and another scar.

At 8:00 a.m., I arrived at the surgery center of the familiar medical center that I drove by daily. The parking lot was shared with the heart department and radiation oncology. The surgery entrance was between the two. I felt a cold negativity run through me as we turned into the parking lot. It was a stark reminder of the thirty-eight times I had done the same thing back in 2018. That was when they'd beamed me up just next door.

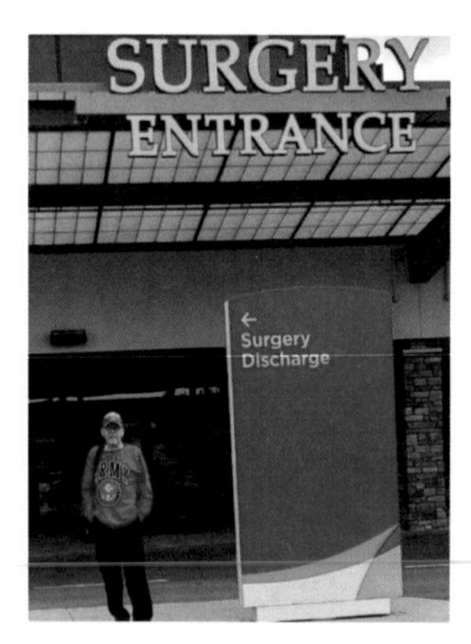

Perry preparing to enter surgery center

I wore warm but loose and comfortable clothing. It was all about getting dressed when I was discharged. I did not want to be wearing anything too complicated. No contacts for surgery day, so my rarely worn prescription glasses were used to be able to see where I was going.

Once I was checked in, Nila sat with me until they called my name. That was when she gave me a hug, a kiss on the cheek, and said, "I love you, babe. You had better come back; I need you."

I knew that the next time I saw Nila, I would be sporting a new five-inch incision and some hidden hardware.

The preparation was similar to all the other times prior to surgery. I took off my crucifix and said a prayer. I donned the open-backed gown and put on my new yellow hospital socks.

The nurse returned and verified my identity again. She made me initial my new bracelet this time. When asked if I wanted heat, I immediately said, "Heck, yeah." The hose was hooked up, and the heated air began to warm my chilly body.

Next, it was time to start my IV. This time we would not be using everyone's favorite vein. It was on the wrong side. This time would be in an accustomed, and typically painful, location. The top of my left hand. Once the IV was started, it was a matter of vitals and awaiting the anesthesiologist. This would be the person to send me on my loopy, relaxing trip while the surgeon cut me open and put me back together. Hopefully, Dr. Stewart could do for me what all the king's horses and all the king's men could not do for Humpty Dumpty.

Once the anesthesiologist stopped by, I knew it was getting close to time to go. But one thing was lacking. Dr. Stewart had not stopped by. Through all of this, I had never met Dr. Stewart. I could not have picked him from a line up if my life depended on it. So, I told the nurse.

The nurse was surprised he had not stopped by.

Actually, three times, they asked, "Are you ready to go?"

Three times, I responded, "I haven't seen Dr. Stewart yet. Isn't he supposed to stop by and draw on me before I go back?" The third time, the nurse literally walked over and looked at my hip to see if I was just not remembering.

Unlike my previous surgeries, I found myself constantly drifting off to sleep. I was tired from lack of sleep and the hip pain that tormented me nightly. Finally, Dr. Stewart made an appearance.

"Do you know what we are doing today?" he asked.

"Yes," I responded, "repair of my left gluteus medius."

"Well said," was his response. He then walked over and gained access to my left hip, where he drew a line that would soon become an incision.

The fourth time the nurse came by and asked, "Are you ready?"

This time my answer was, "Yes. Let's do this."

I struggled to stay awake, even on the ride down the hall to the operating room. Once inside, I was shifted onto the operating table. I was already stupefied. Once the mask was put on my face, I was out.

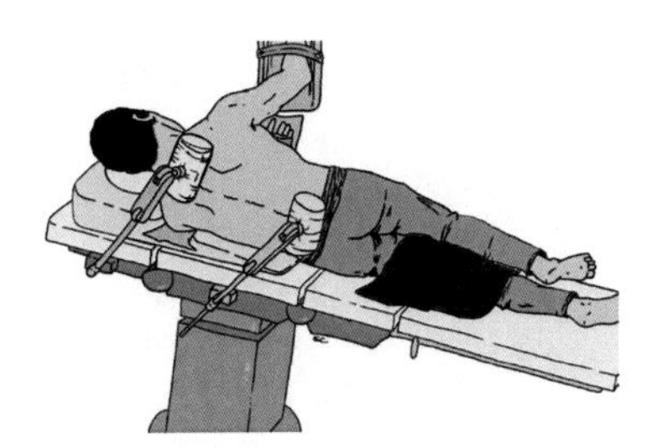

Drawing of right lateral decubitus position by Ezekial Cooper

On the operating table, I was placed in the supine position (on my back with my front facing skyward). After anesthesia was induced, I was turned to the right lateral decubitus position and held in place with pelvic positioners.

My hip was draped in sterile material, and I was given preoperative antibiotics via IV. At this point, Dr. Stewart took an anterolateral approach to the left hip. Unlike a traditional approach where the muscles are cut, the anterior approach allows the surgeon to work between the muscles, keeping them intact.

Next, the skin was sharply incised laterally, centered over the trochanter, and the dissection continued down through subcutaneous tissues to the IT band and tensor fascia. This was split longitudinally down to the long axis of the femur. A Charnley retractor was placed in the opening. A Charnley retractor is a self-retaining hip surgery retractor system that helps to free assisting personnel while providing excellent exposure during hip surgery.

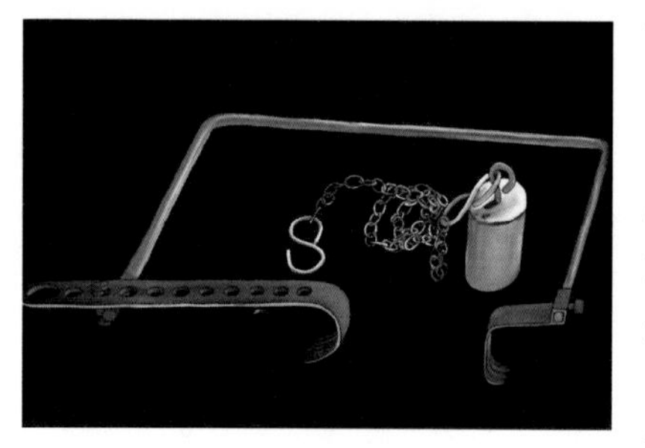

Drawing of Charnley retractor by Ezekial Cooper

The incised area was opened, and the trochanter was noted to be eburnated with a high-grade tear. Eburnation is a degenerative process of bone commonly found in patients with osteoarthritis or non-union fractures. Friction in the joint causes a reactive conversion of the bone to an ivory-like surface at the site of the cartilage erosion.

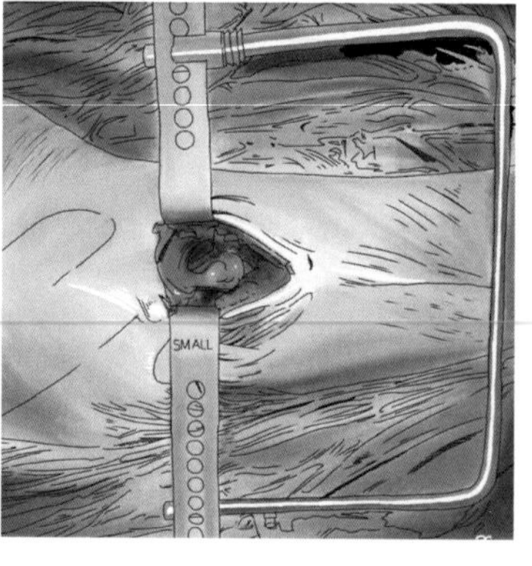

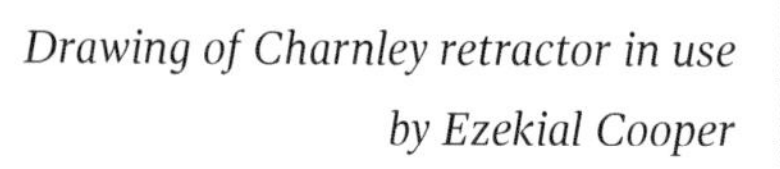

Drawing of Charnley retractor in use by Ezekial Cooper

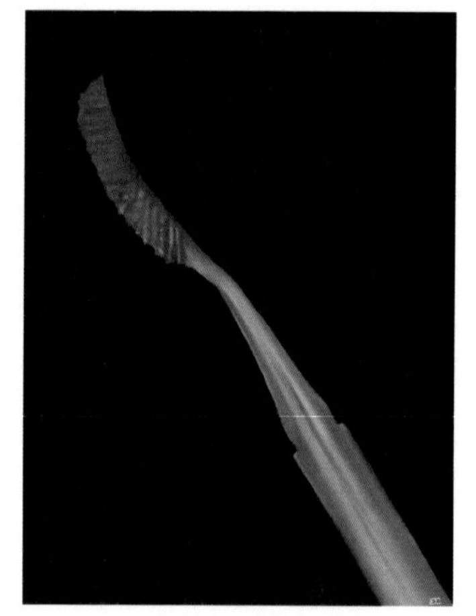

The soft tissue was then further split, opening to the bone and exposing it. A rongeur was utilized to roughen the bone, and the margin of the tear was fully identified.

A rongeur is used in orthopedic surgery to remove bony fragments or soft tissue or to roughen the polished surface of a bone.

Drawing of rongeur tool by Ezekial Cooper

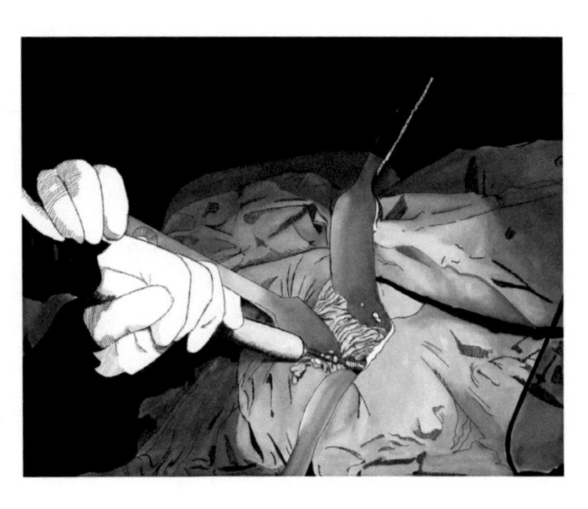

Drawing of rongeur tool in use
by Ezekial Cooper

A Speed-Bridge fixation system was used for the repair. Standard anchor fixation of the tendon creates only a single point of compression directly over the anchor. The Speed-Bridge repair enables an hourglass pattern of fiber tape suture to be laid over the end of the tendon.

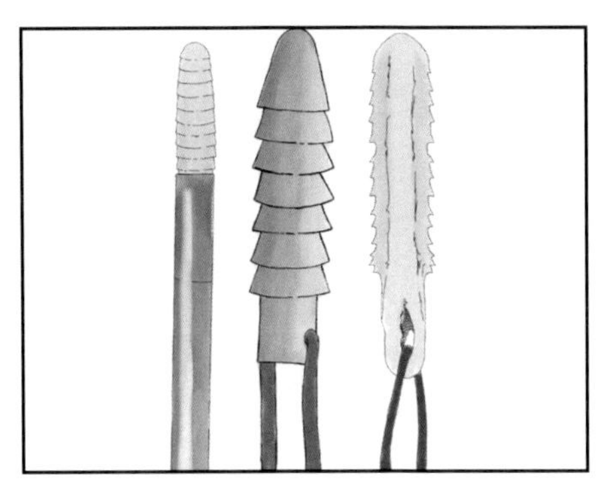

Drawing of anchors used in hip surgery
by Ezekial Cooper

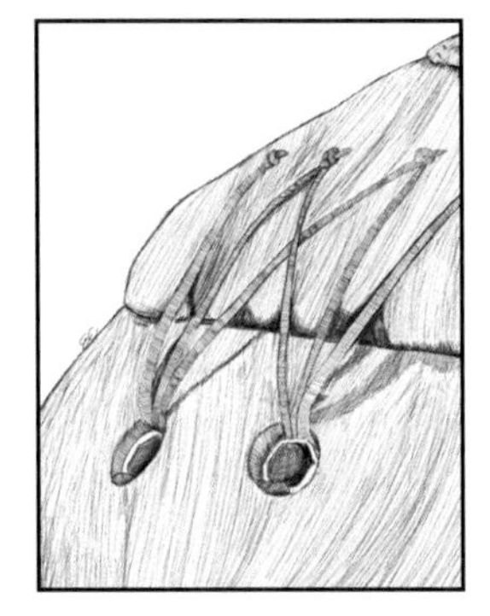

Drawing of Speed-Bridge technique
by Ezekial Cooper

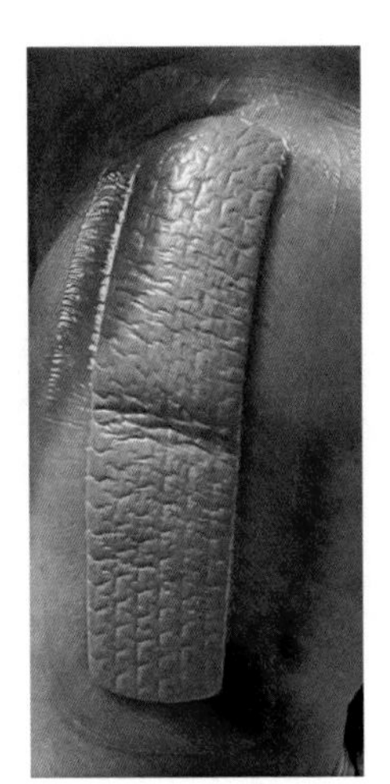

Two anchors were placed into the trochanter. The fiber tape sutures were double loaded and placed through each margin of the abductor (muscle). They were then split and crisscrossed, and a second-row repair was created onto the trochanter. This was then oversewn with a #1 Vicryl suture. Vicryl suture is a synthetic absorbable suture coated with a copolymer plus calcium stearate. It provides two to four weeks of tissue support.

The IT band, tensor fascia, and subcutaneous tissue were closed using Vicryl sutures. The skin was then closed with staple ligatures. Finally, a sterile dressing was applied.

Perry's hip after surgery with sterile dressing

I woke up in the recovery room and immediately knew where I was, although I was still fighting sleep. I wanted to see Nila, and that would require me to appear ready to the nursing staff. So, I made sure they saw me awake and looking around.

When Nila came into the room, I was still sleepy. I found it hard to have any conversation. I just remember saying, "Hey, babe. Here we are again."

I had a green mask on my face that fed oxygen through it. If I did not inhale enough oxygen, the alarm sounded with a loud, obnoxious BEEP, BEEP, BEEP! This would continue until a nurse stopped by, reset the machine, and said, "You need to breathe deeply. Keep breathing deeply for me."

Over and over and over again, like a bad dream, I fell asleep, and the alarm went off, then the nurse would stop by to repeat the procedure. I am sure it was annoying to the nurses to interrupt what they were doing in order to keep coming over and resetting the machine. But it was making me downright angry! It was worse than any snooze going off on an alarm clock. The whole reason I wore a CPAP every night was because I stopped breathing when sitting or lying in a certain posture when asleep. This was the reason the alarm kept sounding and why I could not just take my nap in peace. This continued for thirty minutes.

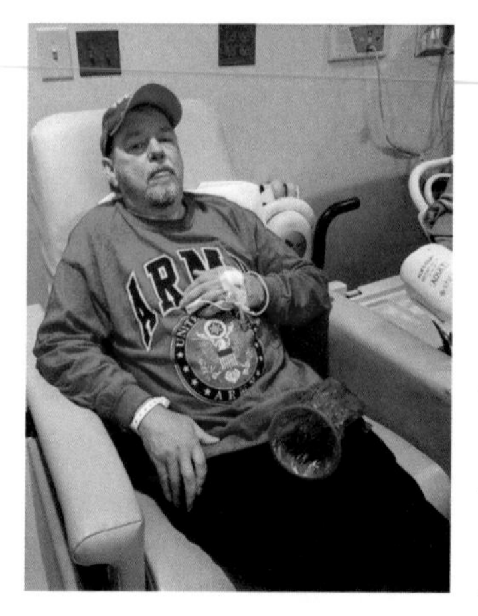

Finally, they came to help me out of bed and give me relief from the green mask that fed oxygen. I was helped into the recliner beside the bed. I was one step closer to going home with Nurse Nila.

Yet we had to wait for what seemed like an eternity. We were waiting for my shiny new silver walker to arrive. It would provide me with a way of getting from place to place. However, I would quickly come to loathe the walker.

Perry post-op hip surgery

Once home, Nurse Nila patiently helped me out of the car and into the house. The dogs were excited to see us and curious about the hospital smells of my incision and clothes. I picked a recliner, and Nila prepared me a place to lie down. There would be time now for a nap until the pain meds wore off. Then I would be significantly limited on how I could sit or sleep.

Just like all the times past, Sparky made sure to get his spot beside me. A sniff of the hip, followed by some gentle licks, as if to let me know that he understood I was damaged before he curled up beside me on the recliner. Hooch was left to lie on the floor in close proximity. Nila had placed a pillow under my right leg to allow it to relax without stressing the surgical area. I placed the CPAP on my face to ensure there would be no dreams of suffocating and immediately fell asleep.

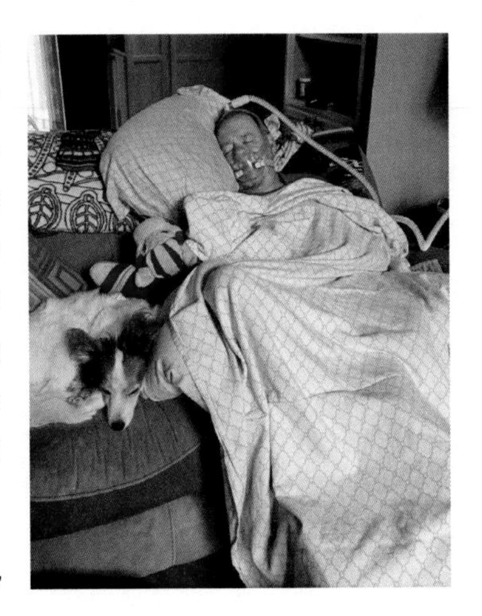

Perry asleep with Sparky and Hooch after hip surgery

I was prescribed 5 mg Oxycodone for pain, prescription-strength aspirin, Zofran for nausea, and a stool softener. The discharge instructions were short, but quite restrictive.

- Must use a walker.
- No abduction exercises (moving leg outward or knees apart).
- Left extremity: Partial weight bearing – 25 percent.
- Right extremity: Weight bearing as tolerated.
- No driving until cleared by Dr. Stewart.
- Change positions every forty-five minutes.
- Apply ice for thirty minutes four times daily.
- Use an incentive spirometer ten times every hour. (This is a handheld breathing device to curb the chances of developing pneumonia).
- Take pain medication thirty minutes before PT.

The first night was miserable. For whatever reason, the pain medication did little to nothing for me. Getting into bed was a whole theatrical event. It was painful and awkward to slide back on the bed and to get my feet onto the top of the mattress. At that point I was perpendicular to the position I needed to be in to sleep.

Once I was fully on the bed, I had to find a way to maneuver my body into a position where my head was on the pillow, not beside it. I learned quickly that some motions were a huge no-go. Pretty much anything besides moving forward was a challenge. I

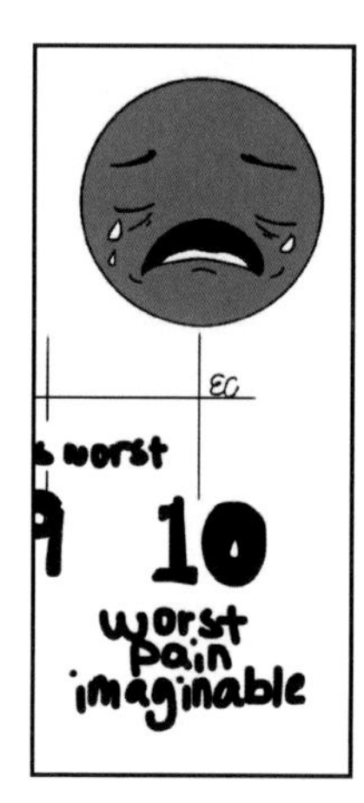

had to keep my knees together and not use my left side to leverage my movements. Twisting, turning, pivoting, and straining were all punished swiftly and forcibly with a number ten emoji.

My body only permitted me to lie in one position, and that was on my back. Both legs had to remain straightened. I crossed my hands on my chest and held my crucifix.

"So, this is what it feels like to lie in a coffin," I thought. "I can't imagine this being very comfortable for eternity."

Drawing of pain emoji by Ezekial Cooper

I already knew some of what was to come. My CPAP did not stay sealed well when I was on my back. When the seal broke, noisy air would blow, and the CPAP became inefficient. That opened the door for troublesome dreams.

The dreams of suffocating came frequently, night after night. Regardless of the dream, there would come a time when I started struggling to breathe. Then, in my dream world, I always tried to make my way outside, thinking my discomfort would ease and air would come easier. I don't really know where those ideas came into my dream-addled brain, but I was always trying to get outside, and each time, it became harder and harder to breathe until, finally, I reached a point of not being able to inhale at all.

In the dreams, my chest and stomach would feel as though they were filled with gas that applied pressure to my lungs and restricted the air from entering. I suppose part of this was from my prior struggles with the paralyzed diaphragm. Then, suddenly, the dreams always ended with me waking up with a gasp and the air from my CPAP blowing noisily from around the seal.

I recall one dream vividly.

It was raining, and I got into the driver's side of a pickup truck. It was not a familiar truck, but in my dream, it belonged to me.

The wipers and defog were on. Between the rain and foggy windows, I could not see outside. Suddenly, I started to struggle to breathe. Some panic set in, as was always the case, and I began telling myself to calm down. "Just relax," I told myself.

Meanwhile, I turned off the heat and lifted my head upward to open my airway to allow more air to enter. But none of these tactics worked. I was unable to inhale more than a fraction of what I needed to live. I was forced to step out of the vehicle, the panic meter rising. I stood next to the truck with my face pointed straight to the sky.

Rain pelted my face, but I needed to breathe the cool, damp air. There was no one around to help me, and the situation was getting dire.

Suddenly, a loud horn rang out. It was then that the realization hit that I was standing in the road, and a large semi was barreling down on me. Before I could move, and before the semi crashed into me, I woke up with a gasp.

This routine occurred so often that I started recognizing what was happening while in my dream! I would literally say (in my dream), "Oh, I know what this is. I need to wake up." And so, I woke myself up.

Sometime in the middle of the first night, I was awakened to pain and burning in my left heel. It was so bad I had to wake Nila.

There was nothing visible, but the burning and pain were immense. It was time for more pain meds, and after taking them, I fell asleep despite the burning pain.

Getting out of bed was just as eventful as getting in. In the middle of the night, I had reached my tolerance for lying in bed and had to relocate. The clock display on the ceiling read 4:25. Little did I know that this would be the normal routine, around the clock, for the next several weeks.

Slowly and methodically, I spun myself around into the perpendicular position that had my feet pointing at my walker beside the bed. Nila helped me to carefully set my feet off the mattress. Again, any slight movement left or right, or any separation of my legs was met with immediate pain. Nila knew the exact moment because I could not contain myself from yelling out in response.

I grabbed the sheet and mattress cover to pull myself up into a sitting position. I hardly had the strength. From there I would latch on to the walker and make my way to the nearest recliner.

This was the routine for me, day and night, for the next three weeks. I was sorely discouraged to realize how slow the progress was and how long the pain lingered.

Twelve days after surgery was my follow-up appointment with Dr. Stewart. Nila chauffeured me to the appointment. Once back in the room, we anxiously awaited the doctor's arrival. The sterile bandage would be removed, and we would get our first look at the incision.

Dr. Stewart arrived and gave us the details of what he had found.

"When I got in to look at the damage, it was worse than I had originally thought," he began to explain. On the paper cover of the bed, he drew the gluteus medius. Then he took his pen and just started marking across it, over and over as he explained. "Seventy-five percent of this muscle was shredded. Some parts were so bad you could see the bone through it. I had to sew in two rows of fabric sutures and attach them to two anchors I placed in your femur. Then, I sewed a patch over the area for greater strength and stability."

"How could this have happened to me without me knowing when I did it?" I asked.

He answered, "These things often happen over time. Imagine laying a rope over the corner of a brick and just sawing back and forth."

This instantly made me think of the many times I had been bent over or squatting, doing some type of physical work. I would raise up and feel a "pop" in my back left hip. I would always tell Nila, "Uh-oh, that wasn't good." I now knew it was likely another fiber of my gluteus medius shredding.

Dr. Stewart explained, "You will be on the walker for six weeks. After that time, the walker goes away, and you will go right into an aggressive PT program."

He then removed the bandage and revealed the five-inch incision with sixteen staples. Next, he grabbed a pair of pointed pliers and removed the staples. Lastly, he placed butterfly bandages on the incision where the staples had been removed.

I mentioned to Dr. Stewart that the pain medication had done little to give me relief. I was always nervous about mentioning pain medication. Thanks to all the abusers, it had become very difficult for people like me, who really needed the relief, to get anything. Dr. Stewart never offered to prescribe anything else, and I did not push the issue. Instead, he recommended I take one 500 mg Tylenol with two 200 mg ibuprofen. Little did he know that I had already been taking this combination in between times for my Oxycodone.

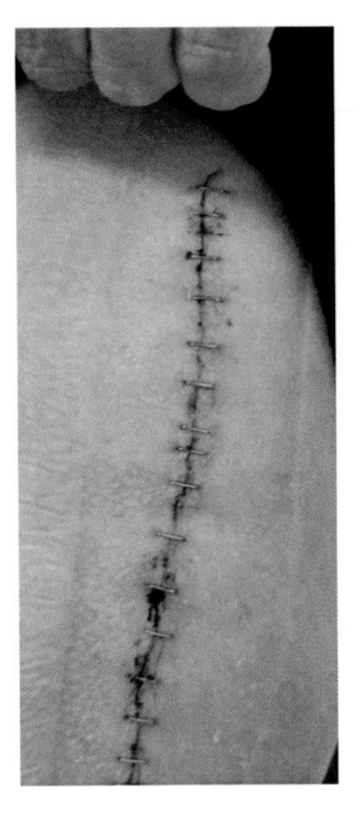

Perry's hip with staples

As the days and weeks came and went, I felt myself stuck in the healing process. It took three weeks before I was able to spend an entire night in bed. I could dress myself, but it was a long, challenging process. The pain was with me constantly. It was impossible to get comfortable.

And my heel was still numb. The burning and aching would wake me. I thought it was because I was having to lie in the same position all night, and my heel was pressed against the mattress. With Nila's help, I was able to place a pillow under my left leg. It supported my leg down to my foot. My left foot hung off the edge of the pillow, and that prevented it from touching the mattress. But this seemed like a Band-Aid. I finally asked Nila to take me to the orthopedic walk-in.

Once I was escorted to a patient room, I explained the problem to the PA seeing me. He ordered an X-ray of my foot.

The X-ray was difficult. I had to get onto the hard table and turn myself around into the correct position. One of the X-rays required me to roll onto my left hip.

"I'm not sure if I can bear to do that," I expressed to the technician.

"How long since your surgery?" she asked.

"Three weeks," I replied.

"Then you should be fine to roll over."

But it was not fine. It was torturous. I wondered if she was even aware of the type of hip surgery I had. Everyone always assumed hip replacement surgery when I told them I had hip surgery.

I made my way back to the room, in far more discomfort and pain than when I left. The PA returned and announced the X-ray was clear. Then he explained his theory for my issue.

"Sometimes during surgery, a nerve is aggravated. This seems to be the case with you. Just keep weight off your heel and give it some time to calm down. This can take a week, a month, or a year. There is no way of knowing."

"Another domino effect from a surgery. This recovery is already incredibly hard, and now I have to deal with the numbness and burning pain in my heel indefinitely," angrily raced through my mind.

June 20 was Father's Day. It was twenty-four days after surgery, with eighteen more before I could ditch the walker. I'd found myself recently sinking into depression and fighting to motivate myself to get out of bed. I did not give up. A Sagittarius does not give up. But it had become a struggle. It was the limited mobility, the fact that I was stuck at home, being alone, not being able to help with housework. I could not drive. It was a struggle just to prepare a sandwich and carry it to the recliner without dropping it. And the pain. The pain followed me everywhere like my shadow, and never took any time off. Eighteen more days seemed like forever.

I was using ice packs more and more as a pain reliever. It helped, but even a small amount of pain tested my mental fortitude after it being relentless for twenty-four days.

The new coater in Calhoun was started, and the crew ran its first trial the week before Father's Day. The second trial was scheduled the following week. I missed both, and this only added to my depressed emotions. Here I was, at home and in a state of recovery again.

I had previously ranked my top worst surgeries. I had number one listed as the diaphragmatic plication. Second was the imperfect surgery by the imperfect doctor on my prostate that resulted in number one. The shoulder surgery was in the top three and as painful and uncomfortable as any. The shoulder surgery also came with PT.

Dr. Stewart once described my surgery as being like rotator cuff surgery, except on the hip. I now fully agree. At least with the shoulder, I did not have to sit or lie on it.

Twenty-six days since surgery and sixteen days until the walker was retired. Last night I had been able to carefully roll onto my left side. The mattress was forgiving, but lying on the side of the surgery was delicate. It felt so wonderful to be off my back, even if it meant coping with some pain. Three minutes after rolling over, I woke up in considerably greater pain. Later that night, I woke up to a different pain, but in the same location. During my sleep, I had managed to roll onto my right side.

At least this was progress. Hopefully, soon, I would be able to sleep comfortably enough on my side to reap the benefits of rest.

A few months ago, Nila had noticed a lump on my spine, about midway on my back. It did not bother me, but we asked Dr. Ballard about it.

Dr. Ballard looked at the lump and then started moving it about. "I don't think it is anything serious," he said. "I am able to move it around. If it developed from the spine, I wouldn't be able to move it like that."

But now the lump was larger, and when I leaned back in a chair, it caused pain. So, Nila and I decided I should go to the doctor and have it checked out.

"I hope this isn't a tumor that has formed from my cancer. If it is, I will not need to wait on a bad report for Mr. Skeleton," was a recurrent thought since the lump first appeared.

It was day thirty-five since surgery. Prior to the procedure I had high hopes of where I would be by that point. But those hopes vanished as I continued the battle of pain and immobility. The night before I had finally been able to roll onto my right side and sleep for less than half an hour. I still could not bear to lie on my left side. No way.

Three times since surgery, I had woken due to pain and sleepily used my left foot to lift my body to rearrange it in bed. Three times I had been punished and had paid for the action over the following two days.

I only had eight days until I retired from the walker and started PT. On day thirty-five, I pondered my situation.

"How can I ditch the walker if I still have pain? Is it atrophy? Could it be that the anchors that are screwed into my already fractured femur have created additional fractures? Whatever is going on, Mr. Skeleton is very unhappy. I sure hope they didn't let some of those really mean cells escape."

I love the Fourth of July. For years we spent it with Steve and Paula. I was hopeful to be able to do so again this year, but my hip was not allowing it. My gluteus medius burned, and my bones had pain that shot down my leg. I could barely handle sitting in a car long enough to take an occasional ride to the salon. There was no way I could survive five hours to their house.

And so, each day, I got out of bed and made my way to the recliner. I had two pillows stacked to soften the cushion. There I sat on ice packs and wrapped them around my hip to freeze away the pain until I could not stand the freeze any longer.

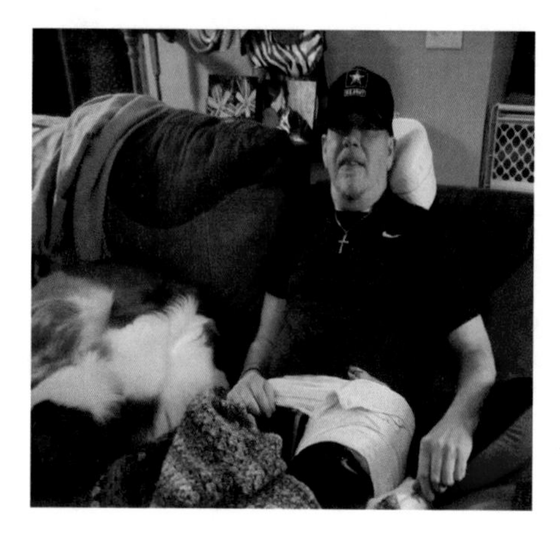

Perry with ice pack

Shane decided to come visit and hang out with me. He could help tremendously and allow me to continue healing. I was thankful for the company. Loneliness and a feeling of worthlessness had crept into my life. My motivation was diminished, and the bed called for me to come and forget about the day. I knew the bed would provide some respite from the suffering.

I imagined the bed calling to me each time I limped past the bedroom. "Come in and lie down. Don't you remember that sleeping is when your body heals? Come heal yourself, and when you wake up, it will be time to walk again."

On June 23, one week prior to day thirty-five, I went to my walk-in medical care facility. I had tried to make an appointment to see Deanna, but she was booked through July! So, I just walked in and hoped to get her.

Sure enough, Deanna saw my name and walked into the room. It was wonderful catching up. She had been keeping tabs on me and knew about almost everything that had happened since I last saw her. What a wonderful person. I have really been blessed to have some special medical people in my life since cancer. She is right there at the top.

After catching up on all things in our lives, Deanna examined the lump on my back. She echoed what Dr. Ballard had said about the lump moving around and not being attached. She knew I was concerned about a lump on my spine and that I knew what it likely meant if it were attached.

When we discussed my bone scans and the January 13 results, there was a serious expression on her face as she listened. I explained about the chemo and stopping it. I told her about the two most recent scans being negative. But her eyes did not hide her serious expression, even though she was wearing a surgical mask.

"The five recognized stages of grief are denial, anger, bargaining, depression, and acceptance. I am in acceptance, right?" I questioned. "It feels like everyone thinks I am in denial. If I am yet to go through anger and depression, I will need more paper to write all of the morbid thoughts."

The outcome of my examination was to contact a general surgeon to schedule removing the lump. I was not sure if that meant another bracelet, but it would definitely mean another scar.

On day thirty-six following my hip surgery, I received a text from the surgeon's office. It appeared I would acquire my next scar on July 19, only eighteen days away.

July 5 was day 40 following my surgery. It was also the day of my appointment with Dr. Famoyin. It was great to be back to some normalcy following the past year's trials, which had included COVID complications. Do not mistake what I am saying. COVID-19 was still out there, but Nila and I had been fully vaccinated, along with 57 percent of the rest of the United States. This meant she could go to all my appointments again.

Dr. Famoyin was surprised to see me with a walker. He stopped us on the way to our room to inquire. He knew of my hip pain complaints over the prior months. But he did not know I'd had surgery since last we met.

The visit went well, and we did a lot of laughing, especially when Nila told him how she thought I got my injury.

"Go ahead and tell him about falling, Perry," she teased.

"I may have fallen on the rock patio one day," I timidly shared with the doctor.

"Tell him how many times, Perry," Nila continued to tease. I did not respond, and at this point, Nila had piqued Dr. Famoyin's interest.

Nila then walked over and stood next to Dr. Famoyin and repeatedly said, "Ten times he fell. Ten times. Not once or twice, but ten times. He would bend over to pick up his cornhole bags and just keep going into a tumble. Ten times," she finished explaining.

"What in the world made you fall ten times?" the doctor asked with a curious grin.

"Alcohol may have been involved. I may have been self-medicating," I shyly answered. The room erupted in laughter, and we moved on.

We discussed my bone scans and the fact that I had two consecutive scans that were negative.

"I think I was right, Doc. I think SCC made the call prematurely," I said. Dr. Famoyin responded honestly. "It seems they must have needed to make quota during COVID. I did not have the luxury of being paid that way. I just had to go home and cry when my business was hit by COVID," he shared in confidence. I believe he was exactly right.

So, we discussed my future treatments and testing. My abdominal CT scan would be in three days. My next bone scan was in August. My next Lupron would be in a week and a half. I would have a blood lab drawn before leaving. All these test results would be monumental for me and my future.

On day forty-two following hip surgery, I limped my way into the orthopedics office on my walker. I visited with Dr. Stewart for a good amount of time and explained how painful the recovery had been. There was a look of surprise on his face as I spoke.

After checking me out, he told me I could trade the walker in for a cane, put full weight on my leg, and start PT.

When we left, Nila and I stopped by the pharmacy and picked up a cane. Of course, I got a blue one. Nila headed to the salon, and I headed to Mountain Forest for my CT scan.

I checked into Mountain Forest, acquired another bracelet, and had the CT scan performed. When I left, I headed to PT. This was the place I had gone years earlier to rehab from my frozen shoulder surgery. There I was assigned to David Lilly as my therapist again. It was like stepping back in time to see Dave again. I wondered if the other therapist working still wore shirts that read "I will fight the good fight" on the back.

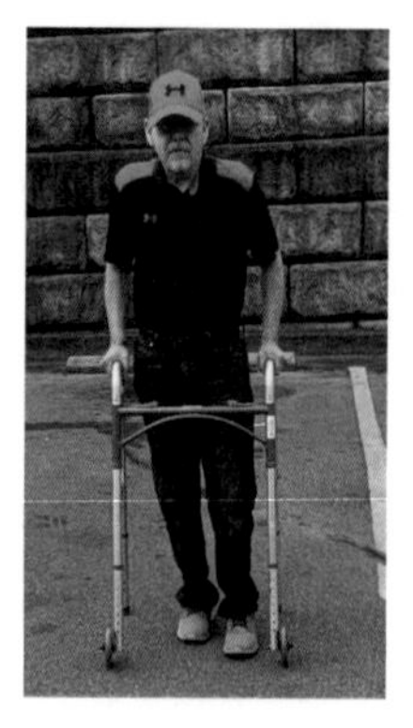

Perry with walker

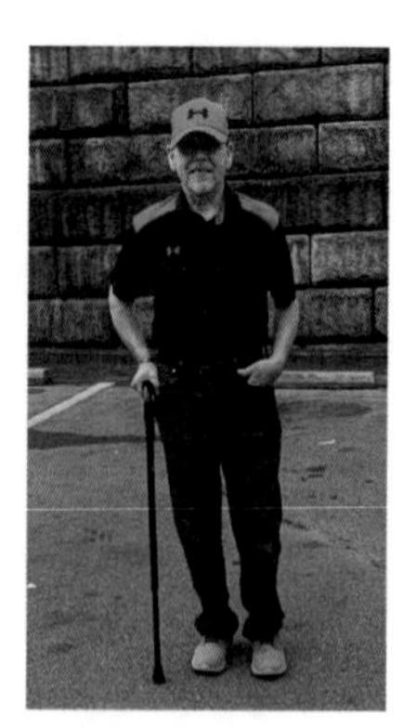

Perry with cane

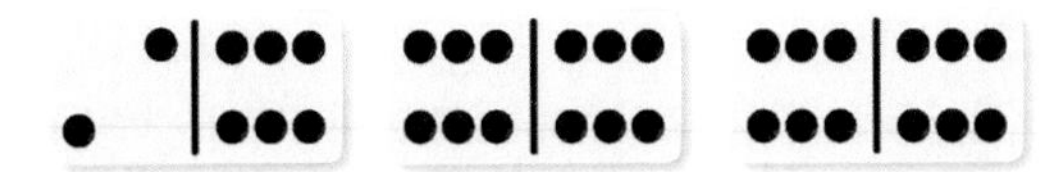

Chapter 32

MADE OF SCARS PART III

It was July 11, 2021, and my newest scar had mostly healed from my sixteenth surgery. I wasn't experiencing much trouble with my gluteus medius muscle, surprisingly. But my hip and leg bone remained frequently angry. I still could not sleep on either side without being awakened by sharp pains around the trochanter and femur on my left side. And I could only hope that PT would fix me.

It was also the four-year anniversary since Deanna called me with an unnerving sense of urgency and despair in her voice. Deanna had informed me that my PSA was high. I had prostate cancer. Truth be known, I'd probably had it for several years prior to that day.

"I am still alive after four years. I am not sure how all of that equates to the grim 35 percent prediction, but I am not dead. I do not feel like I am dying. I feel blessed and alive. But the blue pig can change that in August."

Next on the agenda for me was PT. In true Sagittarian fashion, I set myself up for a major test immediately following being released from the walker. I would be flying to Detroit, Michigan, on the twelfth to participate with my boss and coworkers working a booth at Foam Expo for three days. Was I up for it? Likely not. Was I going to suck it up and motor through it? Absolutely.

The trip to Detroit turned out to be a good measuring stick to determine how far I still had to go for my hip to be normal again. I was fortunate to have wheelchair assistance through the airport. I was able to limp through the exhibitions at the show and work the booth. When you consider dinner, my days were fifteen-hours plus.

The domino effect was in play as my knee and ankle ached. After not using my left leg for six weeks, walking took a toll on them. Each day my ankle would swell, reminiscent of the ankle sprains from my basketball and softball days. My knee and foot were weak.

But I ignored the pain, took some OTC meds, and motored on. I wanted to show the team that I was making a spectacular comeback. Doing that was the real test!

Upon returning home, I still had not heard the results of my CT scan. I went to Quality of Life on July 15 for my quarterly Lupron shot and hoped to find out the results.

"It is always the same. What does it mean when there is no news? Is it a good sign? Is something wrong, and they want to see me in person? Has anyone even reviewed the report? My cancer could have spread, and no one may even know."

I inquired about the results upon arrival at Quality of Life. But no one could find a copy of the report. I also called my chiropractor. They were supposed to receive a copy. Again, no news.

This led me to make a trip back to Mountain Forest. There I was able to obtain a copy. I sat down in the waiting area and began reading the report. I found myself scanning rather than reading.

"I don't see the word metastasis. Nothing about an unusual spot. What other medical terms might they have used to describe my cancer showing up on a vital organ?"

But the report was 100 percent positive. I breathed a sigh of relief and called Nila to share the good news.

The next day I showed up for therapy. David Lily took me back and explained the visit was an "evaluation for insurance to determine if I required PT." What a joke. I am referring to the insurance requirement, of course.

"Perhaps I should just email some pictures of my incision and a video of my struggling limp. I could also send my surgical report detailing my shredded gluteus medius and how Dr. Stewart could see the bone through parts of it. And then there were the two anchors installed in my femur."

During the evaluation, there were three times when David asked me to perform a function, and his reaction to my attempt was, "Wow! Have you seen yourself try to do that?"

I left feeling confident that David's assessment would justify my PT.

Next on the agenda, my new general surgeon was going to remove the cyst located on my back, around the spinal area. It had gotten progressively larger and made it very uncomfortable to lean back in a chair or the seat of a car.

"Tumors on the spine are typical when cancer metastasizes. Deanna and Dr. Ballard both said they believe it is not attached to the spine, and I believe them. But is it malignant or benign? I hope it does not take days and days to get the results. Another test, another morbid thought, another period anxiously awaiting results, and another scar."

My surgery was scheduled for July 19. By this time, the latest Lupron shot was really being felt. I was back to having major hot flashes at a rate of ten per day. My energy was knocked back down, and I found myself needing 5-Hour Energy shots to give me a boost by 2:00 p.m. each day.

The surgeon checked out the lump and immediately knew two things:

1. This was a common sebaceous cyst that was harmless.
2. The location over my spine made it apparent why I wanted it removed.

I lay facedown on the chair, which had been reclined to a horizontal position. The doctor cleaned the area and draped fabric material across my back.

"You are going to feel a series of pricks and stings. I am going to numb the area," the doctor explained. The numbing process began and felt like a small bee stinging me. Then, I felt nothing.

"It is going to feel like I am pulling and tugging on this area. Once I cut it open, I will remove the cyst and make sure to clean out the area," the surgeon continued with the play-by-play communication.

After a few minutes of feeling exactly what he had described, it was time for a few stitches and a bandage.

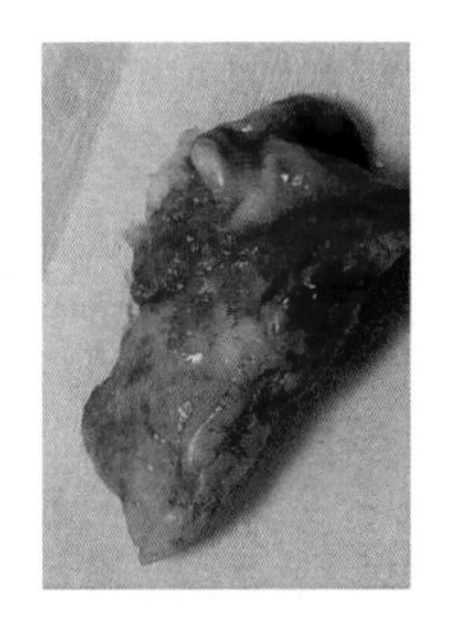

Sebaceous cyst removed from back

"These stitches are located under the skin," he explained. "They will dissolve on their own. Give it twenty-four hours, and you can remove the bandage and take a shower."

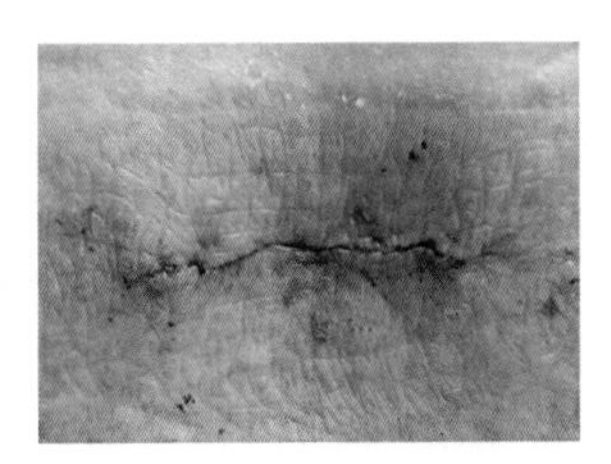

The cyst was intertwined with skin and football shaped. The area was very sore for the first few days but eventually calmed down. With my seventeenth surgery behind me, the next thing on my list was the August bone scan.

Scar from sebaceous cyst

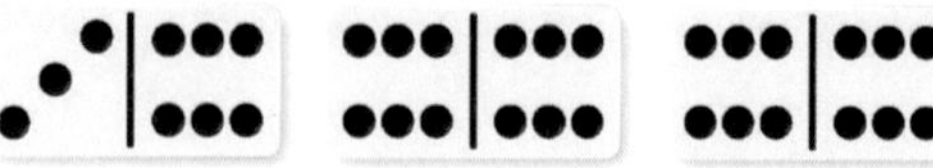
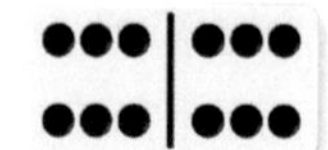

Chapter 33

MADE OF SCARS PART IV

My next bone scan was scheduled for August 18, 2021. I would be returning to the same medical center where my radiation and other scans had been performed. I knew the blue pig would be waiting. Every scan was important to me. But this one had special importance. If negative, I might no longer have them quarterly. Dr. Famoyin might schedule them annually. If my PSA was still undetectable, I could possibly be taken off Lupron again. I would continue moving forward in reverse!

I was finally approved for PT. The first couple of visits were easy for me. Three-pound weights on my feet and rotate clockwise and counterclockwise thirty times. Then the weights were placed on my ankles to do leg lifts. All of this happened while a TENS unit was affixed to my lower back and left leg, just above the knee, while a heating pad was wrapped around my hip. Next were some squats, and on to the step bike for ten minutes.

"You can also use your hands if you want," David explained.

"No, thanks," I replied.

In my mind, a voice said, "A true Sagittarius wouldn't cheat and use his arms to make it easier on his legs. Your arms are fine; just exercise that hip."

And so, I sat there, arms crossed, and worked my legs. As the time was running out, I realized I wasn't that far from making a complete lap on the digital screen. I pressed harder and faster. As the clock ticked closer to the ten-minute mark, I ramped up the speed more and more, trying to complete a lap.

I finished therapy with an ice pack on my hip. The cold was a welcome feeling.

"Five, seven, or ten minutes?" David asked.

"Ten," I responded without hesitation.

I chuckled when David responded with, "Oh, a tough guy, huh?"

After therapy I felt really well. It was a wonderful feeling to have exercised. Anyone who goes to the gym knows what that feeling is like.

But when it came to bedtime, it was an enraged Mr. Skeleton that crawled into bed. All night I kept the TENS unit on me. Three different times I put an ice pack on my hip. I don't even recall what OTC medications I took, but I am quite sure they surpassed the recommended dosage.

Around 4:00 a.m., I placed my final ice pack across my hip and dialed up the TENS unit. The bedroom had been filled with the sounds of me moaning, groaning, and asking God to please give me relief. Sometime afterward, I fell asleep. I awoke again at 5:30 a.m. The ice pack was used up, the TENS unit had turned off, and my hip was aching. This time it was not because of the anchors in my femur or the reconstructed glute; it was because my hip felt frozen to the touch. I conceded the rest of the night and got out of bed.

It was seventy-one days after hip surgery. The same routine repeated through the first few therapy sessions. I backed off slightly to help prevent another pain-filled night. But more was added to my routine. I often pondered going in search of some street drugs like prescription hydrocodone, just to give me some relief. It seemed ironic to think of buying prescription drugs illegally. I would be like the drug addicts who made it so difficult for someone like me, who really needed them, to get a script from my doctor. So, I didn't.

On Monday, August 2, 2021, I was at my last appointment with Dr. Famoyin before my next bone scan. There was a print on the wall in the lab of his office that always spoke to me.

The print that hung in the lab didn't have an author's name. It always reminded me of something Dr. Famoyin would say.

It read, *"If the storms should come, then we shall just dance in the rain."*

Dr. Famoyin entered and greeted me as usual. He asked me how I was feeling. I completely disregarded the fact that my life was, once again, consumed with pain and suffering. So, I told him I felt great. This was true, minus the surgery. I had to share with him that I had taken a fall a week prior.

"I was in my yard, and the dogs got into a spat. My brain said to run and break it up, but my hip refused to cooperate," I explained. "I made sure to turn while falling so I would not land on the surgery side. The fall resulted in separated ribs on my right side," I said.

Dr. Famoyin had been writing notes the whole time. When I finished, he laid the pen down and began shaking his head and laughing in disbelief.

Dr. Famoyin looked up at me and said, "You are Superman! Where are you flying to next?" I laughed and imagined Superman as a kid, wearing a red towel around his neck and pretending to fly.

As we walked out of the office, he turned to me and said once again, "You only have three or four lives left, you know?"

I responded by saying, "Once you read my book, you may say even less than three or four."

I walked along beside the doctor, laughing and cutting up, straight to the lab for my blood draw. Everyone's favorite vein had developed scar tissue and required some additional force to penetrate now. After the blood draw, I checked out and made my next appointment, which would be my first appointment after my bone scan. When the receptionist gave me the date, I just stood and stared into space. "Mr. Muse, is September 13 at 9:00 a.m. all right?"

But there was a more severe consequence to the fall that reared its ugly head just days later. It was at an accelerated rate that I began to seize up. All of my joints seemed to rust, and I once again felt like the Tin Man from *The Wizard of Oz*, caught in the rain with no one to apply much-needed oil. I tried increasing my prednisone, but to no avail. Within two short days, I was barely able to walk or drive.

This led me first to my local medical care facility, where they discovered blood in my urine. The doctor was certain it was kidney stones, but the CT scan showed otherwise. This was when I decided to go back to Dr. Famoyin.

Dr. Famoyin realized the injury was a contused right kidney. He explained that my kidney would reduce functionality during the healing process, and my left kidney would have to make up the difference.

But after explaining to Dr. Famoyin about my head-on car accident, and the severe damage inflicted to my left kidney, he had a new opinion.

"You are in serious trouble. Do you understand?" he asked. "You are in very serious trouble," he repeated. "Your left kidney cannot increase function due to the damage you suffered in the accident. Your right kidney is at a reduced level of function," he continued. "And now your blood is not being filtered adequately. I will send you for an infusion. You must drink a lot of water and cranberry juice to help flush your kidneys. If you are not better tomorrow, I will have no choice but to hospitalize you," he concluded.

As we walked down the hallway, he made an observation. "Do you see how you are walking and unable to stand straight? This is exactly how someone looks just before dialysis," he explained.

I got my infusion and made it back home. I followed the doctor's orders to the letter. That evening I felt almost normal again! The infusion cocktail worked wonders. But two days later, I needed Alanna to drive me back to see Dr. Famoyin again. We were about to begin a long weekend, and I feared what might happen when my only choice of doctors would be limited to the emergency room.

I was unable to walk and could barely get out of the car when we arrived. This time I needed a wheelchair to get to the patient room and then the infusion room.

Fortunately, I made it through the weekend and started to see signs of recovery. Although my kidney was still sore, the rust was minimal in my joints. The water and cranberry juice were helpful. The infusions kept me from the hospital.

This was just another domino effect in my mind. The damage to my gluteus medius needed surgery. For six weeks after surgery, I could not put weight on my left leg. This, along with the surgical repair and anchors, caused extreme weakness in my left leg. In going from the walker to the cane, I did not have the balance and strength to carry myself, and so I fell. The fall resulted in separated ribs, a cracked rib, and a kidney contusion that nearly hospitalized me. I had avoided another close call.

For days to come, I pondered my appointment on the thirteenth.

The morbid thoughts were triggered. I deliberated internally, "Should I change my appointment from the thirteenth? The last time I had bone scan results on the thirteenth, I ended up down in a hole. Do I want to wait that long after the scan? I do not. I need to be sitting in front of the good doctor to hear my results. I may still end up down in a hole, but he will be there to comfort me either way."

September 13, 2021, was also the night Nila and I had purchased tickets to see a band we really liked, Theory of a Deadman. Odd to have picked a band with that name on the thirteenth, now that I think about it. The song that we had been listening to a lot was "Medicate." When you put all of it together with the comment Dr. Famoyin made saying, "You are Superman!" it was eerily coincidental. One of the lyrics in the song says:

Superman is a hero
But only when his mind is clear though
He needs that fix like the rest of us
So he's got no fear when he saves that bus

I finally made a trip to our Calhoun plant, after my visit with Dr. Famoyin and PT, to see the new production coater run. It was uplifting to experience all the people who wanted to see me and ask how I was doing.

Kanita had worked at the Calhoun location for over twenty-five years. She was beloved by our customers and employees alike. Kanita could write her own book. It would be one of tragedy, triumph, kindness, and inspiring resilience.

As we talked, I explained the details of the hip surgery. Then I shared the accident in my yard that led to the separated ribs. What she said next caught me completely off guard.

Kanita said, "Dang, Perry, you have thirteen lives!"

Whoever says thirteen lives? Of all the numbers, it was thirteen again. Doesn't everyone say nine lives because of the myth that is related to cats' ability to always land on their feet?

I later walked into Kanita's office and sat down to discuss how she came to say thirteen.

She was initially rueful. "I have no idea why that came out of my mouth," she confessed. "I didn't mean it in a bad way. I don't even know why I said it," she shared apologetically.

It was then that I shared with her how often the number thirteen had been at play since having cancer. I opened the manuscript on my phone and read to her from chapter 24, Building a Boat. The very first two words in the chapter were "Unlucky 13."

I read the first two paragraphs of chapter 24 to her. After listening intently, Kanita said, "Well, I was meant to say that. It is all part of a bigger plan and was meant to happen."

I agreed and told her, "Well, you have officially made the book now."

Perhaps thirteen wasn't unlucky. Perhaps it was another sign. Either way, I scheduled an additional appointment for the day following my bone scan to get the results sooner and in person.

Today was day seventy-three since my surgery. I had begun taking a one-quarter cut of a muscle relaxer to be able to rest better and ignore the pain longer. I was getting stronger, but the pace was like that of a Sulcata Tortoise. The PT regimen made me hurt in new places. Walking on the cane, coupled with my falls, kept my ribs aggravated on the right side of my body.

The other day, Nila had said to me, "Everything that hurts isn't cancer." She was right. But how did I tell the difference? Any pain in my rib made the dark voice remind me of the tiny sclerotic lesion on my right third rib.

"Have more lesions formed? Remember the guy at Famoyin's office stating that more lesions have appeared over the past year? Why doesn't it seem to be healing if it is something else? Is this just an indication of what the blue pig will reveal in eleven more days?"

I was home alone, preparing dinner and doing a small amount of housework. When I sat down for a break, I opened my horoscope.

Daily / Weekly / Monthly
Sagitarrius
11/22 to 12/21
Alias: The Archer
August 7, 2021

You had the sense recently that some big and important aspect of your life was changing for the better. Since then, Sagittarius, you have probably seen signs of this, which validated what you felt. And yet, you are still having to work through some of the same old problems and dramas, and you are beginning to wonder if your initial feelings of hope were realistic. They are! What you are going through now is just the clearing away of old debris and the tying up of loose ends. Once you get through this, you will begin to see real signs of change.

The kidney contusion and ribs caused me to miss PT for almost two weeks.

Visit number four to PT was on day seventy-eight following surgery. I increased my time on the bike to twelve minutes and my steps per minute (SPM) was up from forty-five to sixty.

Dave had added the cross trainer, which was a cross between steps up and steps forward. Initially I was only able to bear five minutes before my glutes started burning. But on this day, I was able to do ten minutes at fifty SPM.

Next, I worked out with the TRX straps, doing squats. I increased my previous sets by one, going from three to four sets of ten squats.

My last exercise consisted of doing high steps on a trampoline. I marched in place, raising my thighs to a horizontal position. This lasted three minutes. The big breakthrough on this exercise was being able to do it hands free for the first time! This was quite an accomplishment and was proof I was gaining strength and balance.

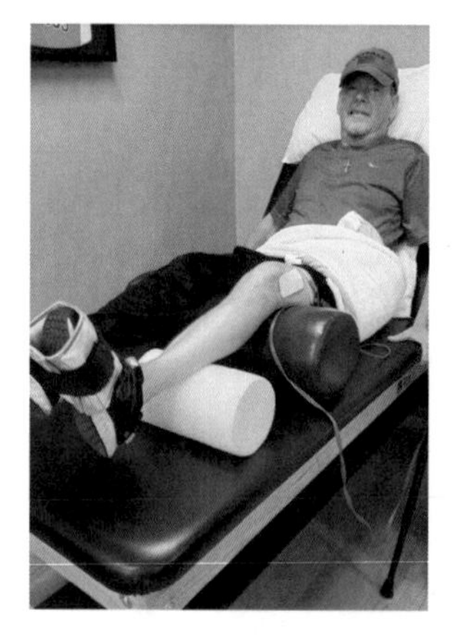

Physical therapy #1

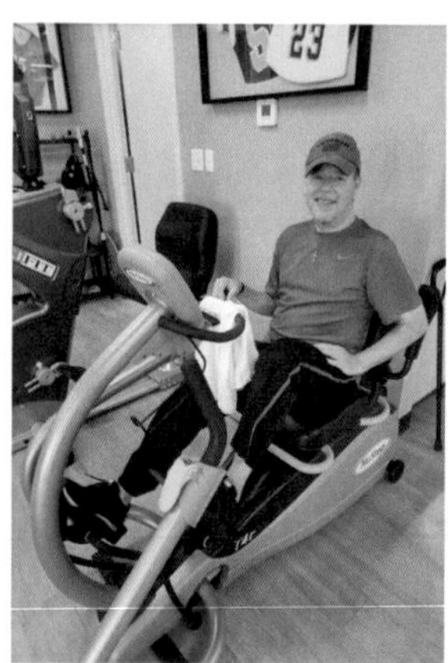

Physical therapy #2

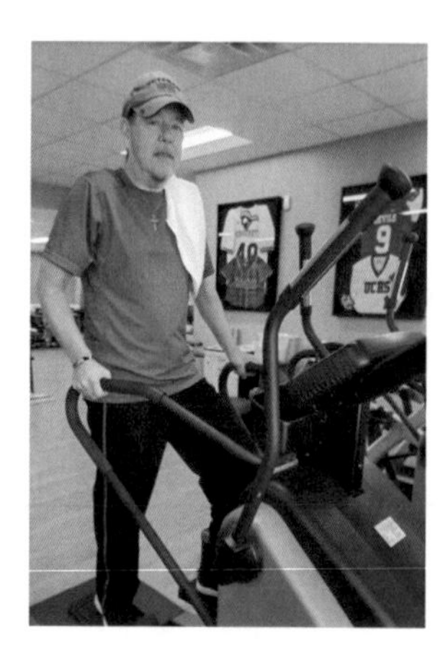

Physical therapy #3

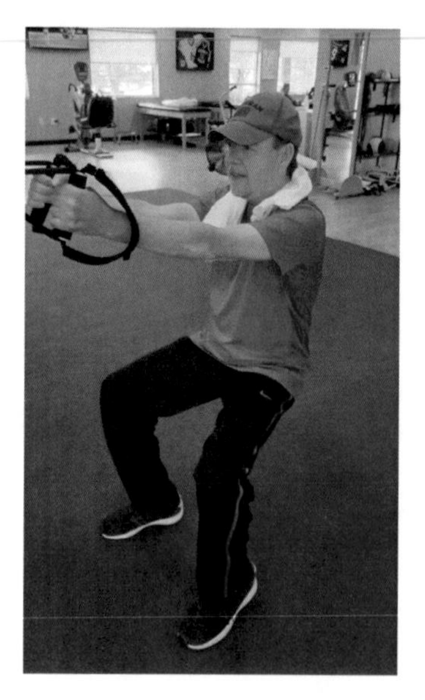

Physical therapy #4

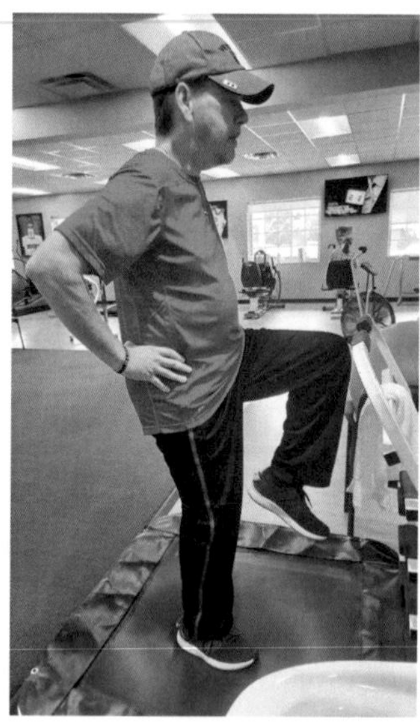

Physical therapy #5

I left therapy walking better and feeling encouraged with the progress. This added to the excitement of this already being a special day for Nila and me. It was the one-year anniversary of our grooming salon being open for business. I went straight to the salon and gave each employee a handwritten thank-you card that also contained a fifty-dollar bonus.

Life was good, and I was able to tell my body was healing. My next event was, of course, seeing what the blue pig had in store for me next week.

The anxiety was especially high this time, leading up to the bone scan. I tried to focus all my energy on working and getting stronger. I made two trips to the Georgia facility in two weeks to work and oversee some new trials. But what I did not consider was the alone time on the ride. Four-plus hours each way, with no one else in the car.

Try as I might, the morbid thoughts were my sole company.

"If the test is negative, I am going to get Sparky certified and begin therapy team work again. If the test is positive, I wonder what chemo treatment they will put me on. If it is negative, I want to get the new project started and finished in Calhoun. That is a two-year project. If positive, who do I tell, and when? If it is negative, I want to plan another trip with Nila after our Bahamas trip with Steve and Paula in November. If it is positive, how will I not ruin everyone's good time?" These thoughts seemed to constantly run in a holding pattern in my mind.

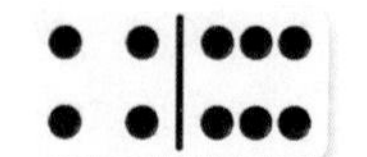 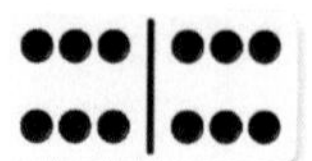 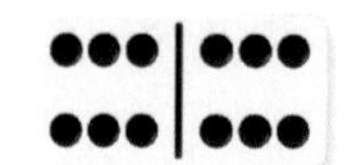

Chapter 34

MADE OF SCARS PART V

August 18, 2021, finally arrived. I made my way to the medical center for my visit with the blue pig. This time I avoided the urge to look over at the radiation oncology entrance. Even though I could see it vividly in my mind, I did not want to experience the sadness that came from seeing it.

After passing through the COVID protocol area, I went to the waiting area for radiology. It was only a few minutes before I was called back. This time I was taken to a secondary waiting area. While waiting, I took the time to say a long prayer.

Mostly I prayed for those who were stuck in Afghanistan after the United States abruptly pulled out of the country. I was thankful for feeling well and for my family. I prayed for others that were on my list for various reasons. I asked God to help me be a better Christian.

Next, I worked on an email. I wanted to get scheduled to have me and Sparky tested to be a therapy team. I missed therapy work and wanted to help others. Just as I finished, my name was called.

The technician took me back and retrieved the blue pig. Then he began prepping my IV needle.

"What story will you have to tell, Mr. Blue Pig?" I pondered as I stared at the container that held the radiopharmaceutical that would find its way into Mr. Skeleton over the next three hours.

The technician tried several times to puncture through the scar tissue on everyone's favorite vein, but I eventually had to ask that he stop. He apologized and wrapped the arm. Next was the same spot on my left arm. There wasn't any scar tissue, but the vein rolled and dodged the needle, as though playing a game with the technician. Eventually, success.

He wrapped my left arm and gave me instructions. I already knew the routine but listened intently.

"Stay hydrated and come back in three hours," he instructed.

It was only 9:00 a.m., but I had already collected another bracelet and two new scars.

I returned to the medical center at 12:15 p.m. I met the same technician and started the familiar routine. I emptied my pockets, removed my belt, grasped my crucifix, and said a prayer before removing it as well.

My last stop before the CT scan room was to empty my bladder. I knew this would be required, plus I had just finished my fourth bottle of water.

It was very quiet as I lay in the dimly lit room on the table. I had been wrapped snugly and the large flaps secured by Velcro. The machine slowly began to move. The quiet and darkness ushered me to sleep. When I awoke, it was from a pain in my abdomen. My bladder had refilled.

I closed one eye and focused intently on the ceiling, using the computer screen as a reference to judge movement. The table I lay on moved incredibly slowly through the scanner. A few minutes later I was still moving slower than a snail's pace through the scanner ring. At this point, the pain was becoming a serious concern.

It was already a chore for me to hold my urine, and I had often been embarrassed when it accidentally slipped out. My bladder was so full right then that I thought I was going to soak my jeans.

The machine finally stopped.

"Come on, man," I repeated in my mind.

"Hey," I said in an above-normal volume. There was no response. The pain intensified.

"HEY," I repeated louder. I could hear the technician talking. Finally, I yelled, "HEY!"

This got his attention, and he hurried to where I was.

"My bladder is full again, and I am about to pee on myself," I shared with a sense of urgency. The technician removed the Velcro and told me I was finished. But I could not raise myself up. The pain was too great, and the strain would surely overwhelm the dam and release the flood. The technician held out his arm and helped me up. I felt very fortunate that the restroom was only about twenty-five feet away. Once I started urinating, I thought it was never going to end. The relief was intoxicating. Note to self: next time, no drinking between the blue pig and the scan.

The following day I was back at the orthopedic facility. Alvin, the PA, said I was progressing well. My ROM was good, and the scar had healed well. I told him about the persistent pain in one spot on my hip and expressed that I thought I would be past the pain by now.

Alvin pressed on the side of my hip and quickly found the spot. I hadn't realized how sore it was to the touch until that moment. Alvin suggested it was likely inflammation of the bursa aggravating my bursitis. He also explained that the IT band was involved in the surgery and runs directly across the bursa.

I was told to buy some Voltaren gel. It was now offered over the counter but could only be obtained with a prescription not long ago. I was instructed to return in four weeks, and if it wasn't significantly better, he would consider a steroid shot into the bursa. The last thing Alvin said was, "Just remember that there was tissue involved in the surgery that could take nine months to a year to fully heal." I was not expecting to hear that.

Next was PT. After a good hard workout, I went home and took care of some calls and emails for Foam Products. Then I showered and headed to meet Nila at Dr. Famoyin's office. After studying it for a few minutes, I decided to wear blue.

Daily / Weekly / Monthly

Sagitarrius

11/22 to 12/21

Alias: The Archer

Thursday August 19, 2021

Somtimes you tend to expect the worst just so you won't be disappointed. If this is ingrained in you - especially when you are chasing a dream that is really important to you - then you need to reset your brain and come up with a better way to operate. Although expecting the the best can certainly result in disappointment now & then, it can't possibly be any worse than living in a state of mind where you are always feeling less than hopeful. Try expecting the best a little at a time, Sagittarius, and you should see more of the best in your life.

I headed to meet Nila and find out the results of my bone scan. Anxiety sometimes tries to transform into fear. I caught myself preparing for how I would react if the news were bad. Before leaving, I just couldn't resist the urge to check my horoscope.

As I drove to meet Nila, I contemplated what my horoscope had said. I had told God that it was in His hands and His control. So why worry, right?

I decided God was speaking to me again through my horoscope app and felt a sense of relief. As I sat at a red light, I quietly said, "Thank you, Lord." When I looked at the car beside me, a sticker in the back window made me laugh out loud.

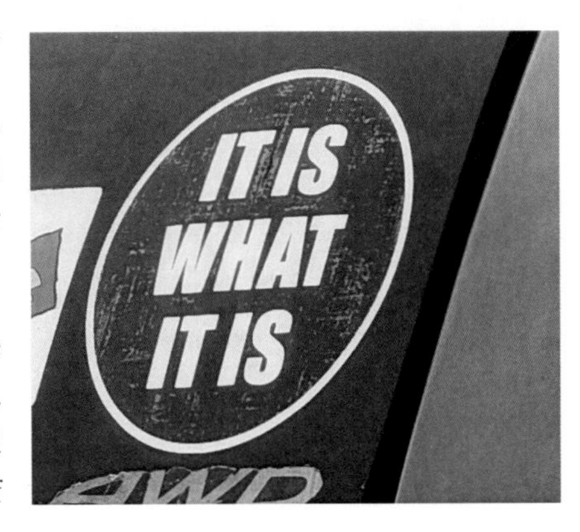

Random sign on a car

I met Nila at Quality of Life at 3:00 p.m. sharp. I laughed when I noticed she had worn her blue Skechers and a blue Under Armour top. We hugged and went inside.

I was concerned we would find out the report had not been sent over yet. Dr. Famoyin was not at the office, and we would see Sara, another wonderful, caring part of my journey.

After checking my vitals, we were taken to room 1. Nila and I were both jittery and held hands while we waited.

Sara walked into the room and greeted us.

"How are you doing today?" she asks.

Nila answered, "Just fine."

Simultaneously, I answered, "Nervous and anxious."

Sara immediately understood why and, before she even got seated, said, "It's all good. Nothing to worry about. I will go over it with you, but it is a good report."

"Three in a row!" I wanted to yell. "It's been seven months since we were given the devastating diagnosis on January 13. 'Your cancer has spread into your bones and is now incurable' were the morbid words. Since that day, I have had three consecutive bone scans that have said I am clear. Mr. Skeleton is still safe. Thank you, Lord. I have work to do and won't disappoint you."

My next appointment with Dr. Famoyin was September 13. This was when we would talk about my schedule for the future. Perhaps I would be put on a less frequent schedule for bone scans. Maybe even taken off Lupron again. At least until my PSA rose again.

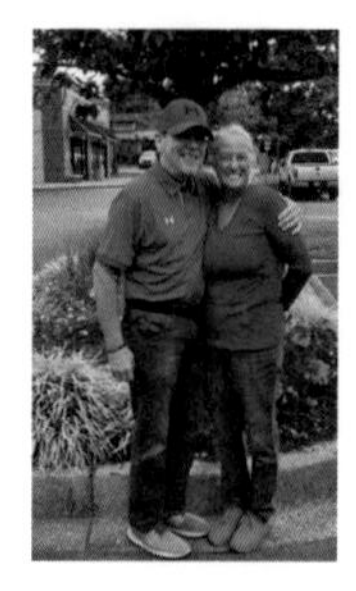

"We don't want to kill the patient trying to treat the cancer," were the doctor's words that often popped up in my mind.

The relief and happiness were indescribable. I called my boss Erik to share the news. That evening we went to dinner with Alanna and Cory to celebrate.

Perry & Nila wearing all blue following bone scan results

On day one hundred and twelve following my hip surgery, I retired the cane and began walking unassisted. I had developed peroneal tendonitis in my foot. This was the result of not walking on it for so long, then walking and exercising, then stopping, and starting back. This required me to wear a boot for a couple of weeks. Another domino in my journey.

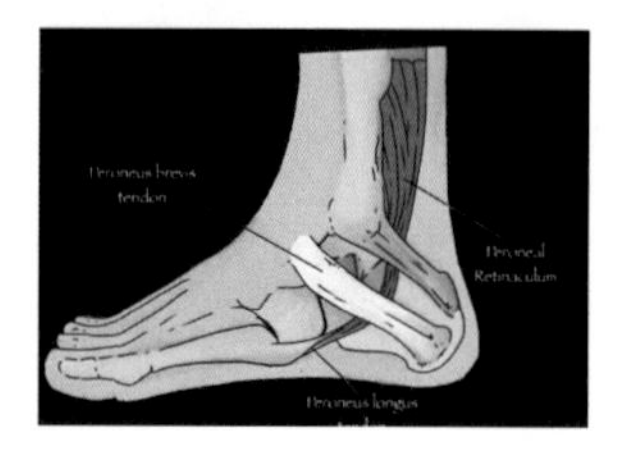

Drawing of foot and peroneal tendons by Ezekial Cooper

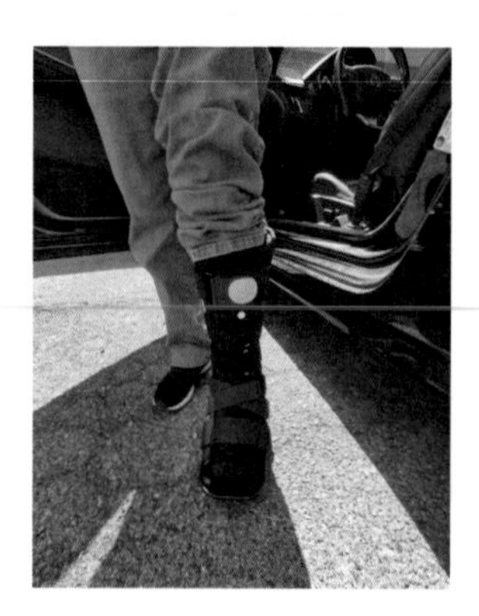

The bone scan, and awaiting the results, will be routine for the remainder of my life. Each time, we will deal with the anxiety leading up to the scan and then the emotional roller coaster waiting to hear the results, actually wondering if we will hear the words, "This is consistent with bone metastasis." If that day arrives, I will be glad I made time to build my boat. Dr. Famoyin will be hard at work on my quality of life.

Perry wearing a boot on left foot

I spent my whole life working. I am grateful to say that since jumping into the workforce at age thirteen, I have never had an unemployment check. I was always working for the day when I could quit and relax in my senior years, only to find, after my cancer diagnosis, that life might decide to retire me first.

I have fought four years, trying to protect Mr. Skeleton from cancer. That will continue forever. But if the cancer ever moves there, it appears it will be Mr. Skeleton that eventually kills me.

I try not to dwell on the end. But I do pay attention to movies and other people's stories. I do recall those friends and family I visited who were dying from cancer and their solemn end of life. The images and memories are forever burned into my brain.

My prediction if Mr. Skeleton is invaded: "I expect my anemia to worsen. That will start the domino effect of organ or brain problems. There will likely be tumors and pain. Oh yes, I am almost guaranteed more pain. There may not be an emoji for that level of pain. The morphine will become abundant, and one day, I will lose consciousness to escape the pain, and with it, my awareness of reality."

Everyone dies at some point. We all know that. Consider there are 7.9 billion people on earth at this very moment. In one hundred and thirty years, they will all be dead.

So, my mindset has been more about the time I have remaining, whether I end up dying of cancer or something else.

When I was a youth, I was somewhat of a delinquent. As a young adult, I was arrogant, ungrateful, and often angry. But once I married Nila and had a family, my view of life changed. Loving someone and having a family is life changing. I am sure this is true for many. I have often thought of dying throughout my life, sometimes because of the death of another, or sometimes because I was secretly terrified, recalling that I had somehow escaped death on more than one occasion.

And so, for decades, I have pondered dying and meeting God. I think of all the bad things I have done and said to people. I think of the unnecessary little lies. I think of taking when I should have been giving, stealing when I should have been buying. I am embarrassed to have thought I alone was responsible for my blessings and good fortune.

I cannot go back and change what I have done in the past. Unfortunately, there are those who may not forgive and forget my trespasses. For that I am truly ashamed and sorry.

There is a picture that hung in the patient room at Quality of Life that always inspired me. The picture had a quote by Maria Robinson. It read, "*Nobody can go back and start a new beginning, but anyone can start today and make a new ending.*"

And so, for half of my life or more, I have worked to be a better person. To create a better ending. It is difficult to change habits. It takes commitment. I have often backslid and found myself indulging in old ways. All I can do is put as much time and distance between the period in my life that I did regretful things and the time when I die. All I can do is be thankful for my blessings and try to be a positive influence on my family and friends. The longer I am allowed to live, the longer I must be a good father, friend, husband, grandfather, sibling, son, and coworker. And I pray for forgiveness from those I have wronged. After all, forgiveness is all I can wish for since I cannot teleport back in time for a redo. Cancer did not give me this mission I am on. Cancer just made me more laser focused on it.

While awaiting one of my scans, I noticed a quotation on the wall in front of me. Again, I ask, "Can God write a horoscope in an app? Can God write a profound quotation?" Probably not in the literal sense, although He created the amazing human body. I believe things happen as they are meant to. Perhaps when my life became threatened, I just started paying a little more attention. The quotation by Ben Herbster became a positive affirmation of the path I had chosen.

"The greatest waste in the world is the difference in what we are and what we could become."

Will there be conversations about me with grandchildren, friends, or other family as time passes once I am deceased? Will my children and grandchildren even read my book? Who knows? Someone asked me, "What made you decide to write a book?" My response was simple. "I wanted to share information that may be helpful to others dealing with cancer or other medical issues. I wanted to inspire others to fight the good fight and find positivity in the most negative situations. Also, I was once told that if you want your story to be told accurately, you have to write it yourself."

My mom had a vision of me where I was standing before many, many people and preaching to them. I called it a dream once, and she corrected me, saying, "It was more than a dream, Perry. It was a vision sent to me." Perhaps my life and this book are that vision coming to fruition. Perhaps this is how I can touch others and provide inspiration, faith, strength, and knowledge.

I was watching Dr. Charles Stanley one Sunday morning on television. During his sermon, he said, "People ask me, how will God judge me? What if I haven't been as good of a Christian as I should have been? What will God do?" I tell them, "The first thing He is going to do is love you. Then He will judge you based on your life and reward you accordingly. Some may receive greater rewards than others, but the first thing God will do is love you."

My mom always told me that I would stand before God one day. My life would flash before my eyes, and I would be judged on the life that I lived and the person I had been.

I often imagine that I am standing before God, my life passing before us like a movie and feeling ashamed of some of those earlier years. In my thoughts, I fear God will form His judgment long before we are even halfway.

In my mind, I imagine looking to God and saying, "God, please keep watching. I promise it will get better."

1) Claw hammer bounced off rock (stitches)

2) Bicycle wreck with sister (stitches)

3) Rifle scope (stitches)

4, 5, 6) Tonsillectomy, adenoids, sack of gravel

7, 8) Torn bicep, torn labrum surgery

9) Diaphragmatic plication surgery

10) Appendectomy surgery

11) Thumb surgery

12) Dupuytrens surgeries

13, 14) Rotator cuff surgery

15) Dog bite (stitches)

16) Broken window (stitches)

17) Motorcycle wreck surgery

18, 19, 20) Prostatectomy surgery

21) Gluteus medius surgery

22) Dog bite (stitches)

23) Box cutter (stitches)

24) Horse wreck (stitches)

25) Dog bite (stitches)

26) Go-cart wreck (stitches)

27) Dog bite

28) Cyst surgery 1 and 2

29) Ankle surgery

30) Nail in foot (stitches)

31) Ruptured kidney

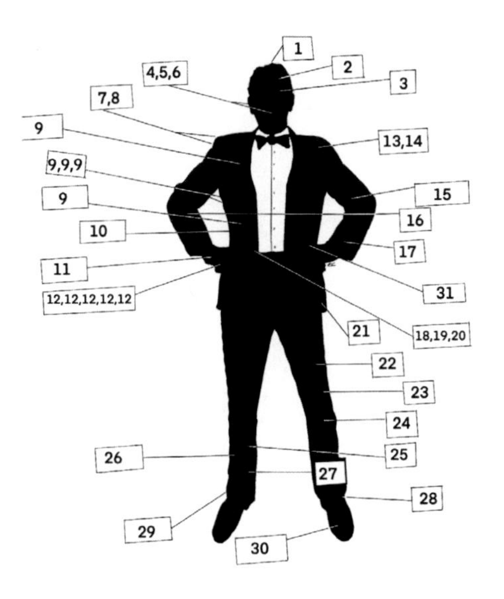

Drawing of silhouette by Ezekial Cooper

This song accurately depicts a big part of who I am. I can definitely relate to the lyrics, and I understand them from a personal perspective.

MADE OF SCARS

Stone Sour 2006

GLOSSARY OF TERMS

A

Abdominal Distension: Abdominal distension refers to the swelling of the abdomen. The distension is caused by either air (gas) or fluid collection. *(Medindia)*

Acid Reflux: Acid reflux is when some of the acid content of the stomach flows up into the esophagus, into the gullet, which moves food down from the mouth. *(Medical News Today)*

Adenocarcinoma: Cancers that start in glandular tissues that make mucus or fluid, such as the lung, breast, prostate, or colon. Adenocarcinomas are considered a specific type (subtype) of carcinomas. *(Hopkins Medicine)*

Adenoidectomy: Adenoidectomy is the surgical removal of the adenoid for reasons which include impaired breathing through the nose, chronic infections, or recurrent earaches. *(Cleveland Clinic)*

Adenopathy: Adenopathy is any disease or inflammation that involves glandular tissue or lymph nodes. The term is usually used to refer to lymphadenopathy or swollen lymph nodes. *(Medical News Today)*

Adhesive Capsulitis: A condition affecting the shoulder, making it painful and stiff with loss of mobility. *(Focus Medica)*

Anemia: A condition in which the blood is deficient in red blood cells, in hemoglobin, or in total volume. *(Merriam-Webster Medical dictionary)*

Anesthesiologist: Anesthesiologists are doctors who specialize in using medication to keep you from feeling pain during surgery. *(WebMD)*

Anterolateral: Situated or occurring in front and to the side. *(Merriam-Webster Medical dictionary)*

Appendicitis: Inflammation of the appendix, a finger-shaped pouch present at the lower right side of the abdomen. Starts with a dull pain in the middle or right side of the abdomen and moves down to the lower right abdomen. *(Focus Medica)*

Atelectasis: A condition where lungs collapse partially or completely. Mild cases show no signs and symptoms but might develop breathing difficulty when it spreads. *(Focus Medica)*

Ativan: Ativan is a prescription medicine used to treat the symptoms of anxiety disorders. Ativan may be used alone or with other medications. Ativan belongs to a class of drugs called Antianxiety Agents, Anxiolytics, Benzodiazepines, Anticonvulsants, Benzodiazepine. *(RX Professional)*

Autoimmune Disorder: A disorder caused by a reaction of an individual's immune system against the organs or tissues of the body. Autoimmune processes can have different results: slow destruction of a particular type of cell or tissue, stimulation of an organ into excessive growth, or interference in function. *(Free Medical Dictionary)*

Axillary: Pertaining to the armpit, the cavity beneath the junction of the arm and the body. *(Medicinenet.com)*

B

Barrett's Esophagus: Abnormal change of the cells present in the lower portion of the esophagus (food pipe) due to acid reflux, which causes the lining to thicken and inflamed. *(Focus Medica)*

Biopsy: Obtaining a sample of tissue for laboratory analysis. *(Focus Medica)*

Blake Drain: BLAKE drains are a special type of silicon, radiopaque drain used post-open-heart surgery to help patients recover by removing excess fluid around the lungs. *(Hunker.com)*

Blastocyst Stage: In humans, blastocyst stage of development occurs during the first- and second-week following fertilization (GA week 3 and 4) and is described initially as Carnegie stage 3. This stage is followed by blastocyst hatching and implantation. *(Embryology)*

Blue Pig: Lead storage containers used to store radioactive materials. When preparing radiopharmaceuticals, doses are drawn from a vial into a syringe while using a tungsten syringe shield. After the dose has been drawn into the syringe, the radioisotope vial may be stored in a lead storage container (Blue Pig) or tungsten vial shield. *(Nuclear-shields.com)*

Bone Mineral Density: A test to measure bone strength by measuring the density of minerals, especially calcium in the bone using X-rays or CT scan. *(Focus Medica)*

Bone Scan: An imaging test of skeletal system used to diagnose metabolic problems of the bones using X-rays. *(Focus Medica)*

BRCA Gene Mutation: A BRCA mutation occurs when the DNA that makes up the gene becomes damaged in some way. When a BRCA gene is mutated, it may no longer be effective at repairing broken DNA and helping to prevent breast cancer. *(Nationalbreastcancer.org)*

Bronchitis: Bronchitis is an inflammation of the lining of your bronchial tubes, which carry air to and from your lungs. People who have bronchitis often cough up thickened mucus, which can be discolored. Bronchitis may be either acute or chronic. Often, developing from a cold or other respiratory infection, acute bronchitis is very common. chronic bronchitis, a more serious condition, is a constant irritation or inflammation of the lining of the bronchial tubes, often due to smoking. *(healthline.com)*

Bursa: The fluid filled sacs that cushion the joints. *(Focus Medica)*

Bursitis: An inflammation of bursae, the fluid filled sacs that cushion the joints. This causes pain, swelling and stiffness around the joint. *(Focus Medica)*

C

C Reactive Protein (CRP): A protein present in blood serum in various abnormal states (such as inflammation or neoplasia).
(Merriam-Webster Medical dictionary)

Cancerous Lesions: In cancer terminology, lesion is another term for tumor. *(infobloom.com)*

Cartlidge: A usually translucent somewhat elastic tissue that composes most of the skeleton of vertebrate embryos and except for a small number of structures.
(Merriam-Webster Medical dictionary)

Catheter: A flexible tube inserted through a narrow opening into a body cavity, particularly the bladder, for removing fluid. *(Oxford Dictionaries)*

Cetirizine: Cetirizine is an antihistamine used to relieve allergy symptoms such as watery eyes, runny nose, itching eyes/nose, sneezing, hives, and itching.
(First Databank)

Charnley Retractor: A self-retaining hip surgery retractor system helps to free assisting personnel while providing excellent exposure during hip arthroplasty and hip fracture surgery.
(*surgicalinstruments.com)*

Chemotherapy: Treatment that uses drugs to stop the growth of cancer cells, either by killing the cells or by stopping them from dividing. Chemotherapy may be given by mouth, injection, or infusion, or on the skin, depending on the type and stage of the cancer being treated.
(cancer.gov)

Chronic Obstructive Pulmonary Disease (COPD): A chronic inflammatory lung disease that causes obstructed airflow from the lungs. Symptoms include breathing difficulty, cough, mucus (sputum) production and wheezing. It's typically caused by long-term exposure to irritating gases or particulate matter, most often from cigarette smoke. *(Mayo Clinic)*

Colonoscopy: An exam used to detect changes or abnormalities in the large intestine (colon) and rectum. During a colonoscopy, a long, flexible tube (colonoscope) is inserted into the rectum. A tiny video camera at the tip of the tube allows the doctor to view the inside of the entire colon. *(Mayo Clinic)*

Computed Tomography (CT scan): A computerized tomography (CT) scan combines a series of X-ray images taken from different angles around your body and uses computer processing to create cross-sectional images (slices) of the bones, blood vessels and soft tissues inside your body. CT scan images provide more-detailed information than plain X-rays do. *(Mayo Clinic)*

Continuous Positive Airway Pressure (CPAP): A machine to pump air under pressure into the airway of the lungs. This helps keep the windpipe open during sleep. The forced air delivered by CPAP (continuous positive airway pressure) prevents episodes of airway collapse that block the breathing in people with obstructive sleep apnea and other breathing problems. *(Medline Plus)*

Contrast: A substance injected into the body that illuminates certain structures that would otherwise be hard to see on the radiograph. *(Free Medical Dictionary)*

Corticosteroids: Any of a group of steroid hormones produced in the adrenal cortex or made synthetically. There are two kinds: glucocorticoids and mineralocorticoids. They have various metabolic functions, and some are used to treat inflammation. (*Free Medical Dictionary)*

D

Decadron: Used to treat conditions such as arthritis, blood/hormone disorders, allergic reactions, skin diseases, eye problems, breathing problems, bowel disorders, cancer, and immune system disorders. It is also used as a test for an adrenal gland disorder (Cushing's syndrome). *(First Databank)*

Dialysis: A blood purifying treatment given when kidney function is not optimum. *(Focus Medica)*

Diaphragm: A sheet of internal skeletal muscle in humans and other mammals that extends across the bottom of the thoracic cavity. The diaphragm is the most important muscle of respiration, and separates the thoracic cavity, containing the heart and lungs, from the abdominal cavity: as the diaphragm contracts, the volume of the thoracic cavity increases, creating a negative pressure there, which draws air into the lungs. *(Wikipedia)*

Diaphragmatic Plication: A surgical procedure that has been performed since the 1920s for the treatment of diaphragmatic paralysis. Diaphragmatic paralysis is a serious problem for individuals suffering from the respiratory abnormalities, reduced energy levels, and sleep disturbances that are commonly associated with the disorder. *(Medscape)*

Double Lumen: A type of endotracheal tube which is used in tracheal intubation during thoracic surgery and other medical conditions to achieve selective, one-sided ventilation of either the right or the left lung. *(Wikipedia)*

Dual Energy X-Ray Absorptiometry (DXA): The gold standard for diagnosing osteoporosis (OP). It uses X-rays at two energy levels and works on the principle that, as X-rays pass through body tissues, they are attenuated to a different extent in different tissue types. *(RACGP.org)*

Duodenum: The duodenum, the first and shortest section of the small intestine, is a key organ in the digestive system. *(verywellhealth.com)*

Dupuytrens Contracture: A condition in which one or more fingers bend in towards the palm due to the development of fibrous connective tissue between the tendons of the finger. *(Focus Medica)*

Dyspnea: Shortness of breath. *(WebMD)*

E

Eburnated: A degenerative process of bone commonly found in patients with osteoarthritis or non-union of fractures. Friction in the joint causes the reactive conversion of the sub-chondral bone to an ivory-like surface at the site of the cartilage erosion. *(Wikipedia)*

Edema: Swelling caused due to excess fluid accumulation in the body tissues. Edema can occur in any parts of the body. *(Focus Medica)*

Electric Cauterizing Unit: Uses high-frequency electrical energy to cut tissue or coagulate bleeding. The preferential conduction of electrical energy by blood vessels facilitates coagulation. *(sciencedirect.com)*

Electrocardiogram (EKG): Records the electrical signals in your heart. It's a common and painless test used to quickly detect heart problems and monitor your heart's health. *(Mayo Clinic)*

Electrolytes: Minerals in your blood and other body fluids that carry an electric charge. *(Medline Plus)*

Embryonic Stem Cells (ESCs): An immortal extension of short-lived pluripotent cells that exist in a preimplantation embryo. *(sciencedirect.com)*

Endoscope: An instrument which can be introduced into the body to give a view of its internal parts. *(Dictionary)*

Endothoracic Fascia: The endothoracic fascia is the layer of loose connective tissue deep to the intercostal spaces and ribs, separating these structures from the underlying pleura. This fascial layer is the outermost membrane of the thoracic cavity. The endothoracic fascia contains variable amounts of fat. *(Wikipedia)*

Esophageal Sphincter: A bundle of muscles at the top of the esophagus. The muscles of the UES are under conscious control, used when breathing, eating, belching, and vomiting. They keep food and secretions from going down the windpipe. *(WebMD)*

Esophagogastroduodenoscopy: A test to examine the lining of the esophagus, stomach, and first part of the small intestine (the duodenum). *(Medline Plus)*

Extraprostatic Extensions: A medical term associated with a higher risk of recurrence and metastasis and lower cancer-specific survival after radical prostatectomy. *(radiopaedia.org)*

F

Fatigue: Extreme tiredness resulting from mental or physical exertion or illness. (*Dictionary)*

Ferritin: A blood protein that contains iron. A ferritin test helps your doctor understand how much iron your body stores. *(Mayo Clinic)*

Flexeril: Cyclobenzaprine is used short-term to treat muscle spasms. It is usually used along with rest and physical therapy. *(First Databank)*

Flonase: Used to relieve seasonal and year-round allergic and non-allergic nasal symptoms, such as stuffy/runny nose, itching, and sneezing. (*First Databank)*

Fluoroscopy: An imaging modality that uses x-rays to allow real-time visualization of body structures. During fluoroscopy, x-ray beams are continually emitted and captured on a screen, producing a real-time, dynamic image. This allows for dynamic assessment of anatomy and function. *(healthgrades.com)*

Forced Vital Capacity: FVC is used to evaluate your lung function. It measures the effect that your lung disease has on your ability to inhale and exhale. *(verywellhealth.com)*

G

Gastroesophageal Reflux Disease (GERD): When stomach acid frequently flows back into the tube connecting your mouth and stomach (esophagus). This backwash (acid reflux) can irritate the lining of your esophagus. *(Mayo Clinic)*

Gleason Score: Most of the prostate cancer cases diagnosed today have Gleason grades of 5, 6, or 7. The more aggressive forms of prostate cancer have scores of 8, 9, or 10. *(prostate-cancer.com)*

Glenohumeral Debridement: Procedure used to remove tissue in the shoulder joint that has been damaged from arthritis, overuse, or injury. The physician uses a small camera, called an arthroscope, which is inserted into the shoulder joint. *(omahashoulder.com)*

Gluteus Medius: The function of the gluteus medius muscle is to work with other muscles on the side of your hip to help pull your thigh out to the side in a motion called hip abduction.4 The gluteus medius also serves to rotate your thigh. For example, when walking and lifting your left leg up and forward, the right gluteus medius is contracting to keep your body level. Failure for this to happen may result in gait abnormalities and tipping sideways while walking. *(verywellhealth.com)*

H

Hematocrit: A hematocrit test is part of a complete blood count (CBC). Measuring the proportion of red blood cells in your blood can help your doctor make a diagnosis or monitor your response to a treatment. A lower-than-normal hematocrit can indicate: 1. An insufficient supply of healthy red blood cells (anemia) 2. A large number of white blood cells due to long-term illness, infection, or a white blood cell disorder such as leukemia or lymphoma. *(Mayo Clinic)*

Hematologist Oncologist: A doctor who specializes in treating cancers of the blood. They have extra training in the blood system, lymphatic system, bone marrow, and cancers. *(WebMD)*

Hemoglobin: A red protein responsible for transporting oxygen in the blood of vertebrates. Its molecule comprises four subunits, each containing an iron atom bound to a heme group. *(Dictionary)*

Hepatitis C: A viral infection that causes inflammation of liver that leads to liver inflammation. *(Focus Medica)*

Hepatitis C Antibody Test (HCV): Recommended initially to screen hepatitis C infection. The doctors may recommend additional tests to check the severity of the liver damage before the medications. *(Focus Medica)*

Hiatal Hernia: A condition in which the upper part of the stomach bulges through an opening in the diaphragm. *(Focus Medica)*

Hip Abduction: The movement of the leg away from the midline of the body. The hip abductors are important and often forgotten muscles that contribute to our ability to stand, walk, and rotate our legs with ease. *(healthline.com)*

Hyaluronic: Hyaluronic acid is a substance that is naturally present in the human body. It is found in the highest concentrations in fluids in the eyes and joints. *(WebMD)*

Hydrocodone: A class of medications called opiate (narcotic) analgesics. It works by changing the way the brain and nervous system respond to pain. *(medlineplus.gov)*

I

Incentive Spirometer: A handheld device that helps your lungs recover after a surgery or lung illness. Your lungs can become weak after prolonged disuse. *(healthline.com)*

Infraspinatus Muscle: In human anatomy, the infraspinatus muscle is a thick triangular muscle, which occupies the chief part of the infraspinatus fossa. As one of the four muscles of the rotator cuff, the main function of the infraspinatus is to externally rotate the humerus and stabilize the shoulder joint. *(Wikipedia)*

Intratendinous Insertional Tear: Tear in the muscles or tendons surrounding the shoulder joint. This causes pain in the shoulder, especially on movement. *(Focus Medica)*

Iron Infusion: A procedure in which iron is delivered to your body intravenously, meaning into a vein through a needle. This method of delivering medication or supplementation is also known as an intravenous (IV) infusion. Iron infusions are usually prescribed by doctors to treat iron deficiency anemia. *(healthline.com)*

IT Band: The iliotibial band (IT band) is a thick band of fibers that begins at the iliac crest (the border of the most prominent bone of the pelvis) in the pelvis and runs on the lateral or outside part of the thigh until it attaches into the tibia (shinbone). *(emedicinehelp.com)*

IV: A device that is used to allow a fluid (such as blood or a liquid medication) to flow directly into a patient's veins. *(merriam-webster.com)*

K

Kidney Contusion: Often called a kidney bruise, occurs following blunt trauma or direct impact to the lower back. This trauma leads to bleeding inside of the kidney. It may also cause pain, tenderness, and discoloration of the skin. Your back muscles and rib cage protect your kidneys. *(healthline.com)*

L

Labrum: A piece of fibrocartilage (rubbery tissue) attached to the rim of the shoulder socket that helps keep the ball of the joint in place. When this cartilage is torn, it is called a labral tear. *(hopkinsmedicine.org)*

Laparoscopic Surgery: Also called minimally invasive surgery, band aid surgery, or keyhole surgery, is a modern surgical technique in which operations are performed far from their location through small incisions elsewhere in the body. *(Wikipedia)*

Lateral Decubitus Position: A position in which a patient lies on his or her side and which is used especially in radiography and in making a lumbar puncture. *(merriam-webster.com)*

Leukemia: A type of cancer which affects the production and function of blood cells. This causes swollen lymph nodes, recurrent nosebleeds, tiredness, frequent infections, weight loss, bleeding, and bone pain. *(Focus Medica)*

Lung Parenchyma: Although often used to refer solely to alveolar tissue, term describes any form of lung tissue including bronchioles, bronchi, blood vessels, interstitium, and alveoli. *(The Free Dictionary)*

Lupron: A prescription hormone medicine used in the palliative treatment of advanced prostate cancer. *(drugs.com)*

Lymph Nodes: Each of several small swellings in the lymphatic system where lymph is filtered, and lymphocytes are formed. *(Dictionary)*

M

Magnetic Resonance Imaging (MRI): Provides precise details of your body parts, especially soft tissues, with the help of magnetic fields and radio waves. *(Focus Medica)*

Mandibular Tori: A bony growth in the mandible along the surface nearest to the tongue. Mandibular tori are usually present near the premolars and above the location of the mylohyoid muscle's attachment to the mandible. In 90% of cases, there is a torus on both the left and right sides. *(Wikipedia)*

Mean Platelet Volume: A measure of the average size of your platelets, a type of blood cell that helps prevent bleeding. *(verywellhealth.com)*

Mediastinal: A membranous partition between two body cavities or two parts of an organ, especially that between the lungs. *(Dictionary)*

Meniscus: A C-shaped piece of soft and fibrous cartilage, also known as fibrocartilage, that provides shock absorption and cushion to your knee. It is also wedge-shaped which improves joint congruency, further adding to knee stability. *(Jacksonville Orthopedic Institute)*

Mesenteric: A membranous fold attaching an organ to the body wall. *(The Free Dictionary)*

Metastasis: The word used to describe a cluster of cancer cells in one area that arose from a cancer in another region of the body. Cancer that has spread in this way is called metastatic cancer. *(verywellhealth.com)*

Methylation: Chemically speaking, methylation is the process of adding methyl groups to a molecule. A methyl group is a chemical structure made of one carbon and three hydrogen atoms. Since methyl groups are chemically inert, adding them to a protein (the process of methylation) changes how that protein reacts to other substances in the body, thus affecting how that protein behaves. *(revolutionhealth.com)*

Morphine: A pain medication of the opiate family that is found naturally in a dark brown, resinous form, from the poppy plant (Papaver somniferum). It can be taken orally or injected. It acts directly on the central nervous system (CNS) to increase feelings of pleasure and warm relaxation and to reduce pain. *(Wikipedia)*

Myositis: Inflammation of the muscles that are used to move the body. Caused due to infection, injury, or autoimmune disease. *(Focus Medica)*

N

Naturopathic: These are also called naturopathic doctors (ND) or Doctor of Naturopathic Medicine (NMD). They usually attend an accredited four-year, graduate-level school. They learn the same basic sciences as conventional medical doctors (MD). *(WebMD)*

Nerve Block: Procedures that can help prevent or manage many different types of pain. They are often injections of medicines that block pain from specific nerves. They can be used for pain relief as well as total loss of feeling if needed for surgery. *(hopkinsmedicine.com)*

Nodule: A growth of abnormal tissue. Nodules can develop just below the skin. They can also develop in deeper skin tissues or internal organs. The thyroid gland and lymph nodes may develop nodules as well. *(healthline.com)*

NSAIDS: Nonsteroidal anti-inflammatory agents (usually abbreviated to NSAIDs) are a group of medicines that relieve pain and fever and reduce inflammation. *(drugs.com)*

O

Orthopedic: The branch of medicine dealing with the correction of deformities of bones or muscles. *(Dictionary)*

Osteoarthritis: Inflammation of one or more joints. It is the most common form of arthritis that affects joints in the hand, spine, knees, and hips. *(Focus Medica)*

Osteopenia: Reduced bone mass due to a decrease in the rate of osteoid synthesis to a level insufficient to compensate normal bone lysis. The term is also used to refer to any decrease in bone mass below the normal. *(The Free Dictionary)*

Osteoporosis: A condition when bone strength weakens and is susceptible to fracture. It usually affects hip, wrist, or spine. *(Focus Medica)*

Oxycodone: An opioid pain medication sometimes called a narcotic. Oxycodone is used to treat moderate to severe pain. *(drugs.com)*

Oxycontin: An opioid pain reliever used to treat moderate to severe pain. Includes OxyContin side effects, interactions, and indications. *(drugs.com)*

P

Paraaortic: The periaortic lymph nodes (also known as lumbar) are a group of lymph nodes that lie in front of the lumbar vertebrae near the aorta. These lymph nodes receive drainage from the gastrointestinal tract and the abdominal organs. *(Wikipedia)*

Patulous: Spreading widely from a center. *(Merriam-Webster Dictionary)*

Pericardial Effusion: A condition with the accumulation of too much fluid in the pericardium, a sac surrounding the heart. Mild cases are not harmful, but sometimes it may affect the functioning of the heart. *(Focus Medica)*

Peroneal Tendonitis: A common cause of pain around the back and outside of the foot due to injury or damage to the tendons. The peroneal tendons are strong, cord-like structures that link the peroneal muscles of the calf to the bones of the foot. Tendonitis occurs when microtears cause tendon damage and inflammation. *(healthline.com)*

Phrenic Nerve: The phrenic nerve is a pair of nerves, the right and left phrenic nerves, that activate contraction of the diaphragm that expands the thoracic cavity. *(sciencedirect.com)*

Rongeur: Surgical instrument with a sharp edge scoop shaped tip. Rongeur is used for gouging out bone fragments and soft tissue. *(surgical123.com)*

Rotator Cuff: Your rotator cuff is made up of muscles and tendons that keep the ball (head) of your upper-arm bone (humerus) in your shoulder socket. It also helps you raise and rotate your arm. *(WebMD)*

S

Scars: A scar is usually composed of fibrous tissue. Scars may be formed for many different reasons, including as a result of infections, surgery, injuries, or inflammation of tissue. *(hopkinsmedicine.org)*

Sciatic Nerve: The sciatic nerve is a peripheral nerve. Its nerve roots emerge from the lower spine and combine to form the sciatic nerve. As the sciatic nerve runs down the leg, it divides into several smaller branches along the way. Many of its branches provide nerve stimulation to the muscles in the legs. Sensory nerves throughout the leg and foot travel up the leg to merge with the sciatic nerve. *(verywellhealth.com)*

Sclerotic Lesion: An unusual hardening or thickening of your bone. They can affect any bone and be either benign (harmless) or malignant (cancerous). In general, they're slow growing. Both benign and malignant sclerotic lesions are usually classified by their number and size: than cancerous ones and tend to be smaller as well. *(healthline.com)*

Sebaceous Cyst: A swelling in the skin arising in a sebaceous gland, typically filled with yellowish sebum. Also called wen. *(Dictionary)*

Sedimentation Rate (SED Rate): The speed at which red blood cells settle to the bottom of a column of citrated blood measured in millimeters deposited per hour and which is used especially in diagnosing the progress of various abnormal conditions (as chronic infections). *(Merriam-Webster Medical dictionary)*

Shoulder Impingement: A painful condition that happens when the tendons and soft tissues around your shoulder joint become trapped between the top of your upper arm bone (the humerus) and the acromion, a bony projection that extends upward from your scapula (shoulder blade). *(healthline.com)*

Shoulder Manipulation: A procedure to relieve shoulder stiffness and poor range of motion. This procedure may be suggested if other treatment does not help. The other treatments may include exercise, medicine, and physical therapy. Shoulder manipulation breaks away scar tissue that keeps your shoulder from moving properly. *(drugs.com)*

Sleep Apnea: A sleep disorder where breathing is interrupted repeatedly during sleep. Characterized by loud snoring and episodes of stop breathing. *(Focus Medica)*

Pleural Cavity: The space that lies between the pleura, the two thin membranes that line and surround the lungs. The pleural cavity contains a small amount of liquid known as pleural fluid, which provides lubrication as the lungs expand and contract during respiration. *(verywellhealth.com)*

Pleurisy: Inflammation of the pleura, thin layer of tissue that lines the lungs and chest wall. This can cause severe chest pain that worsens during breathing. *(Focus Medica)*

Pneumonia: An infection of the air sacs in one or both the lungs. Characterized by severe cough with phlegm, fever, chills, and difficulty in breathing. *(Focus Medica)*

Polymyalgia Rheumatica (PMR): An inflammatory disorder typically seen in older adults that causes widespread aching, stiffness, and flu-like symptoms. It is more common in women than men and is seen more often in Caucasians than any other race. *(arthritis.org)*

Polyp: A colon polyp is a small clump of cells that forms on the lining of the colon. Most colon polyps are harmless. But over time, some colon polyps can develop into colon cancer, which is often fatal when found in its later stages. *(Mayo Clinic)*

Post-Traumatic Stress Disorder (PTSD): A mental health condition that's triggered by a terrifying event — either experiencing it or witnessing it. Symptoms may include flashbacks, nightmares, and severe anxiety, as well as uncontrollable thoughts about the event. *(Mayo Clinic)*

Prednisone: Prednisone is used to treat conditions such as arthritis, blood disorders, breathing problems, severe allergies, skin diseases, cancer, eye problems, and immune system disorders. *(First Databank)*

Prolia: Used to treat bone loss (osteoporosis) in people who have a high risk of getting fractures. *(First Databank)*

Prostate: The prostate helps make some of the fluid in semen, which carries sperm from your testicles when you ejaculate. *(WebMD)*

Prostate Specific Antigen (PSA): A protein manufactured exclusively by the prostate gland; PSA is produced for the ejaculate where it liquifies the semen and allows sperm cells to swim freely; elevated levels of PSA in blood serum are associated with benign prostatic hyperplasia and prostate cancer. *(Merriam-Webster Medical Dictionary)*

Prostatectomy: Surgery to remove part or all of the prostate gland. *(Mayo Clinic)*

Psoriasis: A chronic skin disease which results in scaly, often itchy areas in patches. *(Focus Medica)*

Pulmonary Function Tests (PFTs): A group of tests that assess how well the lungs work by measuring lung volume, capacity, rates of flow, and gas exchange. *(Focus Medica)*

Pulmonary Specialist: A pulmonologist, or pulmonary disease specialist, is a physician who possesses specialized knowledge and skill in the diagnosis and treatment of pulmonary (lung) conditions and diseases. *(healthcommunities.com)*

Punctate: Marked with points or dots; having minute spots or depressions. *(Dictionary)*

R

Radionuclide: A chemical substance, called an isotope, that exhibits radioactivity. *(The Free Dictionary)*

Radiopharmaceutical: A drug, compound or other material labeled or tagged with a radioisotope, which is used to diagnose or treat cancer and manage pain of bone metastases. (The Free Dictionary)

Recombinant Immunoblot Assay (RIBA): A blood test that detects antibodies to the hepatitis C virus (HCV). *(Focus Medica)*

Red Blood Cell Count (RBC): An RBC count is the number of red blood cells per a particular volume of blood. It may be reported in millions of cells per microliter (mcL) of blood or in millions of cells per liter (L) of blood. The "normal" range can sometimes vary depending on whose blood is being tested. *(verywellhealth.com)*

Renal Mass: The word renal means kidney. The words "tumor" and "mass" mean abnormal growths in the body. A renal mass, or tumor, is an abnormal growth in the kidney. Some renal masses are benign (not cancerous) and some are malignant (cancerous). One in four renal masses are benign. Smaller masses are more likely to be benign. *(urologyhealth.org)*

Restless Leg Syndrome: A disorder that causes an overwhelming urge to move legs, usually associated with unpleasant sensations often during sleep and relieved by movement. *(Focus Medica)*

Rheumatoid Arthritis: A usually chronic autoimmune disease that is characterized especially by pain, stiffness, inflammation, swelling, and sometimes destruction of joints —abbreviation R.A. *(Merriam-Webster Medical dictionary)*

Rheumatoid Factor (RF): An immune system protein that attacks healthy cells in the body. High RF levels in the blood can indicate an autoimmune condition, such as rheumatoid arthritis. *(Medical News Today)*

Rheumatologist: A board-certified internist or pediatrician who is qualified by additional training and experience in the diagnosis and treatment of arthritis and other diseases of the joints, muscles, and bones. After four years of medical school and three years of training in either internal medicine or pediatrics, rheumatologists devote an additional two to three years in specialized rheumatology training. *(hss.edu)*

Speedbridge Fixation: An innovative soft-tissue fixation device used in the treatment of Achilles injuries. While standard anchor fixation of the tendon creates only a single point of compression directly over the anchor, the SpeedBridge repair enables an hourglass pattern of FiberTape® suture to be laid over the distal end of the tendon. This -4anchor construct enables a true knotless repair and a greater area of compression for the tendon, improving stability such that immediate postoperative weightbearing and range of motion is possible. *(Arthrex.com)*

Spirometry: A simple test used to help diagnose and monitor certain lung conditions by measuring how much air you can breathe out in one forced breath. It's carried out using a device called a spirometer, which is a small machine attached by a cable to a mouthpiece. *(nhs.uk)*

Sternomanubrial: Sometimes referred to as the sternomanubrial joint, is the articulation between the upper two parts of the sternum, the manubrium and sternal body. *(radiopaedia.org)*

Steroid Shot: Steroid injections are man-made drugs very similar to cortisol, a hormone your body makes in your adrenal glands. "Steroid" is short for corticosteroid, which is different from the hormone-related steroid compounds that some athletes use. You may hear them called cortisone injections, cortisone shots, steroid shots, or corticosteroid injections. *(WebMD)*

Subacromial Decompression: A surgical procedure conducted to treat sports injuries, such as impingement syndrome. *(infobloom.com)*

Subcortical Cyst: A fluid-filled sac that forms in the bone just beneath the cartilage of a joint such as the hip, knee, or shoulder. *(verywellhealth.com)*

Subcutaneous: The subcutaneous tissue layer of skin plays a number of important roles in the body, as outlined below. Of particular importance, it connects the dermis to the muscles and bones in the body with the help of specialized connective tissue. It also assists the function of the dermis by providing support to the blood vessels, lymphatic vessels, nerves, and glands that pass through it to reach the dermis. The subcutaneous tissue is essential because of its role in padding the body. *(new-medical.net)*

Subfascial: Situated, occurring, or performed below a fascia. *(treehozz.com)*

Supine Position: The supine position is one of the four basic patient positions. The three other positions are prone, lateral, and lithotomy. In supine position, the patient is face up with their head resting on a pad positioner or pillow and their neck in a neutral position. *(steris.com)*

T

Tens Unit: A battery-powered device that delivers electrical impulses through electrodes placed on the surface of your skin. *(clevelandclinic.org)*

Tensor Fascia: A fusiform muscle enclosed between two layers of fascia lata with a length of 15cm approximately and overlying the gluteus minimus and some part of the gluteus medius. Its myotomes are fourth lumbar nerve root. *(physio-pedia.com)*

Testosterone: Testosterone is a hormone found in humans, as well as in other animals. In men, the testicles primarily make testosterone. *(healthline.com)*

Tonsillectomy: The surgical removal of the tonsils, two oval-shaped pads of tissue at the back of the throat — one tonsil on each side. *(Mayo Clinic)*

Trigger Finger: Surgical repair of trigger finger involves releasing the A1 pulley by cutting the fibers with a needle through the skin or by making an incision with a scalpel. Is This an Emergency? If you are experiencing serious medical symptoms, seek emergency treatment immediately. *(healthfully.com)*

Trochanter: One of the bony prominences toward the near end of the thighbone (the femur). There are two trochanters: The greater trochanter - A powerful protrusion located at the proximal (near) and lateral (outside) part of the shaft of the femur. *(medicinenet.com)*

T-Score: The t score determines the ratio of differences between two groups or samples, as well as the differences within a group or sample. The DEXA scan or ultrasound will give you a number called a T-score, which represents how close you are to average peak bone density. *(health.havard.edu)*

U

Ultrasound: A medical test that uses high-frequency sound waves to capture live images from the inside of your body. It's also known as sonography. *(healthline.com)*

Urologist: A doctor in the field of medicine that focuses on diseases of the urinary tract and the male reproductive tract. *(healthline.com)*

Uvula: The uvula is the little fleshy part that hangs down from the soft palate of your mouth, and one of its purposes is to stop food from going up your nose when you swallow. Just like a tiny, disgusting doggy door, it swings up and down, blocking the path to your nose as the food races past, funneling it down into your esophagus. *(sciencealert.com)*

V

Vicryl Suture: A synthetic, absorbable suture commonly applied to wounds or incisions in interior body tissues. Within the body, polyglycolic acid, the main component of a Vicryl™ sutures, is broken down by a process known as hydrolysis. *(infobloom.com)*

Volteran Gel: Used to treat joint pain caused by osteoarthritis in the hands, wrists, elbows, knees, ankles, or feet. Voltaren Gel may not be effective in treating arthritis pain elsewhere in the body. *(drugs.com)*

X

Xanax: Alprazolam is used to treat anxiety and panic disorders. *(First Databank)*

X-Ray: Painless test which produces images of structures in body, especially bones using high energy electromagnetic waves. *(Focus Medica)*

Xtandi: Enzalutamide is used to treat prostate cancer. *(First Databank)*

Z

Zofran: This medication is used alone or with other medications to prevent nausea and vomiting caused by cancer drug treatment (chemotherapy) and radiation therapy. It is also used to prevent and treat nausea and vomiting after surgery. *(First Databank)*

Zometa: This medication is used to treat high blood calcium levels (hypercalcemia) that may occur with cancer. Zoledronic acid is also used with cancer chemotherapy to treat bone problems that may occur with multiple myeloma and other types of cancer (such as breast, lung) that have spread to the bones. *(First Databank)*

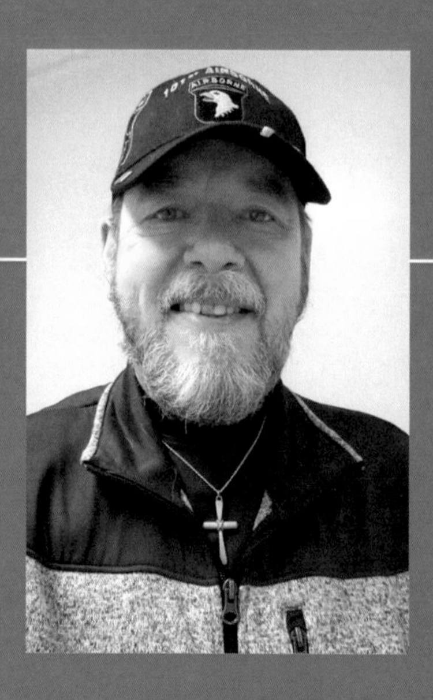

PERRY MUSE is a U.S. Army veteran, businessperson of more than 30 years, entrepreneur, artist, husband, father, and author. He has been listed in the Who's Who of Music and the Who's Who of Business Leaders. Perry is also a lifelong survivor of death-defying accidents. In 2017 he was diagnosed with stage 4 cancer. This life-changing event required him to reach deep inside and find courage, faith, and to become an expert intellect about his conditions and treatments. Perry's writing is entertaining, funny, extremely educational, and most importantly, all unbelievably true. Today he lives in Johnson City, Tennessee, with his wife and three dogs.

MORBID THOUGHTS AND THE DOMINO EFFECT

PERRY MUSE

MORBID THOUGHTS AND THE DOMINO EFFECT
Passing Thoughts During Cancer

Published by Gatekeeper Press
2167 Stringtown Rd, Suite 109
Columbus, OH 43123-2989
www.GatekeeperPress.com

Library of Congress Control Number: 2022936814

ISBN (paperback): 9781662925627
eISBN: 9781662925634

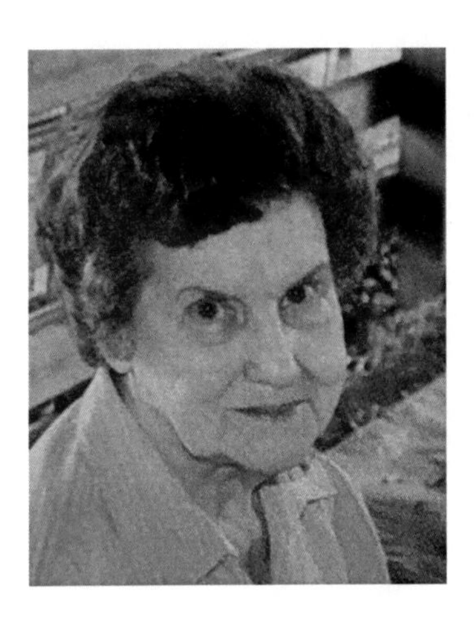

In loving memory of my mother